T0227260

Dual Energy CT: Applications in Head and Neck and Neurologic Imaging

Editors

REZA FORGHANI
HILLARY R. KELLY

NEUROIMAGING CLINICS OF NORTH AMERICA

www.neuroimaging.theclinics.com

Consulting Editor
SURESH K. MUKHERJI

August 2017 • Volume 27 • Number 3

ELSEVIER

1600 John F. Kennedy Boulevard • Suite 1800 • Philadelphia, Pennsylvania, 19103-2899

http://www.neuroimaging.theclinics.com

NEUROIMAGING CLINICS OF NORTH AMERICA Volume 27, Number 3
August 2017 ISSN 1052-5149, ISBN 13: 978-0-323-53243-3

Editor: John Vassallo (j.vassallo@elsevier.com)
Developmental Editor: Casey Potter

Neuroimaging Clinics of North America (ISSN 1052-5149) is published quarterly by Elsevier Inc., 360 Park Avenue South, New York, NY 10010-1710. Months of issue are February, May, August, and November. Business and editorial offices: 1600 John F. Kennedy Blvd., Suite 1800, Philadelphia, PA 19103-2899. Business and editorial offices: 6277 Sea Harbor Drive, Orlando, FL 32887-4800. Periodicals postage paid at New York, NY, and additional mailing offices. Subscription prices are USD 365 per year for US individuals, USD 581 per year for US institutions, USD 100 per year for US students and residents, USD 415 per year for Canadian individuals, USD 740 per year for Canadian institutions, USD 525 per year for international individuals, USD 740 per year for international institutions and USD 260 per year for Canadian and foreign students and residents. To receive student/resident rate, orders must be accompanied by name of affiliated institution, date of term, and the *signature* of program/residency coordinator on institution letterhead. Orders will be billed at individual rate until proof of status is received. Foreign air speed delivery is included in all *Clinics* subscription prices. All prices are subject to change without notice. POSTMASTER: Send address changes to *Neuroimaging Clinics of North America*, Elsevier Health Sciences Division, Subscription **Customer Service, 3251 Riverport Lane, Maryland Heights, MO 63043. Telephone: 1-800-654-2452 (U.S. and Canada); 314-447-8871 (outside U.S. and Canada). Fax: 314-447-8029. E-mail: journalscustomer service-usa@elsevier.com (for print support); journalsonlinesupport-usa@elsevier.com (for online support).**

Reprints. For copies of 100 or more of articles in this publication, please contact the Commercial Reprints Department, Elsevier Inc., 360 Park Avenue South, New York, NY 10010-1710. Tel.: 212-633-3874; Fax: 212-633-3820; E-mail: reprints@elsevier.com.

Neuroimaging Clinics of North America is covered by *Excerpta Medical/EMBASE,* the RSNA Index of Imaging Literature, *MEDLINE/PubMed (Index Medicus),* MEDLINE/MEDLARS, SciSearch, Research Alert, and Neuroscience Citation Index.

PROGRAM OBJECTIVE

The goal of Neuroimaging Clinics of North America is to keep practicing radiologists and radiology residents up to date with current clinical practice in radiology by providing timely articles reviewing the state of the art in patient care.

TARGET AUDIENCE

Practicing radiologists, radiology residents, and other healthcare professionals who utilize neuroimaging findings to provide patient care.

LEARNING OBJECTIVES

Upon completion of this activity, participants will be able to:
1. Review the uses and applications of dual energy CT.
2. Discuss the use of dual energy CT in the evaluation of head and neck disorders.
3. Recognize emerging and upcoming applications of dual energy CT.

ACCREDITATION

The Elsevier Office of Continuing Medical Education (EOCME) is accredited by the Accreditation Council for Continuing Medical Education (ACCME) to provide continuing medical education for physicians.

The EOCME designates this enduring material for a maximum of 15 *AMA PRA Category 1 Credit*(s)™. Physicians should claim only the credit commensurate with the extent of their participation in the activity.

All other healthcare professionals requesting continuing education credit for this enduring material will be issued a certificate of participation.

DISCLOSURE OF CONFLICTS OF INTEREST

The EOCME assesses conflict of interest with its instructors, faculty, planners, and other individuals who are in a position to control the content of CME activities. All relevant conflicts of interest that are identified are thoroughly vetted by EOCME for fair balance, scientific objectivity, and patient care recommendations. EOCME is committed to providing its learners with CME activities that promote improvements or quality in healthcare and not a specific proprietary business or a commercial interest.

The planning committee, staff, authors and editors listed below have identified no financial relationships or relationships to products or devices they or their spouse/life partner have with commercial interest related to the content of this CME activity:

Giorgio Ascenti, MD; Margaret N. Chapman, MD; Hugh D. Curtin, MD; Tommaso D'Angelo, MD; Anjali Fortna; Bezhad Forghani, M.Eng; Rajiv Gupta, MD, PhD; Ranliang Hu, MD; Shahmir Kamalian, MD; Hillary R. Kelly, MD; Peter Komlosi, MD, PhD; Hirofumi Kuno, MD, PhD; Mark Levental, MD; Eric Liao, MD; Silvio Mazziotti, MD, PhD; Suresh K. Mukherji, MD, MBA, FACR; Atul Padole, MD; Almudena Pérez-Lara, MD, PhD; Lorne Rosenbloom, MD, PhD; Osamu Sakai, MD, PhD; Kotaro Sekiya, DDS, PhD; Ashok Srinivasan, MD; Karthik Subramaniam; Ahmed M. Tawfik, MBBCH, MSc, MD; John Vassallo; Thomas J. Vogl, MD; Katie Widmeier; Amy Williams; Gary Wing, PhD.

The planning committee, staff, authors and editors listed below have identified financial relationships or relationships to products or devices they or their spouse/life partner have with commercial interest related to the content of this CME activity:

Andreas Michael Bucher, MD is a consultant/advisor for Boston Scientific Corporation and Bayer AG.
Bruno De Man, PhD has an employment affiliation with General Electric.
Reza Forghani, MD, PhD is on the speakers' bureau for, a consultant/advisor for, and has stock ownership in Real Time Medical, and is a consultant/advisor for General Electric.
Michael H. Lev, MD, FAHA is a consultant/advisor for General Electric; Takeda Pharmaceuticals U.S.A Inc; MedyMatch Technology, LTD; and D-Pharm, and has stock ownsership in General Electric.
Stuart R. Pomerantz, MD is a consultant/advisor for General Electric.
Julian L. Wichmann, MD is on the speakers' bureau for General Electric and Siemens USA.
Max Wintermark, MD, MAS is a consultant/advisor for General Electric.

UNAPPROVED/OFF-LABEL USE DISCLOSURE

The EOCME requires CME faculty to disclose to the participants:
1. When products or procedures being discussed are off-label, unlabelled, experimental, and/or investigational (not US Food and Drug Administration [FDA] approved); and
2. Any limitations on the information presented, such as data that are preliminary or that represent ongoing research, interim analyses, and/or unsupported opinions. Faculty may discuss information about pharmaceutical agents that is outside of FDA-approved labelling. This information is intended solely for CME and is not intended to promote off-label use of these medications. If you have any questions, contact the medical affairs department of the manufacturer for the most recent prescribing information.

TO ENROLL

To enroll in the *Neuroimaging Clinics of North America* Continuing Medical Education program, call customer service at 1-800-654-2452 or sign up online at http://www.theclinics.com/home/cme. The CME program is available to subscribers for an additional annual fee of USD $235.

METHOD OF PARTICIPATION

In order to claim credit, participants must complete the following:

1. Complete enrolment as indicated above.
2. Read the activity.
3. Complete the CME Test and Evaluation. Participants must achieve a score of 70% on the test. All CME Tests and Evaluations must be completed online.

CME INQUIRIES/SPECIAL NEEDS

For all CME inquiries or special needs, please contact elsevierCME@elsevier.com.

NEUROIMAGING CLINICS OF NORTH AMERICA

THE CLINICS ARE AVAILABLE ONLINE!
Access your subscription at:
www.theclinics.com

NEUROIMAGING CLINICS OF NORTH AMERICA

Contributors

CONSULTING EDITOR

SURESH K. MUKHERJI, MD, MBA, FACR
Professor and Chairman, Walter F. Patenge
Endowed Chair, Department of Radiology,
Michigan State University, Chief Medical
Officer and Director, Health Care Delivery,
Michigan State University Health Team,
East Lansing, Michigan

EDITORS

REZA FORGHANI, MD, PhD
Associate Chief, Department of Radiology,
Clinical Investigator, Segal Cancer Centre and
Lady Davis Institute for Medical Research,
Jewish General Hospital, Assistant Professor,
McGill University, Montreal, Quebec, Canada

HILLARY R. KELLY, MD
Assistant Professor, Departments of
Radiology, Massachusetts General Hospital
and Massachusetts Eye and Ear Infirmary,
Harvard Medical School, Boston,
Massachusetts

AUTHORS

GIORGIO ASCENTI, MD
Section of Radiological Sciences, Department
of Biomedical Sciences and Morphological and
Functional Imaging, University of Messina,
Messina, Italy

MARGARET N. CHAPMAN, MD
Department of Radiology, Boston Medical
Center, Boston University School of Medicine,
Boston, Massachusetts

HUGH D. CURTIN, MD
Chief, Department of Radiology,
Massachusetts Eye and Ear Infirmary,
Professor of Radiology, Harvard Medical
School, Boston, Massachusetts

TOMMASO D'ANGELO, MD
Section of Radiological Sciences, Department
of Biomedical Sciences and Morphological and
Functional Imaging, University of Messina,
Messina, Italy; Department of Diagnostic and
Interventional Radiology, University Hospital
Frankfurt, Frankfurt, Germany

BRUNO DE MAN, PhD
GE Global Research, Niskayuna, New York

BEHZAD FORGHANI, M.Eng
Reza Forghani Medical Services Inc,
Cote St-Luc, Quebec, Canada

REZA FORGHANI, MD, PhD
Associate Chief, Department of Radiology,
Clinical Investigator, Segal Cancer Centre and
Lady Davis Institute for Medical Research,
Jewish General Hospital, Assistant Professor,
McGill University, Montreal, Quebec, Canada

RAJIV GUPTA, MD, PhD
Associate Professor, Department of
Radiology, Massachusetts General Hospital,
Harvard Medical School, Boston,
Massachusetts

RANLIANG HU, MD
Assistant Professor, Department of Radiology
and Imaging Sciences, Emory University,
Atlanta, Georgia

SHAHMIR KAMALIAN, MD
Division of Emergency Radiology,
Department of Radiology, Massachusetts
General Hospital, Instructor, Harvard Medical
School, Boston, Massachusetts

HILLARY R. KELLY, MD
Assistant Professor, Departments of
Radiology, Massachusetts General Hospital
and Massachusetts Eye and Ear Infirmary,
Harvard Medical School, Boston,
Massachusetts

PETER KOMLOSI, MD, PhD
Department of Radiology, University of
Pittsburgh, Pittsburgh, Pennsylvania

HIROFUMI KUNO, MD, PhD
Department of Radiology, Boston Medical
Center, Boston University School of Medicine,
Boston, Massachusetts; Department of
Diagnostic Radiology, National Cancer Center
Hospital East, Kashiwa, Chiba, Japan

MICHAEL H. LEV, MD, FAHA
Director of Emergency Radiology and
Emergency Neuroradiology, Division of
Emergency Radiology, Department of
Radiology, Massachusetts General Hospital,
Professor, Harvard Medical School, Boston,
Massachusetts

MARK LEVENTAL, MD
Chief, Department of Radiology, Jewish
General Hospital, Associate Professor,
McGill University, Montreal, Quebec,
Canada

ERIC LIAO, MD
Clinical Lecturer, Division of Neuroradiology,
Department of Radiology, University of
Michigan Health System, Ann Arbor,
Michigan

SILVIO MAZZIOTTI, MD
Section of Radiological Sciences,
Department of Biomedical Sciences and
Morphological and Functional Imaging,
University of Messina, Messina, Italy

ANDREAS MICHAEL BUCHER, MD
Institute for Diagnostic and Interventional
Radiology, Johann Wolfgang Goethe
University Hospital, Frankfurt am Main,
Germany

ATUL PADOLE, MD
Research Fellow, Department of Radiology,
Massachusetts General Hospital, Boston,
Massachusetts

ALMUDENA PÉREZ-LARA, MD, PhD
Head and Neck Imaging Fellow, Department of
Radiology, Jewish General Hospital, McGill
University, Montreal, Quebec, Canada

STUART R. POMERANTZ, MD
Director of Neuroradiology CT, Division of
Neuroradiology, Department of Radiology,
Massachusetts General Hospital, Instructor,
Harvard Medical School, Boston,
Massachusetts

LORNE ROSENBLOOM, MD
Assistant Professor, Department of Radiology,
Jewish General Hospital, McGill University,
Montreal, Quebec, Canada

OSAMU SAKAI, MD, PhD
Departments of Radiology,
Otolaryngology–Head and Neck Surgery,
and Radiation Oncology, Boston Medical
Center, Boston University School of
Medicine, Boston, Massachusetts

KOTARO SEKIYA, DDS, PhD
Department of Diagnostic Radiology,
National Cancer Center Hospital East,
Kashiwa, Chiba, Japan

ASHOK SRINIVASAN, MD
Associate Professor, Division of
Neuroradiology, Department of Radiology,
University of Michigan Health System,
Ann Arbor, Michigan

AHMED M. TAWFIK, MBBCH, MSc, MD
Associate Professor, Department of Diagnostic
and Interventional Radiology, Faculty of
Medicine, Mansoura University, Mansoura,
Egypt

THOMAS J. VOGL, MD
Professor, Director, Institute for Diagnostic and
Interventional Radiology, Johann Wolfgang
Goethe University Hospital, Frankfurt am Main,
Germany

GARY WING, RT
Department of Radiology, Jewish General
Hospital, McGill University, Montreal, Quebec,
Canada

JULIAN L. WICHMANN, MD
Department of Diagnostic and Interventional
Radiology, University Hospital Frankfurt,
Frankfurt, Germany

MAX WINTERMARK, MD, MAS
Department of Radiology, Stanford
University School of Medicine, Stanford,
California

Contents

There are increasing applications of dual-energy computed tomography (CT), a type of spectral CT, in neuroradiology and head and neck imaging. In this 2-part review, the fundamental principles underlying spectral CT scanning and the major considerations in implementing this type of scanning in clinical practice are reviewed. In the first part of this 2-part review, the physical principles underlying spectral CT scanning are reviewed, followed by an overview of the different approaches for spectral CT scanning, including a discussion of the strengths and challenges encountered with each approach.

There are increasing applications and use of spectral computed tomography or dual-energy computed tomography (DECT) in neuroradiology and head and neck imaging in routine clinical practice. Part 1 of this 2-part review covered fundamental physical principles underlying DECT scanning and the different approaches for scanning. Part 2 focuses on important and practical considerations for implementing and using DECT in clinical practice, including a review of different images and reconstructions produced by these scanners and important and practical issues, ranging from image quality and radiation dose to workflow-related aspects of DECT scanning, that routinely come up during operationalization of DECT.

This article reviews the physical principles of dual-energy material decomposition and its current implementation. Clinical applications of dual-energy material decomposition including differentiation of calcification from hemorrhage and iodinated contrast from hemorrhage are highlighted, and their applications to neuroimaging are reviewed.

Dual-energy computed tomography (CT) has the potential to improve detection of abnormalities and increase diagnostic confidence in the evaluation of a variety of neurologic conditions by using different x-ray energy–dependent absorption behaviors of different materials. This article reviews the virtual monochromatic imaging applications of dual-energy CT, particularly material decomposition algorithms to improve lesion conspicuity, define lesion-normal tissue interface using different reconstruction techniques, and discuss miscellaneous emerging applications of dual-energy CT for neuroimaging, with an emphasis on their potential clinical utility.

Dual-energy computed tomography (DECT) has become an increasingly widespread and useful component of the neuroimaging armamentarium, offering automated bone removal, metallic artifact reduction, and improved characterization of iodinated contrast enhancement. The application of these techniques to CT neuroangiography enables a number of benefits including more efficient 3D postprocessing, contrast dose reduction opportunities, successful differentiation of hemorrhage from contrast staining following thromboembolic recanalization therapy, improved detection of active contrast extravasation in the setting of intracranial hemorrhage, and more precise characterization of atheromatous steno-occlusive disease.

There are multiple emerging applications of dual-energy computed tomography (DECT) for the evaluation of pathology in the head and neck, in particular head and neck squamous cell carcinoma. Studies suggest that DECT image sets reconstructed as supplements to routine diagnostic images may improve lesion visualization, determination of tumor extent, and identification of invasion of critical anatomic structures. This article reviews the evidence for the use and potential advantages of supplementary DECT reconstructions for the evaluation of head and neck squamous cell carcinoma. A summary of potentially useful reconstructions and a suggested approach for multiparametric DECT evaluation of head and neck cancer based on current evidence are presented.

There is recent interest in the use of dual-energy computed tomography (CT) in head and neck imaging, and the results are encouraging. This article reviews dual-energy CT applications as complementary tools to conventional CT scanning in the evaluation of cervical lymphadenopathy. The article cites the most relevant studies and highlights their results. Single-source and dual-source dual-energy applications including virtual noncontrast images, linear and nonlinear image blending, monochromatic images, iodine quantification, and spectral Hounsfield unit attenuation curve analysis are reviewed. Future directions and research suggestions are discussed in brief.

Dual-energy computed tomography (DECT) and its specific algorithms and applications have been increasingly recognized in clinical practice as a valuable advance in technology beyond what is possible with the established postprocessing capabilities of single-energy multidetector computed tomography, mainly because of its potential benefits regarding image quality and contrast. DECT may represent an alternative approach to purely attenuation-based imaging of the head and neck, because it provides a material-specific visualization based on spectral information. With this approach, owing to its physical properties, iodine can be assessed as a potential "biological tracer" to improve depiction of tumor conspicuity and grade of invasion.

Capturing the energy-dependent x-ray attenuation of different tissues, dual-energy computed tomography offers multiple benefits in the imaging of the spine, such as bone and iodinated contrast removal, monosodium urate imaging, and robust reduction of beam-hardening artifacts. The emerging new applications of this technique include bone marrow imaging in acute trauma and myeloinfiltrative disorders, improved bone density determination, and noninvasive assessment of spinal gout.

Conventional computed tomography (CT) uses a polychromatic energy beam to offer superb anatomic detail of the head and spine. However, technical challenges remain that can degrade the diagnostic image quality of these examinations. Dual-energy CT analyzes the changes in attenuation of soft tissues at different energy levels, from which different reconstructions can be made to yield the optimal contrast-to-noise ratio, reduce beam-hardening artifact, or evaluate tissue composition. In this article, selective applications of the dual energy CT technique are discussed, highlighting a powerful tool in the diagnostic CT evaluation of the head, neck, and spine.

There is increasing use of dual-energy computed tomography (DECT) for the evaluation of head and neck pathologic entities. Optimal DECT utilization requires familiarity with the appearance of normal tissues variants, and pathologic entities on different DECT reconstructions that may be used in clinical practice. The purpose of this article is to provide a practical, pictorial review of the appearance of normal anatomic structures and different neoplastic and nonneoplastic head and neck pathologic entities on commonly used DECT reconstructions.

Almudena Pérez-Lara, Mark Levental, Lorne Rosenbloom, Gary Wing, and Reza Forghani

There is increasing use and popularity of dual-energy computed tomography (DECT) in many subspecialties in radiology. This article reviews the practical workflow implications of routine DECT scanning based on the experience at a single institution where a large percentage of elective neck CTs are acquired in DECT mode. The article reviews factors both on the production (technologist) and on the interpretation (radiologist) side, focusing on challenges posed and potential solutions for seamless workflow implementation.

Reza Forghani, Ashok Srinivasan, and Behzad Forghani

In the last article of this issue, advanced analysis capabilities of DECT is reviewed, including spectral Hounsfield unit attenuation curves, virtual monochromatic images, material decomposition maps, tissue effective Z determination, and other advanced post-processing DECT tools, followed by different methods of analysis of the attenuation curves generated using DECT. The article concludes with exciting future horizons and potential applications, such as the use of the rich quantitative data in dual energy CT scans for texture or radiomic analysis and the use of machine learning methods for generation of prediction models using spectral data.

Foreword
Dual-Energy Computed Tomography: Applications in Neurologic, Head, and Neck Imaging

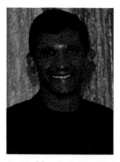

Suresh K. Mukherji, MD, MBA, FACR
Consulting Editor

Dual-energy computed tomography (CT) is the most exciting innovation in CT since the introduction of helical acquisition. The ability to create iterative MeV maps and quantitatively analyze the data provides new opportunities for clinical care and scholarly pursuits. This issue of *Neuroimaging Clinics* is dedicated to dual-energy CT and covers a wide range of clinical applications in the brain, spine, and head and neck.

The beauty of this issue is the focus on practical applications that can quickly be integrated into clinical practice. I want to express my gratitude to all of the authors for their wonderful contributions to this outstanding issue.

I also want to thank Drs Reza Forghani and Hillary Kelly for guest editing this issue. They are two "superstars" in Head and Neck and Neuroradiology. These are truly special individuals, and I only wish I had 50% of their intellect and energy. I was delighted when they accepted this invitation to guest edit, and they have delivered a product that exceeded my wildest expectations. I also know the future of our subspeciality is in "good hands" with such talented individuals. Thank you, Hillary and Reza, for your energy, drive, and leadership!

Suresh K. Mukherji, MD, MBA, FACR
Department of Radiology
Michigan State University
Health Care Delivery
Michigan State University Health Team
846 Service Road
East Lansing, MI 48824, USA

E-mail address:
mukherji@rad.msu.edu

Neuroimag Clin N Am 27 (2017) xv
http://dx.doi.org/10.1016/j.nic.2017.05.002
1052-5149/17/© 2017 Published by Elsevier Inc.

Preface

Dual-Energy Computed Tomography in Neuroradiology and Head and Neck Imaging: State-of-the-Art

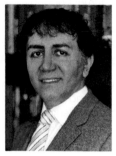 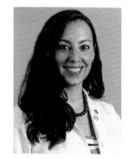

Reza Forghani, MD, PhD   Hillary R. Kelly, MD

Editors

Dual-energy computed tomography (DECT) was first attempted in the 1970s, but because of technical challenges, it was not until 2006 that the first DECT system was made clinically available. In the decade since its introduction into the clinical arena, the applications and clinical indications of DECT have exponentially increased. Although neuroradiologic applications initially lagged behind some other subspecialties, it is becoming increasingly apparent that DECT can be applied to a wide range of indications in the brain, spine, and the head and neck, with the potential to increase diagnostic confidence, efficiency, and accuracy. Modern DECT scanning platforms allow for simultaneous or near simultaneous image acquisition at two different energy spectra, generating data sets that can be postprocessed to provide tissue characterization and material differentiation that cannot be obtained using single-energy computed tomography. In neuroradiologic and head and neck imaging, these advanced capabilities and the multitude of possible reconstructions bring to mind MR imaging sequences.

As with any advance in imaging technology, widespread adoption with translation from the research realm to the clinical arena requires careful consideration with respect to resource management, education, technical support, reproducibility, and workflow efficiency. In preparing this issue, we recruited a group of international experts in an attempt to comprehensively cover all aspects of DECT for the practicing neuroradiologist. The first two articles provide a detailed overview of the physical principles that underlie DECT, compare and contrast the DECT systems currently available commercially, and address important technical considerations for implementation and use of these systems in clinical practice. These articles are followed by detailed reviews of the current and potential future applications of DECT in neuroimaging and head and neck imaging, covering a wide array of potential oncologic and nononcologic applications. Practical considerations, including use in routine clinical practice and workflow implementation, as well as potential emerging applications such as texture analysis and advanced tissue

Neuroimag Clin N Am 27 (2017) xvii–xviii
http://dx.doi.org/10.1016/j.nic.2017.05.001
1052-5149/17/© 2017 Published by Elsevier Inc.

neuroimaging.theclinics.com

characterization, are also discussed in detail in dedicated articles.

We hope that this issue will serve as an excellent resource for both radiologists currently using DECT and those hoping to incorporate DECT into their daily practice. Although the topic can initially seem technically daunting, it is clear that DECT has the potential to help us as radiologists provide more confident and accurate diagnoses, with the possibility of significantly impacting patient management.

We sincerely thank all of the authors for accepting our invitations, for their fantastic work in this issue, as well as for their efforts to advance the field. We would also like to express our gratitude to Dr. Suresh K. Mukherji for the opportunity to guest edit this issue of *Neuroimaging Clinics*. Lastly, this issue would not have been possible without the support and patience of John Vassallo, Associate Publisher, and Casey Potter, Developmental Editor, at Elsevier. We are extremely proud of what we have accomplished with this issue, hope that it will stimulate interest in expanding the use of DECT in clinical practice, and look forward to comments and feedback from the readers.

Reza Forghani, MD, PhD
Department of Radiology
Segal Cancer Centre
Lady Davis Institute for Medical Research
Jewish General Hospital & McGill University
Room C-212.1
3755 Cote Ste-Catherine Road
Montreal, Quebec H3T 1E2 Canada

Hillary R. Kelly, MD
Department of Radiology
Massachusetts General Hospital
Harvard Medical School
55 Fruit Street, GRB-273A
Boston, MA 02114, USA

Department of Radiology
Massachusetts Eye and Ear Infirmary
Harvard Medical School
243 Charles Street
Boston, MA 02114, USA

E-mail addresses:
rforghani@jgh.mcgill.ca (R. Forghani)
hillary.kelly@mgh.harvard.edu (H.R. Kelly)

Dual-Energy Computed Tomography

Physical Principles, Approaches to Scanning, Usage, and Implementation: Part 1

Reza Forghani, MD, PhD[a],*, Bruno De Man, PhD[b], Rajiv Gupta, MD, PhD[c]

KEYWORDS

- Dual-energy CT • Spectral CT or multienergy CT • Dual-source CT • Fast kVp switching
- Gemstone spectral imaging • Layered or sandwich detectors • Photon counting
- Virtual monochromatic images

KEY POINTS

- Spectral computed tomography (CT) material differentiation relies on differences in energy-dependency of the attenuation of different materials.
- The photoelectric effect has a strong energy dependence, and the attenuation due to the photoelectric effect is highly dependent on the atomic number (Z) of the element.
- Elements with a high atomic number, such as iodine, that have a strong energy dependence can be exploited for spectral CT scanning.
- Current commercially available spectral CT scanners are dual-energy CT scanners that may consist of 1 or 2 tubes, or use specialized layered detectors for spectral separation.
- Multienergy scanning systems, such as photon counting scanners, are under development but not yet commercially available for routine clinical use.

INTRODUCTION

Dual-energy computed tomography (DECT) or spectral computed tomography (CT) is an advanced form of CT that uses different X-ray spectra to enhance material differentiation and tissue characterization. Current commercially available clinical systems use 2 different photon spectra for scanning, and therefore, the term DECT is sometimes used interchangeably with spectral CT. However, it is noteworthy that the term spectral CT could also encompass more

Disclosures: R. Forghani has acted as a consultant for GE Healthcare and has served as a speaker at lunch and learn sessions titled "Dual-Energy CT Applications in Neuroradiology and Head and Neck Imaging" sponsored by GE Healthcare at the 27th and 28th Annual Meetings of the Eastern Neuroradiological Society in 2015 and 2016 (no personal compensation or travel support for these sessions). B. De Man is CT Business Portfolio Leader and Manager of Image Reconstruction Laboratory, GE Global Research. R. Gupta declares no relevant conflict of interest.
[a] Department of Radiology, Segal Cancer Centre and Lady Davis Institute for Medical Research, Jewish General Hospital, McGill University, Room C-212.1, 3755 Cote Ste-Catherine Road, Montreal, Quebec H3T 1E2, Canada; [b] GE Global Research, One Research Circle, KWC1300B, Niskayuna, NY 12309, USA; [c] Department of Radiology, Massachusetts General Hospital, Harvard Medical School, 55 Fruit Street, Boston, MA 02114, USA
* Corresponding author.
E-mail address: rforghani@jgh.mcgill.ca

Neuroimag Clin N Am 27 (2017) 371–384
http://dx.doi.org/10.1016/j.nic.2017.03.002

advanced systems capable of discrimination between more than 2 spectra, such as the photon counting scanners currently under investigation and development. Therefore, strictly speaking, the terms are not synonymous and DECT is a subset of spectral CT.

Applications of DECT for clinical use were initially explored in the 1970s.[1–7] However, the technological and computational advances necessary for implementation of DECT and successful introduction into the clinical arena were not yet made. Therefore, attempts for implementation were temporarily abandoned, just to be revived later with the introduction of the first DECT system in the clinical arena in 2006.[8,9] DECT scanning, as the name implies, is based on image acquisition with 2 different energy spectra. The data obtained are then combined in order to generate images for routine clinical interpretation or for more advanced material characterization. The objectives of this 2-part review are to provide an overview of the (1) physical principles behind spectral CT scanning and material differentiation, (2) major spectral CT acquisition systems available clinically, and (3) basics of implementation and use of the technology in clinical practice.

FUNDAMENTAL PRINCIPLES OF SPECTRAL COMPUTED TOMOGRAPHIC SCANNING AND MATERIAL CHARACTERIZATION
Overview

With conventional, single-energy computed tomography (SECT), a polychromatic beam is emitted by a single source (X-ray tube), passes through the patient resulting in attenuation of the beam, and is captured by an array of detector cells. The resulting projection data, after preprocessing and reconstruction via sophisticated computer algorithms, is rendered into CT slices that are used for diagnostic interpretation. With DECT, on the other hand, projection data are obtained at 2 different energy spectra instead of one, and the information acquired is then blended to create images for routine diagnostic interpretation. More advanced tissue analysis and material characterization are also feasible with these data sets.

The key advantage of DECT over SECT is that by acquiring data at 2 different energy spectra, it is possible to use sophisticated computer algorithms to combine the different energy data in order to evaluate tissue attenuation at different energies rather than at a single effective energy. Because different types of materials and tissues may attenuate X-rays differently at different energies depending on their elemental composition,

DECT may be used to perform tissue characterization beyond what is possible with conventional SECT. For successful DECT scanning and material characterization, the following fundamental considerations related to the scanner type and tissues being characterized must be taken into account.

Fundamentals of Dual-Energy Computed Tomography Scanning: Factors Related to the Scanner

For acquiring the projection data, the scanner must use different energy spectra and separately record the high- and low-energy measurements. This has been implemented in the clinical setting in multiple ways. One way is through simultaneous use of 2 different imaging chains, each with its own dedicated source and detector. Another way to accomplish this is via a single X-ray source that is capable of fast switching between 2 energy levels and a detector with very fast readout capability; technical innovations in modern X-ray source technology—taking advantage of the high-voltage controls for X-ray generation—enable this capability. In yet another design, it is possible to acquire high- and low-energy data sets by use of specialized detectors that have 2 different scintillator layers, one for high energy and the other for low energy, built into them. Various methods for acquiring dual-energy data sets are discussed in detail later in this article.

For the purposes of material differentiation, it would be ideal for each of the 2 different energy X-ray beams to be composed of monochromatic energies. However, with current X-ray tube technology used in the clinical setting, it is not possible to generate monochromatic X-ray spectra. Therefore, clinical DECT scanners use polychromatic X-ray sources but attempt to have as little overlap between the different energy spectra as possible. **Fig. 1** shows a typical X-ray spectrum at 80 kilovolt peak (kVp) and 140 kVp, including inherent X-ray tube filtration, generated with the XSpect simulator.[10] For DECT systems relying on different tube voltages for spectral separation, the standard peak energies used for scan acquisition are typically at 80 and 140 kVp. For some dual-source scanner models, 90 or 100 kVp with a filter may be used instead of 80 kVp, especially for scanning heavier patients. Alternatively, energies lower than 80 kVp, for example, 70 kVp, may also be used with some models or for specialized applications such as in pediatric imaging. For the high-energy acquisitions, 150 kVp may be used instead of 140 kVp with some models. Protocols may also vary depending on the scanner vendor or the specific application under consideration.

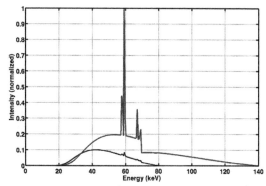

Fig. 1. Typical X-ray spectrum for X-ray tube voltages of 80 kVp and 140 kVp, including inherent X-ray tube filtration (generated with the XSpect simulator). The peaks represent characteristic lines of a tungsten anode, and the continuous spectrum is the result of bremsstrahlung. This example illustrates the polychromatic nature of the X-ray beams used for DECT scanning. For DECT scanning, it is desirable to achieve as much separation as possible between the low-energy and high-energy spectra. In addition, the tube voltage used must not be too low or too high. If it is too low, it will be excessively absorbed by the body, yielding little information; if it is too high, it will not yield useful information because of poor tissue contrast. In routine DECT, 80-100 kVp (low-energy spectrum) and 140-150 kVp (high-energy spectrum) are commonly used settings for this purpose, although there may be variations depending on the scanner model, filters used, or the specific clinical application at hand. (*Courtesy of* Reza Forghani, MD, PhD, Montreal, Quebec, Canada and Bruno De Man, PhD, Niskayuna, NY.)

The reason for the choice of energies is that typically, at peak energies less than approximately 80 kVp, too few photons are generated and, in addition, a large proportion of photons would be absorbed by the body, and therefore, not generate any clinically useful information.[1,11] For the high-energy acquisitions, voltages higher than 140 kVp (or 150 kVp for some models) are typically not available on all DECT scanners. Furthermore, such high energies may result in higher dose and too little soft tissue contrast, limiting applications in the clinical setting, although they could still be useful for specialized applications and for discriminating between low Z and high Z materials (discussed in greater detail in the following section).

Fundamentals of Dual-Energy Computed Tomography Scanning: Factors Related to the Materials or Tissues Being Evaluated

Beyond the specific technique used for image data acquisition, factors related to the materials or tissues of interest must be taken into account for successful clinical application of DECT (**Box 1**). It is important to understand the basis of DECT material characterization as well as the strengths and limitations of this technique. X-ray attenuation is governed by 2 main processes, with a third process only contributing a negligible amount. At the typical tube voltages used in CT, Compton scattering accounts for the greatest contribution to the overall attenuation. Compton

---

Box 1
Physical basis of material characterization and differentiation using dual-energy computed tomography

- DECT material differentiation relies on *energy dependence* of CT attenuation for different materials.
- Compton scatter and photoelectric effect are the main processes accounting for attenuation during CT scanning.
- Whereas the Compton effect is minimally dependent on photon energy, the photoelectric effect is strongly X-ray energy dependent.
- Because of its strong energy dependency, the photoelectric effect is key for material differentiation based on spectral properties with DECT.
- The photoelectric effect is also highly dependent on the atomic number (Z) of the element being imaged.
- Elements with a high atomic number, such as iodine (Z = 53) and calcium (Z = 20), have strong spectral properties and can be readily differentiated from low-Z materials (such as H, C, N, and O); this property forms the basis of multiple clinical applications for DECT scanning.
- To distinguish different materials or tissues based on their spectral properties, there must be a sufficient difference in their atomic number (Z) or effective atomic number.

scattering is a function of both the electron density of the tissue and the tube voltage and spectrum. The electron density of the tissue is the dominant factor, as Compton effect is only minimally dependent on photon energy.[9]

The other important physical process accounting for CT attenuation is the photoelectric effect. This effect, which is strongly dependent on the atomic number or Z (ie, the number of protons within the nucleus) of the elements that constitute the tissue under consideration, is particularly important for spectral CT.[12] Photoelectric interactions are strongly energy dependent, and as a result, key for DECT material characterization. The third physical process, Rayleigh or coherent scatter (related to the electrons), only accounts for a very small percentage of interactions and attenuation and is typically considered negligible in conventional absorption-based CT.

For elements or tissues to be distinguishable based on their spectral properties, there must be sufficient difference in their atomic number or Z. Understanding the impact of such elemental or tissue properties is critical when planning applications of DECT in any research or clinical setting. As an example, common elements found in the human body, such as hydrogen (Z = 1), carbon (Z = 6), nitrogen (Z = 7), and oxygen (Z = 8), have low, very

similar atomic numbers. As a result, these materials do not have sufficient component of photoelectric interactions: their attenuation is relatively low and very similar to each other at different energies, precluding reliable differentiation based on their spectral properties (Fig. 2).[1,13]

Elements with high atomic numbers and large differences in their atomic numbers, on the other hand, have a stronger energy dependence and can be distinguished from lower-Z materials using DECT. Among these elements, one of the prime candidates that is of clinical interest is iodine (Z = 53) (see Fig. 2). Most clinically used CT contrast agents are iodine based and are widely used for a variety of indications that include oncologic imaging and angiography. Iodine's strong energy dependence can therefore be exploited in a variety of settings in which contrast-enhanced CT scans are obtained for material characterization, iodine quantitation, and improving diagnostic evaluation using DECT. Among the elements that are intrinsic to the human body and have a relatively high atomic number, calcium (Z = 20) is another prime candidate. This element has been used in a variety of clinical applications in body imaging and head and neck imaging. These applications are covered in greater detail in subsequent articles in this series.

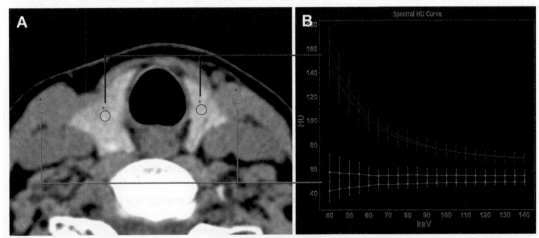

Fig. 2. Example of tissues with weak and strong spectral characteristics based on their elemental composition. Axial non-contrast-enhanced CT image of the neck acquired in dual-energy mode using a fast kVp switching scanner is shown (A). Region of interest analysis was performed comparing the spectral Hounsfield unit attenuation curves of muscle (green) to that of the thyroid gland (blue) (B). Most of the soft tissue in the human body, including muscle, is composed of low-Z materials such as oxygen (Z = 8), carbon (Z = 6), and hydrogen (Z = 1). As a result, there is little energy dependency of measured attenuation of muscle on an uninfused study (B; green curves). The thyroid gland, on the other hand, contains iodine (Z = 53) with strong energy dependence due to photoelectric effect. Note the marked energy-dependent increase in its attenuation at low energies approaching the K-edge of iodine (33.2 keV) (B; blue curves). Because most clinically used CT contrast agents are iodine based, iodine's strong energy dependence can be exploited in a variety of clinical settings.

OVERVIEW OF CURRENT AND EMERGING DUAL-ENERGY COMPUTED TOMOGRAPHIC SYSTEMS

The first DECT scanner approved for clinical use, a dual-source CT scanner, was introduced into the market in 2006. This scanner was followed a few years later by a CT scanner with fast kVp switching and fast detector technology. Since then, multiple scanners based on different dual-energy technologies have become available for clinical use from different vendors. There has also been refinement of different scanner types for optimizing image quality, postprocessing capabilities, radiation exposure, and ease of use. As is the case with any type of high-end technology, this is an evolving area with continued refinements and iterations being introduced. In this section, an up-to-date overview of the major DECT scanner types currently available is provided. The focus is on the fundamentals, such as mode of acquisition, as well as the advantages and disadvantages of each system. Additional information that is specific and pertinent to each scanner type is also provided as needed. It should be noted that for commercially available scanners, depending on the vendor, more than one model or generation of that scanner type may be available. Therefore, even for the same overall design, there may be important variations in the capabilities offered. This article focuses on the fundamentals of each design. A complete description of the variations in different models of the same scanner type is beyond the scope of this article, and interested readers are referred to vendor-provided documentation and literature. This section concludes with a discussion of emerging spectral CT platforms such as photon counting scanners.

Dual-Source Dual-Energy Computed Tomography

As the name implies, a dual-source scanner consists of 2 source and detector combinations[1,2,9,11,14,15] (Siemens AG, Forchheim, Germany) (Fig. 3). The source-detector combinations are at a near perpendicular angle, allowing the same volume to be scanned simultaneously with high- and low-energy spectra. The obvious advantage of this system is that separate tubes are used for generating the high- and low-energy spectra. The use of separate tubes enables independent adjustment of the tube voltage and current and helps optimize separation of the low- and high-energy spectra. Furthermore, the use of separate tubes facilitates balancing the total amounts of quanta emitted from the 2 tubes.

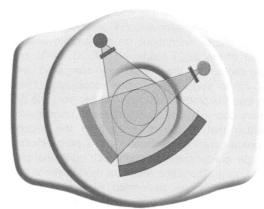

Fig. 3. Dual-source DECT (Siemens AG). Schematic illustration of dual-source detector combination scanners with the 2 imaging chains in a nearly orthogonal configuration, allowing the same slice to be scanned simultaneously at the 2 energies. Yellow is used to illustrate the low-energy spectrum, and blue, the high-energy spectrum. Typically, 80-100 kVp (low energy spectrum) and 140-150 kVp (high energy spectrum) are used depending on the model, but other combinations may be used for specific applications. Because there are 2 separate source-detector pairs, a filter can be placed to harden the high-energy spectrum. For some higher generation dual-source scanners, it is possible to use a higher kVp for the lower spectrum (90 or 100 instead of 80 kVp) in conjunction with a filter. Because of the limited space in the CT gantry, there is only sufficient space for a smaller second detector, which in turns places restrictions on the usable field of view of the dual-energy CT mode, as shown in the illustration. (*Courtesy of* Reza Forghani, MD, PhD, Montreal, Quebec, Canada and Bruno De Man, PhD, Niskayuna, NY.)

Because of the use of 2 X-ray tubes, a filter may be applied to the tube emitting the higher energy spectrum in order to harden the spectrum (ie, reduce associated low-energy quanta from the polychromatic emission). For some scanner models, an additional filter may be available for use with the tube emitting the lower energy spectrum as well. If the second filter is used, acquisitions will typically be performed at 100/140 kVp instead of 80/140 kVp. This enables acquisition of scans with lower image noise for larger patients, whereby 80 kVp may not yield optimal results. An additional advantage of 2 separate tubes is that the combined tubes can provide a higher total X-ray flux in a given amount of time, which is also beneficial for larger patients. The use of separate tubes also allows the application of established SECT technology and algorithms.

Among the disadvantages, one pertains to challenges posed by the limited space in the CT gantry. Because of this, there is only sufficient space for a smaller second detector, which in turns places restrictions on the usable field of view of the DECT mode (eg, 27, 33, or 35 cm, depending on the model) as compared with 50 cm for single-energy mode acquisitions. There is also the problem of cross-scatter from the primary course of one source-detector combination hitting that of the detector from the second source-detector combination at a perpendicular angle, contaminating its data with additional bias and noise. Therefore, technical modifications and optimizations are performed to reduce cross-scatter and corrections applied during image reconstruction (using different methods depending on the scanner model) to mitigate, at least in part, these effects.

This design also results in challenges for post-processing of the projection data. Because the projection data are acquired at different angles, for a given z-axis position, there is an offset of 90°. As a result, there is at least 70 milliseconds (ie, one-quarter rotation time) delay or "temporal skew" between the high and the corresponding low projection measurements. This temporal skew makes it hard to perform material decomposition in the projection domain, especially if there is any patient motion. Hence, the high- and low-energy datasets are separately reconstructed by filtered back projection, and material decomposition is performed afterward in the image domain, which may lead to imperfect elimination of beam hardening and reduced material decomposition accuracy. Last, there are considerable additional hardware requirements for this system compared with the single-source scanners, posing technological challenges and imposing certain limitations on the longitudinal or detector z-coverage of the system because the detector cost could become prohibitive.

Single-Source Dual-Energy Computed Tomography with Rapid kVp Switching: Gemstone Spectral Imaging

This scanner consists of a single source and detector combination[1,16–18] (GE Healthcare, Waukesha, WI, USA) (Fig. 4). With this scanner, the tube voltage follows a square wave form, and projection data are collected for twice the number of view angles, half at high- and the other half at low-tube voltage. This approach is made possible by the fast sampling capabilities of a proprietary, garnet-based scintillator detector with very low afterglow, referred to as Gemstone. During a single rotation, the image acquisition using this scanner is on a view-by-view basis, alternating between low and

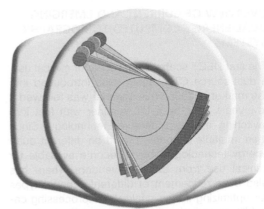

Fig. 4. Single-source DECT with rapid kVp switching: GSI (GE Healthcare). Schematic illustration of this type of a single source-detector combination system. Yellow is used to illustrate the low-energy spectrum, and blue, the high energy spectrum, typically 80/140 kVp. DECT projection data are acquired by very fast switching between low- and high-energy spectra combined with fast sampling capabilities of a proprietary, garnet-based scintillator detector with low afterglow for spectral separation at each successive axial or spiral view. (Courtesy of Reza Forghani, MD, PhD, Montreal, Quebec, Canada and Bruno De Man, PhD, Niskayuna, NY.)

high kVp. Since the temporal skew or the delay between the high and low projections is as low as 50 microseconds, there is excellent spatiotemporal registration, and material decomposition is performed directly in the projection domain, making it quantitatively accurate and robust against any possible patient motion. With current Gemstone spectral imaging (GSI) scanners, axial or helical acquisitions are obtained for the full field of view of 50 cm.

On the source side, the generator and tube used for these scanners are capable of reliably switching between the 80 and 140 kVp voltages, with sampling periods as fast as 50 microseconds. For this approach to be successful, a highly specialized generator capable of very rapid transitions in tube potential as well as very fast electronics and detector materials are required.

Overall, the advantages of rapid kVp switching or GSI DECT systems are excellent temporal registration and a cost-efficient design offering an opportunity to increase the longitudinal detector coverage up to 160 mm. These systems also enable scanning over the entire full field of view of 50 cm. In addition, material decomposition can be performed in the projection space, which helps to reduce beam-hardening artifacts in virtual monochromatic images (VMIs) generated in this manner (VMIs and other DECT reconstructions are discussed in part 2 of this review). If needed, with these systems, additional spectral analysis or reconstruction of different VMIs or maps can also be performed retrospectively in the image space based on the data generated from the original material decomposition and reconstruction from the projection data.

One challenge in the design and implementation of such a system is the issues related to the relative photon flux between the 2 energies. In order to address this challenge, the scanners are designed to balance the flux, with allocation of additional time for the low kVp relative to the high kVp acquisition. Not only does this approach serve to reduce photon starvation conditions, but when complemented by the appropriate choice of rotation speed, it also achieves a more balanced flux state between the 2 energies and neutralizes patient radiation exposure.

Disadvantages of this system include those related to adaptation of the current that can result in a relative reduction of signal from the low-energy spectrum, but this is partly compensated for by the additional time allocated for the low kVp acquisition, as described earlier. Last, in practice, the time profile of the tube voltage has a slightly trapezoidal shape rather than a purely rectangular shape. As a result, the spectral difference is slightly lower than the nominal tube voltages, and this has to be accounted for during image reconstruction.

Layered Detector Dual-Energy Computed Tomography

In the systems discussed so far, spectral energy separation is mainly dependent on design or alterations at the X-ray source and generator level that result in generation of the 2 different energy spectra. With layered detector or "sandwich" detector DECT,[1,2,19,20] on the other hand, spectral separation is achieved at the level of the detector (Philips Healthcare, Andover, MA, USA) (**Fig. 5**). These systems consist of a single source and detector combination. However, they use highly specialized detectors that consist of 2 scintillator layers that have maximal sensitivity for different X-ray photon energies. When seen in a cross-sectional view, the detectors consist of 2 layers of scintillators directly on top of one another, with an optional interlayer filter. The system takes advantage of the polychromatic nature of the X-ray beam, and a single scan is performed at a high energy (120 or 140 kVp). The first or top (inner) layer preferentially absorbs lower-energy photons, by design approximately 50% of the total incident photon flux. The second, bottom (or outer) layer

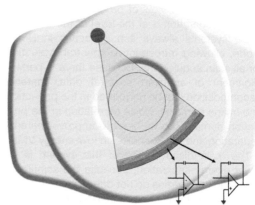

Fig. 5. Layered or sandwich detector DECT (Philips Healthcare). Schematic illustration of this type of a single source-detector combination system in which spectral separation is achieved at the level of the detector. This system takes advantage of the polychromatic nature of the beam produced at the source and highly specialized detectors that consist of 2 layers having maximal sensitivity for different energies. The first layer (*yellow*) preferentially absorbs the low-energy photons, by design approximately 50% of the total incident photon flux. The second layer (*blue*) absorbs the remaining high-energy photons. (*Courtesy of* Reza Forghani, MD, PhD, Montreal, Quebec, Canada and Bruno De Man, PhD, Niskayuna, NY.)

absorbs the remaining photons, which are primarily higher-energy photons. Naturally, this scheme works only because of the polychromatic nature of the X-ray beam generated by a conventional bremsstrahlung tube.

One advantage of this system is its excellent temporal registration. Because energy separation is at the level of the detector and does not rely on different energy spectra generated at the source, there is no time lag between acquisitions of the different energy spectra. Therefore, this system is well suited for material decomposition in the projection domain, which would make it quantitatively accurate and robust for possible patient motion. Along similar lines, there is also perfect spatial registration of the acquired data to create the complete spectral dataset, without the need to compensate for shifting or interpolation that may be seen with systems relying on energy separation at the X-ray source.

The fact that the tube always operates at high kVp results in a high total X-ray power, which is advantageous for larger patients. Because of the detector design with most low-energy photons being absorbed by the first layer, there is in effect "filtration" of those photons and hardening of the spectrum absorbed by the second layer. Similar to the fast kVp switching systems, scanning is performed at the full field of view of 50 cm. Last, because spectral separation is at the level of the detector, these systems always acquire scans in DECT mode, allowing retrospective spectral evaluation for all scan acquisitions. Because there is perfect alignment of acquired spectral data, material decomposition can be performed in the projection and image domains. Noise correlation in the projection domain can be used to improve material separation and reduce noise on low-energy VMIs.

The main disadvantage of this system is its lower energy separation, because the scintillator absorption properties do not offer a sharp distinction between lower- and higher-energy photons. As a result, the material differentiation contrast is decreased unless a higher radiation dose is used. An earlier design choice to mitigate this challenge is to use an interlayer filter between the 2 scintillator layers. The use of an interlayer filter improves the energy separation but also reduces the dose efficiency. The noise level can be balanced between low- and high-energy acquisitions by designing individual-layer thicknesses in order to try and achieve comparable noise levels at the 2 different energies. Because spectral separation is exclusively at the level of the detector, this system does not permit alterations at the source that may optimize the balance between low- and high-energy spectra emitted, unlike the fast kVp switching or dual-source systems. This system does not have the problems of cross-scatter discussed earlier for dual-source scanners, but is susceptible to a different type of cross-scatter between the 2 detector layers. The technical challenges and expense for these systems are related to their specialized detector hardware requirements. Because of the relatively recent introduction of this system in the market, at this time there are fewer studies available that use this DECT technique. As a result, the clinical efficacy of this design when compared with dual-source or fast kVp switching systems is largely unknown. However, this is likely to change with time with more widespread availability and use of this type of scanner.

Single-Source Dual-Energy Computed Tomography with Beam Filtration at the Source: TwinBeam Dual-Energy Computed Tomography

A relatively recent addition to clinically available DECT systems is the TwinBeam DECT scanner[21,22] (Siemens AG) (**Fig. 6**). This system consists of a single source and detector combination, and spectral separation is achieved at the level of the source. However, unlike the fast kVp approach, the beam is prefiltered using 2 different materials and split into high- and low-energy beams. A split filter consisting of gold and tin is placed at the output of the tube, resulting in separation of the beam into a side with a lower-energy spectrum and a side with a higher-energy spectrum. The corresponding halves of the detector are then used for detection of the low- and high-energy spectra (see **Fig. 6**).

Advantages of this system include the ability to image the full field of view, and lesser hardware complexity and lower cost compared with all above systems. TwinBeam may even be incorporated as an upgrade to some scanner models. The main disadvantage is that a different portion of the patient is irradiated by the low- and high-energy spectra. Hence, a helical scan is needed so that each voxel scanned at one energy is eventually also scanned with the other energy. The resulting temporal skew, however, is very high, and there is relatively poor temporal registration between high- and low-energy scans of any given voxel. Another important challenge is that a central 2- to 3-mm portion of the beam will have a mixed energy spectrum due to the finite focal spot size. As a result, that portion of the data cannot be used for material discrimination. There is also potential for cross-scatter originating from one side of the beam contaminating data at the other side of the beam. There are in addition limited ways of balancing the photon flux of the low- and high-energy spectra for optimal spectral differentiation beyond what the X-ray beam filters provide. These systems have become commercially available only recently, and therefore, at this time, there are relatively few clinical studies using this system design. This will undoubtedly change over time and more data on the performance of these systems is likely to emerge with an increase in their availability and use.

Dual-Energy Computed Tomographic Scanning Using Sequential Acquisitions

One of the earliest and technologically most straightforward ways to obtain DECT scans, at least from a hardware standpoint, is by acquiring 2 different scans sequentially.[1,2,6,12] With this approach, the spectral data at 2 different energies are acquired sequentially at the same table position or a range of table positions using different tube voltages (**Fig. 7**). The basic scheme can be optionally enhanced with the use of an additional reconfigurable filter similar to the dual-source or TwinBeam scanners.

The obvious advantage with this approach is that there is little to no significant hardware modification required for scanning, and an established technology can be used for the acquisitions. The

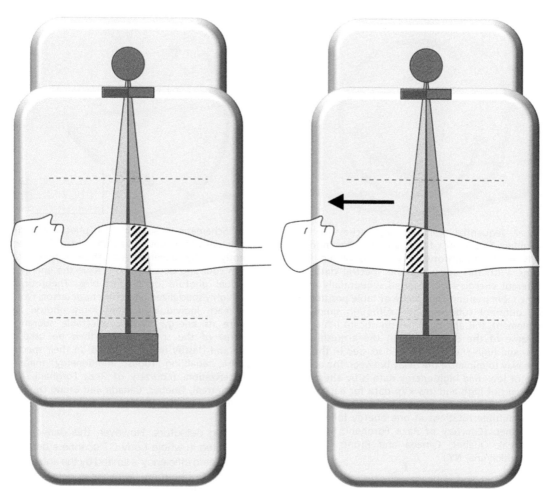

Fig. 6. Single-source DECT with beam filtration at the source: TwinBeam DECT (Siemens AG). Schematic illustration of this type of a single source-detector combination system in which a split filter consisting of gold and tin is placed at the output of the tube, resulting in separation of the beam into low- and high-energy spectra. The corresponding halves of the detector are then used for detection of the low- and high-energy spectra. (*Courtesy of Reza Forghani, MD, PhD, Montreal, Quebec, Canada and Bruno De Man, PhD, Niskayuna, NY.*)

major and significant disadvantage is the temporal skew between the high- and low-energy acquisitions. The inherent delay or temporal skew can pose a limitation on evaluation of any process requiring a high temporal resolution, such as moving organs as may be seen in cardiac imaging. It would also pose a limitation on processes in which there is a change in contrast opacification, such as angiographic acquisitions or even routine studies evaluating tissue enhancement. Furthermore, any patient motion between the different energy acquisitions can result in significant distortion of spectral data. In its simplest form, sequential scans may be obtained with any CT scanner, and the acquired data combined afterward for spectral analysis.

One way to partially mitigate the most significant disadvantage of this system is by minimizing the delay between the acquisition of low- and high-

energy data. This can be achieved by alternating scanning of high and low kVp data for each gantry rotation, instead of scanning the entire volume with multiple rotations at one energy followed by the other (see **Fig. 7**). Partial scanning techniques may also help with temporal resolution for scanning of relatively static organs, but the delays are still too long, and motion misregistration of low- and high-energy data remains a significant problem. The alternating acquisition of different energy data at each gantry position is the approach used by some scanners with DECT capabilities, such as some Aquilion ONE models (Toshiba, Tochigi, Japan) and Revolution EVO (GE Healthcare). Other commercially available CT scanners may also have the option of sequential DECT acquisitions, some limited to that of the entire scanned volume at one energy followed by the other for very limited DECT applications. However, even with the more

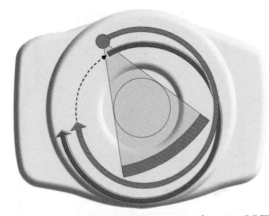

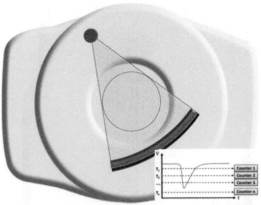

Fig. 7. Sequential scanning approaches to DECT scanning. This is one of the earliest and technologically most straightforward ways to obtain DECT scans. With this approach, the spectral data at 2 different energies are acquired sequentially at the same table position, or a range of table positions using different tube voltages. Although simpler to implement, this approach has significant limitations because of the delay between the acquisition of low- and high-energy data, as discussed in the text. One way to minimize the delay between the acquisition of low- and high-energy data is by alternating scanning of high and low kVp data for each gantry rotation, instead of scanning the entire volume with multiple rotations at one energy followed by the other. (*Courtesy of* Reza Forghani, MD, PhD, Montreal, Quebec, Canada and Bruno De Man, PhD, Niskayuna, NY.)

Fig. 8. Schematic illustration of a photon counting scanner, one of the most advanced spectral CT systems currently under development. These scanners use photon counting detectors to resolve the energy of individual photons or photon bins. Theoretically, these highly specialized and efficient detectors would count each individual incident X-ray photon and measure its energy. Narrow selectable subranges (or bins) of the spectrum can then be used to detect and classify materials based on their spectral response, enabling robust multienergy material characterization. (*Courtesy of* Reza Forghani, MD, PhD, Montreal, Quebec, Canada and Bruno De Man, PhD, Niskayuna, NY.)

refined approaches, major limitations regarding effects of motion and temporal misregistration remain. These factors may limit successful application and use of this technology to certain niche areas.

Emerging Spectral Computed Tomographic Systems

One of the most advanced spectral CT systems currently under investigation and development is the photon counting scanner (**Figs. 8** and **9**).[2,23–34] The principle behind these scanners is the use of photon counting detectors that are used to resolve the energy of individual photons or photon bins. Theoretically, these highly specialized and efficient detectors would count each individual incident X-ray photon and measure its energy range. Narrow selectable subranges (or bins) of the spectrum can then be used to detect and classify materials based on their spectral response, enabling robust multienergy material characterization.

There are multiple potential advantages of such a system. Photon-counting detectors have a higher geometric efficiency than conventional energy-

integrating detectors. However, this cannot fully be exploited in whole-body CT scanners because the geometric efficiency is limited by the antiscatter collimator. Furthermore, with these detectors, an energy threshold may be applied to enable the rejection of false counts that are solely due to measured electronic noise. Hence, the impact of detector electronic noise can be entirely eliminated, or at least significantly reduced. Although electronic noise will still affect the measured energy of true individual photons, it will not alter photon counts.

These systems are conceptually interesting because they provide energy information for each individual photon, and they may have the potential to perform K-edge imaging and detect and classify materials of potential interest at very low concentrations. As such, photon counting has the potential to provide improved spectral material characterization compared with current clinically available approaches. The potential advantages of photon counting systems include improvements in characterization of energy dependency of material attenuation and improved distinction of a material based on its specific K-edge, also referred to as K-edge imaging.

In practice, however, there are challenges that need to be overcome. There is still a substantial overlap between the different energy bins, and it

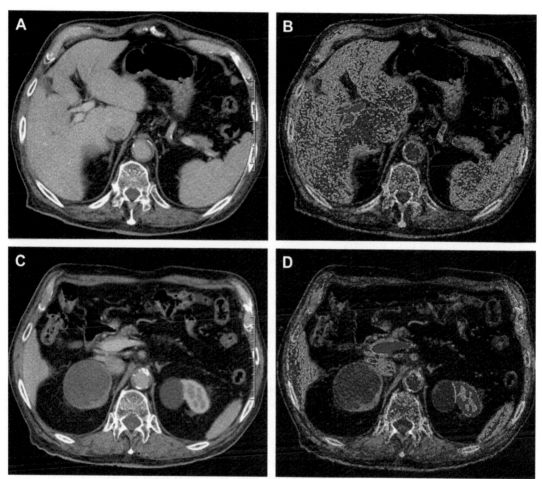

Fig. 9. Examples of abdominal images obtained with a full field-of-view photon-counting CT scanner prototype developed by GE Healthcare and installed at Rabin Medical Center, Israel in 2008. Two different slices are shown in 2 different representations: (*A, C*) monochromatic images at 70 keV and (*B, D*) effective Z images. Different Z numbers are mapped to different colors. The images were obtained with a 32-slice helical scan, 1-second gantry rotation, 140 kVp and 140 mA. (*Courtesy of* Dr Ofer Benjaminov, Rabin Medical Center, Israel; with permission.)

is not yet clear whether the energy separation will be a significant advantage. Another advantage of photon-counting detectors is their smaller cell size, which could offer a substantial increase in spatial resolution. However, this would have to be coupled to a smaller focal spot size and a major X-ray flux, and a dose increase would be required to maintain acceptable image noise at the higher spatial resolution. For example, if all other factors are kept unchanged, a 2-fold improvement in spatial resolution may require a 16-fold increase in radiation dose in order to maintain the same image noise.

The main limitations and challenges of photon counting spectral CT are currently technical in nature. Although photon counting detectors are used in other disciplines such as nuclear medicine, application of this technology for CT

scanning faces significant technological hurdles because of the high exposure rates and photon flux required for CT. These hurdles include pulse pileup effects that can result in loss of counts, or potentially, even "paralyze" the detector. Pulse sharing across multiple detector pixels or K-escape (reemission of a characteristic X-ray) can also occur and result in degradation of the accuracy of the recorded energy. To be effective, photon counting detectors would have to be much faster than currently used CT detectors and avoid prohibitively long scan times. Currently, there are no commercially available photon-counting scanners for clinical use, but different prototypes are available that may one day enable clinical implementation of this exciting technology and open a new era of spectral CT imaging, potentially at a molecular level.

In addition to active investigations and development of photon counting scanners, alternative methods aimed at expanding multienergy evaluation capabilities of spectral CT are also being explored. One example is the adaptation and combination of dual-source and TwinBeam technologies described earlier to perform triple or quadruple beam acquisitions.[35] Another example is the use of multi-kVp imaging, switching the X-ray tube between multiple voltages. These are other examples of exciting opportunities and areas of active research aimed at producing more robust spectral CT platforms in the future. The different types of clinical DECT scanners and spectral CT scanners under investigation or development are summarized in **Table 1**.

Table 1
Different types of spectral computed tomography in clinical use or under development

Commercially available clinical DECT approaches and scanners	
Tube voltage-based DECT scanners	
Dual-source DECT	• Two-source detector combinations at nearly 90° angles • Allow the same volume to be scanned simultaneously at the 2 energies
Single-source DECT with rapid kVp switching (GSI)	• Single source and detector combination • Very fast (submillisecond) switching between low- and high-energy spectra using a single source at each successive axial or spiral view enables DECT acquisition
Detector-based DECT scanners	
Layered or sandwich detector DECT	• Single source and detector combination • Highly specialized dual-layer detectors, each layer having maximal sensitivity for different energies, used for DECT acquisition
Filtration-based DECT scanners	
Single-source DECT with beam filtration at the source (TwinBeam DECT)	• Single source and detector combination • A split filter at the output of the tube results in separation of the beam into low- and high-energy spectra, that in turn are detected by their respective halves of the detector enabling DECT acquisition
Temporally sequential scanning	
Sequential scanning of entire scan volume	• Scan the volumes sequentially at the 2 different energies • In theory possible with any scanner with the use of appropriate software for merging of different energy data
Sequential scanning of each gantry rotation	• Alternating scanning of high and low kVp data for each gantry rotation instead the entire volume • Reduces temporal and spatial misregistration compared with sequential scanning of the entire volume at each energy
Spectral CT approaches and scanners under development	
Dual-source and filtration-based combinations	• Combination of dual-source DECT and split filter placed at the output of one or both tubes • Each source with split filter results in separation of the beam into low- and high-energy spectra detected by their respective halves of the detector • Could potentially enable the acquisition of triple or quadruple energy acquisitions
Photon counting	• Detector-based material differentiation • Narrow selectable subranges (or bins) of the spectrum can potentially be used to detect and classify materials based on their spectral "K-edge" patterns • If successfully implemented, it could represent the most advanced spectral CT system to date, enabling robust multienergy material characterization

SUMMARY

Spectral CT is an exciting and evolving technology that has the potential to change the traditional SECT approach currently used in most clinical settings. DECT provides a new layer of information, previously unavailable using SECT. This new information has the potential to be expanded to elemental or molecular composition analysis far beyond conventional SECT scanning. In this article, the first part of a 2-part review, the fundamental principles underlying spectral CT scanning and different spectral CT systems, both commercially available or under investigation, were reviewed. Such familiarity is essential for those using or planning to use this technology optimally.

Since the advent of DECT systems, there has been a steady increase in the applications of this technology for the evaluation of brain or head and neck abnormality. Concomitantly, there has been a steady increase in the number of commercially available systems. Multiple workflow optimizations are also being implemented to efficiently incorporate this technology into the clinical routine. Various articles in this issue review different applications of DECT and how they are being incorporated into the clinical workflow. Even at this early stage in the development of this technology, it is clear that DECT will play an increasingly important role in neuroradiology and head and neck imaging and further improve the diagnostic evaluation of our patients.

REFERENCES

1. Johnson TRC, Kalender WA. Physical background. In: Johnson T, Fink C, Schönberg SO, et al, editors. Dual energy CT in clinical practice. Berlin: Springer-Verlag Berlin Heidelberg; 2011. p. 3–9.

2. McCollough CH, Leng S, Yu L, et al. Dual- and multi-energy CT: principles, technical approaches, and clinical applications. Radiology 2015;276(3):637–53.

3. Chiro GD, Brooks RA, Kessler RM, et al. Tissue signatures with dual-energy computed tomography. Radiology 1979;131(2):521–3.

4. Genant HK, Boyd D. Quantitative bone mineral analysis using dual energy computed tomography. Invest Radiol 1977;12(6):545–51.

5. Kelcz F, Joseph PM, Hilal SK. Noise considerations in dual energy CT scanning. Med Phys 1979;6(5):418–25.

6. Millner MR, McDavid WD, Waggener RG, et al. Extraction of information from CT scans at different energies. Med Phys 1979;6(1):70–1.

7. Macovski A, Alvarez RE, Chan JL, et al. Energy dependent reconstruction in X-ray computerized tomography. Comput Biol Med 1976;6(4):325–36.

8. Flohr TG, McCollough CH, Bruder H, et al. First performance evaluation of a dual-source CT (DSCT) system. Eur Radiol 2006;16(2):256–68.

9. Johnson TR, Krauss B, Sedlmair M, et al. Material differentiation by dual energy CT: initial experience. Eur Radiol 2007;17(6):1510–7.

10. Dodge CW. A rapid method for the simulation of filtered x-ray spectra in diagnostic imaging systems. Wayne State University; 2008. Available at: http://gateway.proquest.com/openurl?url_ver=Z39.88-2004&res_dat=xri:pqdiss&rft_val_fmt=info:ofi/fmt:kev:mtx:dissertation&rft_dat=xri:pqdiss:3315609.

11. Johnson TR. Dual-energy CT: general principles. AJR Am J Roentgenol 2012;199(5 Suppl):S3–8.

12. Alvarez RE, Macovski A. Energy-selective reconstructions in X-ray computerized tomography. Phys Med Biol 1976;21(5):733–44.

13. Michael GJ. Tissue analysis using dual energy CT. Australas Phys Eng Sci Med 1992;15(2):75–87.

14. Petersilka M, Bruder H, Krauss B, et al. Technical principles of dual source CT. Eur J Radiol 2008;68(3):362–8.

15. Krauss B, Schmidt B, Flohr TG. Dual source CT. In: Johnson T, Fink C, Schönberg SO, et al, editors. Dual energy CT in clinical practice. Berlin: Springer-Verlag Berlin Heidelberg; 2011. p. 10–20.

16. Chandra N, Langan DA. Gemstone detector: dual energy imaging via fast kVp switching. In: Johnson T, Fink C, Schönberg SO, et al, editors. Dual energy CT in clinical practice. Berlin: Springer-Verlag Berlin Heidelberg; 2011. p. 35–41.

17. Kalender WA, Perman WH, Vetter JR, et al. Evaluation of a prototype dual-energy computed tomographic apparatus. I. Phantom studies. Med Phys 1986;13(3):334–9.

18. Xu D, Langan DA, Wu X, et al. Dual energy CT via fast kVp switching spectrum estimation. Paper presented at: Medical Imaging 2009: Physics of Medical Imaging. Lake Buena Vista (FL), March 14, 2009.

19. Vlassenbroek A. Dual layer CT. In: Johnson T, Fink C, Schönberg SO, et al, editors. Dual energy CT in clinical practice. Berlin: Springer-Verlag Berlin Heidelberg; 2011. p. 21–34.

20. Alvarez RE, Seibert JA, Thompson SK. Comparison of dual energy detector system performance. Med Phys 2004;31(3):556–65.

21. Euler A, Parakh A, Falkowski AL, et al. Initial results of a single-source dual-energy computed tomography technique using a split-filter: assessment of image quality, radiation dose, and accuracy of dual-energy applications in an in vitro and in vivo study. Invest Radiol 2016;51(8):491–8.

22. Kaemmerer N, Brand M, Hammon M, et al. Dual-energy computed tomography angiography of the head and neck with single-source computed tomography: a new technical (Split Filter) approach

for bone removal. Invest Radiol 2016;51(10): 618–23.

23. Schlomka JP, Roessl E, Dorscheid R, et al. Experimental feasibility of multi-energy photon-counting K-edge imaging in pre-clinical computed tomography. Phys Med Biol 2008;53(15):4031–47.

24. Shikhaliev PM. Tilted angle CZT detector for photon counting/energy weighting x-ray and CT imaging. Phys Med Biol 2006;51(17):4267–87.

25. Wang X, Meier D, Taguchi K, et al. Material separation in x-ray CT with energy resolved photon-counting detectors. Med Phys 2011;38(3):1534–46.

26. Taguchi K, Iwanczyk JS. Vision 20/20: single photon counting x-ray detectors in medical imaging. Med Phys 2013;40(10):100901.

27. Herrmann C, Engel KJ, Wiegert J. Performance simulation of an x-ray detector for spectral CT with combined Si and Cd[Zn]Te detection layers. Phys Med Biol 2010;55(24):7697–713.

28. Leng S, Yu Z, Halaweish A, et al. A high-resolution imaging technique using a whole-body, research photon counting detector CT system. Proc SPIE Int Soc Opt Eng 2016;9783.

29. Yu Z, Leng S, Jorgensen SM, et al. Initial results from a prototype whole-body photon-counting computed tomography system. Proc SPIE Int Soc Opt Eng 2015;9412.

30. Gutjahr R, Halaweish AF, Yu Z, et al. Human imaging with photon counting-based computed tomography at clinical dose levels: contrast-to-noise ratio and cadaver studies. Invest Radiol 2016;51(7):421–9.

31. Yu Z, Leng S, Jorgensen SM, et al. Evaluation of conventional imaging performance in a research whole-body CT system with a photon-counting detector array. Phys Med Biol 2016;61(4): 1572–95.

32. Iwanczyk JS, Nygard E, Meirav O, et al. Photon counting energy dispersive detector arrays for x-ray imaging. Paper presented at: 2007 IEEE Nuclear Science Symposium Conference Record. Honolulu (HI), October 26, 2007–November 3, 2007.

33. Romman Z, Benjaminov O, Levinson R, et al. Virtual non-contrast ct of the abdomen using a dual energy photon-counting CT scanner: assessment of performance. Paper presented at: Radiological Society of North America 2009 Scientific Assembly and Annual Meeting. Chicago (IL), November 29-December 4, 2009.

34. Benjaminov O, Perlow E, Romman Z, et al. Novel, energy-discriminating photon counting CT system (EDCT): first clinical evaluation—CT angiography: Carotid Artery Stenosis. Paper presented at: Radiological Society of North America 2008 Scientific Assembly and Annual Meeting. Chicago (IL), November 30-December 5, 2008.

35. Yu L, Leng S, McCollough CH. Dual-source multi-energy CT with triple or quadruple X-ray beams. Proc SPIE Int Soc Opt Eng 2016;9783.

Dual-Energy Computed Tomography
Physical Principles, Approaches to Scanning, Usage, and Implementation: Part 2

Reza Forghani, MD, PhD[a],*, Bruno De Man, PhD[b],
Rajiv Gupta, MD, PhD[c]

KEYWORDS

- Dual-energy CT • Virtual monochromatic images • Weighted average images
- Basis material decomposition • Iodine maps • Virtual unenhanced images
- Spectral Hounsfield unit attenuation curves • Workflow

KEY POINTS

- Most clinically used dual-energy computed tomography (DECT) scanners can be used in single-energy or dual-energy mode, except for the layered detector scanners that always acquire data in dual-energy mode.
- DECT scans can be routinely obtained with acceptable doses similar to single-energy CT (SECT), with similar or even slightly better quality (or, conversely, lower dose for the same image quality) in some instances.
- Acquisition in DECT mode also enables generation of additional reconstructions or more sophisticated quantitative analysis not possible with conventional SECT acquisition.
- Commonly used DECT image reconstructions include virtual monochromatic images, weighted average or blended images, and material decomposition maps.
- Workflow friendly implementation is a key consideration and important for implementation of DECT into routine clinical practice.

DUAL-ENERGY COMPUTED TOMOGRAPHY IMPLEMENTATION AND USAGE IN CLINICAL PRACTICE: PRACTICAL CONSIDERATIONS

Different Modes of Acquisition with Current Dual-Energy Computed Tomography Scanners and Implications

Most dual-energy computed tomography (DECT) scanners currently in clinical use, such as dual-source scanners (Siemens AG, Forchheim, Germany) or rapid kilovolt peak (kVp) switching scanners (GE Healthcare, Waukesha, WI), can perform acquisitions in either single-energy computed tomography (SECT) or DECT mode. Indeed, in practice, when the additional information provided by the DECT mode is deemed to be superfluous for the clinical question at hand,

Disclosures: R. Forghani has acted as a consultant for GE Healthcare and has served as a speaker at lunch and learn sessions titled "Dual-Energy CT Applications in Neuroradiology and Head and Neck Imaging" sponsored by GE Healthcare at the 27th and 28th Annual Meetings of the Eastern Neuroradiological Society in 2015 and 2016 (no personal compensation or travel support for these sessions). B. De Man is CT Business Portfolio Leader and Manager of Image Reconstruction Laboratory, GE Global Research. R. Gupta declares no relevant conflict of interest.
[a] Department of Radiology, Segal Cancer Centre and Lady Davis Institute for Medical Research, Jewish General Hospital, McGill University, Room C-212.1, 3755 Cote Sainte-Catherine Road, Montreal, Quebec H3T 1E2, Canada; [b] GE Global Research, One Research Circle, KWC1300B, Niskayuna, NY 12309, USA; [c] Department of Radiology, Massachusetts General Hospital, 55 Fruit Street, Boston, MA 02114, USA
* Corresponding author.
E-mail address: rforghani@jgh.mcgill.ca

these scanners are often operated in the SECT mode. DECT scanning has specific workflow requirements and implications, some of which are discussed later in this article or in an accompanying article in this issue on routine use of DECT scanning for neck imaging. It is therefore to be expected that a proportion of studies performed on such scanners will be performed in SECT mode, and the exact proportion would vary depending on the type of practice and patient population. However, using a DECT scanner *exclusively* in SECT mode does not take advantage of its full capabilities and defeats the purpose of having such a scanner. The only exception to this rule may be the case of a *dual-source* computed tomography (CT) that is primarily devoted to cardiac imaging where the 2 sources are used simultaneously to improve temporal resolution. As a reminder, with most DECT systems, a scan obtained in SECT mode will not be amenable to spectral characterization any more than one acquired using an SECT scanner.

The ability to switch modes of acquisition on these scanners also implies that DECT scanning must be planned and specified beforehand. A practical strategy for efficiently protocoling studies in a radiology department with DECT capability involves developing algorithms for determining which studies should be performed in DECT mode. The decision to acquire scans in DECT mode may be based on a specific referral pattern (eg, all neuro-oncology or head and neck oncology studies), specific highly specialized studies for very selective clinical questions (eg, all studies after intra-arterial interventions for ischemic stroke to distinguish hemorrhage from iodinated contrast), or it may be based on more broad criteria or even routinely based on the body area and/or certain indications (eg, all head CTs; all adult neck studies). These algorithms are likely to evolve as additional studies become available demonstrating applications and potential advantages of DECT technology. However, such algorithms will also likely be significantly impacted by the ease (or lack thereof) of integration into the clinical environment and workflow, in terms of processing effort, time at the CT console, and ability to analyze and reconstruct additional images at the time of clinical interpretation.

One exception to the need for preplanning a DECT scan is the layered or "sandwich" detector scanner (Philips Healthcare, Andover, MA) that is now commercially available. Because spectral separation is based on the detector structure and design, these systems always acquire scans in "DECT mode" and therefore enable

retrospective spectral evaluation for all scan acquisitions. Because of this, with this type of scanner, preselection of scans for acquisition in DECT mode is unnecessary, although it may still be desirable to have preset protocols that determine automatic generation of additional reconstructions of interest for certain scan types and indications.

Radiation Dose and Image Quality

Before implementing DECT for routine clinical use, there are 2 basic requirements. First, images acquired in DECT mode should be at least equivalent to those obtained using standard SECT mode in terms of image quality. Second, the acquisition must be made with an acceptable (preferably, equivalent or lower) patient radiation dose. Once these 2 fundamental requirements are met, the additional postprocessing capabilities made possible by DECT mode are essentially for "free," without any dose or image quality penalty or the need for additional patient scanning (**Box 1**).

Image quality and dose are interrelated, and in effect, for practical purposes, any discussion of one should take the other into consideration. Therefore, strictly speaking, a valid evaluation and comparison of 2 different systems or acquisition modes should be based on a comparison of the dose required to achieve a similar image quality. One way in which image quality can be evaluated is based on image noise, with higher-quality images being less noisy. Image noise may be evaluated subjectively or quantitatively, the latter typically done by measuring the standard deviation (SD) within a region of interest (ROI) either placed on the image just outside a phantom or patient or alternatively within a tissue of interest.[1–4] Other measures of image quality include those related to contrast that can also be evaluated subjectively or quantitatively by different methods.[1–6] It is important to take these factors into account when

---

> **Box 1**
> **Dual-energy computed tomography: essentials**
>
> - Basic DECT reconstructions generated for routine clinical interpretation have *at least* similar quality to conventional SECT images acquired with a similar dose.
>
> - With current clinical scanners, DECT acquisition with an acceptable radiation dose similar to that of SECT is possible on a routine basis.
>
> - Acquisition in DECT mode also enables generation of additional reconstructions or more sophisticated quantitative analysis not possible with conventional SECT acquisitions.

comparing different techniques and radiation dose. For a valid comparison of radiation dose between 2 techniques, the image quality must be similar and vice versa. Task-based image quality analysis methods are gaining interest, especially for the evaluation of iterative reconstruction algorithms, but these are outside the scope of this article.

One specific factor with a significant impact on image noise, and hence on radiation dose, is the image spatial resolution.[7–9] Fundamentally, the image noise, measured by SD, scales with the inverse of the square root of the dose. On the other hand, the image noise scales with the square of the isotropic spatial resolution (assuming the slice thickness and the in-plane resolution change the same way).

$$noise_{STD} \sim \frac{resolution^2_{3D}}{\sqrt{Dose}}$$

Therefore, with all other factors fixed, a dose increase by a factor of 4 would reduce image noise by a factor of 2. However, an isotropic spatial resolution increase by a factor of 2 would increase the image noise by a factor of 4. Hence, in order to keep the noise unchanged, a spatial resolution increase by a factor 2 would require a dose increase by a factor of 16! Intuitively, one might expect that, when the resolution doubles and the voxels are split in 8 equivalent pieces, the dose should increase by a factor of 8. The factor of 16 is because of the complex dependence of noise on spatial resolution and dose, given by the formula above.

Pertaining specifically to DECT, increased radiation dose was a concern during earlier attempts at DECT scanning because of image acquisition at 2 different energies, with some reports indicating a potential for up to ×2.6 increase in radiation dose using sequential DECT scanning compared with SECT.[10] However, with technological improvements and refinements of the current systems in clinical use, this problem has been largely eliminated. A growing number of reports of DECT scans from different body areas in phantoms or patients confirm that DECT scans can be obtained with an acceptable radiation dose for routine clinical use.[1,5,11–15] In a phantom study using 2 different dual-source CT scanners and focusing on the chest, it was reported that DECT scans could be obtained with similar dose and quality as SECT scans.[11] Another study of radiation dose and image quality of neck scans performed using a second-generation dual-source DECT scanner reported that similar image quality could be achieved in DECT mode compared with SECT mode, but with 12% lower radiation dose in DECT mode.[12]

In an early phantom study using a single-source DECT with fast kilovolt peak switching, DECT acquisitions were found to have only a relatively small increase in radiation dose compared with SECT.[13] For a similar image quality as measured by low-contrast detectability, the dose from DECT acquisitions was found to be 14% higher for the phantom acquisition simulating a body examination or 22% higher for the phantom acquisition simulating a head examination.[13] However, in a torso phantom study using a fast kilovolt peak switching scanner, it was reported that DECT virtual monochromatic images (VMIs, discussed later) had a higher contrast and lower noise compared with a 120-kVp SECT acquisition for a given radiation dose.[1] In a study of patient head CTs using a fast kilovolt peak switching scanner, it was reported that an overall similar image quality could be achieved in DECT mode compared with SECT but with 11% lower dose,[14] and another comparison of DECT to SECT head scans also reported favorable image quality at a lower dose using DECT.[15] In the neck, a study comparing DECT and SECT acquisitions performed on the same fast kilovolt peak switching scanner in DECT or SECT mode did not find a significant difference in radiation dose between the 2 groups.[5]

In addition to multiple studies demonstrating feasibility of DECT scans at an acceptable dose comparable to SECT, a few additional broad principles and practicalities need to be considered when doing such a comparison and planning DECT implementation, while abiding by the standard practice to perform studies with radiation doses that are as low as reasonably achievable. One factor to consider is that there can be fairly significant variations in dose with different SECT scanners, even at the same institution, particularly if different model scanners or vendors are compared. The balance of diagnostic quality versus dose also depends on the type of scan, body part, as well as patient demographics and other patient-specific factors. For example, the considerations for an adult patient with head and neck cancer receiving radiation therapy as part of their therapeutic regimen are not the same as routine neck imaging in younger or pediatric patients. Minor differences in radiation dose from a diagnostic CT scan in an adult patient with head and neck cancer are likely to have no significance, and the focus should rather be on obtaining a high diagnostic quality scan that allows for confident diagnosis and staging, which in turn will form the basis for optimal treatment. Last, although beyond the scope of this article, truly deleterious effects of radiation from occasionally performed diagnostic imaging studies in adults, particularly pertaining to cancer risk, are debatable[16,17].

Temporal Resolution

In the context of DECT, 3 time-related parameters are of clinical importance: Total scan time, temporal resolution, and spectral projection delay or skew. The total scan time is the total elapsed time to scan a desired anatomic scan range. It is the time between when the x-ray tube is first activated and when it is switched back off at the end of the complete DECT scan. The clinical significance of total scan time is related to the time of a breath hold, the time during which a patient must hold still during a scan, and the time period over which good contrast opacification must be maintained. Total scan times may range from 100 ms to scan a 16-cm cardiac volume to tens of seconds to scan a full patient body. The total scan time is heavily impacted by the scanner z-coverage and increases for TwinBeam CT (Siemens AG, Forchheim, Germany) (because the helical pitch must be decreased) and sequential DECT modes (because consecutive scans need to be completed).

The temporal resolution is typically defined as the time during which all spectral data for a given image voxel or slice is collected. For most systems, this corresponds to the time of about half a rotation and hence is influenced by gantry speed. The clinical significance of this is the absence of motion artifacts as are sometimes seen primarily in cardiac CT imaging. Note that dual-source CT does not result in a doubling of the temporal resolution in *DECT* mode, because a half rotation is still needed to collect the high- and low-energy projections for both imaging chains. Most vendors offer motion compensation algorithms, which are very powerful in further improving the effective temporal resolution. For TwinBeam CT and sequential scanning, because of the delay between the high- and low-energy measurement of each given slice, the DECT temporal resolution is much poorer, and these DECT approaches are not suitable for cardiac imaging.

The third metric, the spectral skew or the delay between the high- and low-energy measurements for a given projection ray, is unique to DECT and not pertinent to SECT. The spectral skew or delay is primarily important to allow basis material decomposition (BMD) in the projection domain, which in turn offers the cleanest and most accurate elimination of beam hardening or spectral artifacts. The spectral delay also affects the spectral accuracy for fast moving objects, which is independent of the motion artifacts caused by temporal resolution limits. Spectral delay dictates the additional errors and artifacts caused by the motion of an object between the high- and low-energy measurement of a given projection ray.

Here, detector-based DECT systems and fast kilovolt peak switching-based systems have a clear advantage, because their spectral skew is absent or far smaller (<1 ms) than the timespan for most macroscopic biological motion (~10 ms). This temporal skew is really inherent to the scanner design and cannot be controlled through changes in the scan protocol.

Standard and Advanced Dual-Energy Computed Tomography Reconstructions and Basis Material Decomposition

When implementing a DECT program for routine clinical use, one of the basic and fundamental requirements is familiarity with the type of reconstructions that are generated (**Table 1**). This includes a reconstruction that is similar to a standard 120-kVp SECT acquisition that would be used for routine clinical interpretation as well as more advanced reconstructions that may have additional value for diagnostic interpretation. In this section, the most common types of reconstructions that can be generated with DECT scanning are reviewed. More advanced quantitative analysis is discussed in greater detail in a separate article in this issue.

Virtual monochromatic images

The data from the low- and high-energy DECT acquisitions can be combined in a variety of ways to produce images for interpretation. One common type of reconstruction obtained is the VMI. Using sophisticated algorithms, the data from the different energy acquisitions are combined to generate images at any prescribed or predicted x-ray energy level; this image simulates what the actual image would look like if the study was acquired with a monochromatic x-ray beam at that energy. Typical VMI energies with current DECT systems range between 40 and 140 keV, with some dual-source systems allowing higher VMI energy reconstructions up to 190 keV in some investigations evaluating artifact reduction.[18]

Based on data extrapolated from phantom studies and body imaging, 70-keV VMIs are typically considered equivalent to the standard 120-kVp SECT acquisition and are frequently the default setting for routine reconstructions on DECT systems, such as fast kilovolt peak switching scanners (**Fig. 1**).[1,19,20] Indeed, sometimes VMIs may even have a better image quality compared with an SECT acquisition at the same dose. The latter was the case in one study of a torso phantom comparing different energy VMIs from a DECT acquisition and a conventional

Table 1
Overview of dual-energy computed tomography reconstructions

Reconstruction	Description	Comments
VMIs	Low- and high-energy data are combined to generate images at prescribed or predicted energy levels, that is, what the image would look like if the study was acquired with a monochromatic x-ray beam at that energy	• 65 or 70 keV typically considered equivalent to the standard 120-kVp SECT acquisition and used for routine clinical interpretation • Default standard reconstruction type on fast kilovolt peak switching scanners but can be generated with all DECT scanners • Lower limit: 40 keV • Upper limit: 140 keV or higher with some scanners • Different energy VMIs can be used to supplement the 65- or 70-keV reconstructions for specific clinical applications
WA images	Low- and high-energy data are blended in different ways and proportions to produce images for clinical interpretation	• Reconstructions produced on dual-source scanners • 30% blend of low-energy/70% blend of high-energy data typically considered equivalent to the standard 120-kVp SECT acquisition and used for routine clinical interpretation • Similar to the use of different VMI energies, different blends of low- and high-energy data (different proportions, linear vs nonlinear blending) can be used for specific clinical applications
BMD maps	Different energy data are used to identify materials based on their elemental composition and unique spectral characteristics	• Can be used to evaluate the tissue distribution and estimate the concentration of a given material or element (eg, iodine on iodine maps) or create virtual unenhanced images, among others • Can be used for material labeling or classification of materials into predefined groups (eg, uric acid content in renal stones or crystal arthropathy) • DECT is best suited for 2-material decomposition, but 3-material decomposition is also possible by using certain assumptions • For materials to be distinguishable, there must be sufficient differences in their spectral or energy-dependent characteristics

120-kVp SECT acquisition.[1] Image noise was not only lowest on VMIs in the range of 67 to 72 keV compared with other energies, but also lower than an SECT acquisition at a similar dose, supporting their use as conventional SECT equivalent reconstructions and replacements when performing DECT scanning.[1]

To directly evaluate the optimal VMIs for the evaluation of the neck, one study evaluated the signal-to-noise ratio (SNR) of different tissues or neck lesions using a fast kilovolt peak switching scanner.[4] In this study, the SNR was determined by dividing the average density (HU) within regions of interest (ROIs) by the SD within that ROI, with the SD used as a measure of image noise (or an indirect measure of image quality). Although one may use the SD outside the patient as a measure of noise instead, some advocate for using the SD within the tissue itself, arguing that it would be more representative and relevant to the particular structure being evaluated.[2,4] In the aforementioned study of SNR in the neck, normal structures

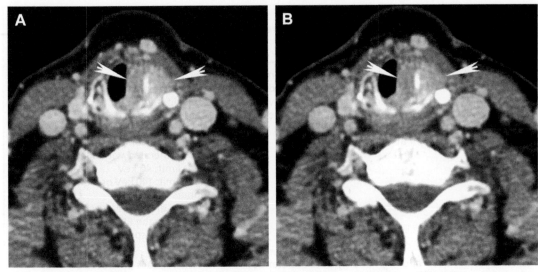

Fig. 1. SECT equivalent VMIs at 65 keV (*A*) and 70 keV (*B*) from a scan of a patient with a left laryngeal cancer (*arrows*) acquired with a fast kilovolt peak switching single source DECT scanner. As discussed in the text, VMIs at these energies are nearly equivalent to a standard 120-kVp SECT acquisition. Quantitatively, there are small differences in tissue attenuation but subjectively they are very similar.

such as muscles at different levels in the neck, normal glandular tissue, and head and neck cancer or pathologic lymph nodes were evaluated. The highest SNR in the soft tissue discrimination range was consistently at 65 keV, closely matched by that of VMIs at 70 or 60 keV.[4]

A subsequent study with a larger number of patients (60) from 2 different institutions also reported similar SNR trends when evaluating the SNR of enhancing part of the tumor in patients with head and neck cancer.[5] Furthermore, consistent with the quantitative SNR results, in a subjective evaluation of the neck CTs including VMI reconstructions at 40, 50, 60, and 65 keV, the 60- and 65-keV VMIs were found to be the most visually appealing and least noisy VMIs. Therefore, at least at one of the author's institutions, the 65 keV is the VMI generated for every neck scan for routine clinical interpretation (see Fig. 1). The SNRs on these reconstructions are close, and as such, the 70-keV reconstructions are acceptable alternatives. The observations supporting routine use of 65-keV VMIs are not unique to the neck. A study of brain CTs also acquired using a fast kilovolt peak switching scanner found that the 65-keV VMIs had the lowest noise for routine brain reconstructions, closely followed by the 70-keV VMIs.[2]

In addition to SECT-equivalent 65- or 70-keV reconstructions used for routine clinical interpretation, VMIs can be reconstructed over a wide range of energies, some of which can be useful for supplementing the 65- or 70-keV images for specific clinical applications.[2–4,6,18,21–26] Specific

clinical applications of different energy VMIs (and other specialized DECT reconstructions) are discussed in multiple articles in this issue and will not be discussed in detail here. However, it is important to understand the basis for these applications, which in one way or another rely on differences in the way different materials or tissues of interest behave at different energies. These differences can be exploited to accentuate differences between certain tissues or lesions and potentially improve overall diagnostic evaluation.

In the first part of this 2-part review, the importance of the photoelectric effect and its energy dependency for spectral material characterization were discussed. Iodine is the main constituent of most CT contrast agents used clinically and has a high atomic number of 53 with strong spectral properties. As such, the energy-dependent changes in attenuation of iodine solutions or contrast-enhanced tissues on infused CT scans well illustrate the expected changes on VMIs at different energies.

To understand the trends in the attenuation of iodine or other elements on different energy VMIs, one needs to understand the basis of the photoelectric effect and its relationship with the K-edge of an element. The photoelectric effect refers to the ejection of an electron from a shell of an atom by an incident photon. The innermost shell (K-shell) has the most strongly bound electrons. The probability of photoelectric interactions generally decreases with higher energies but increases abruptly when the incident photon energy just exceeds the binding electron energy of the K-shell electrons, enabling the ejection of an electron from the K-shell. This energy represents the K-edge for a given element. Therefore, there is a spike in attenuation at the K-edge followed by a rapid drop in the probability of photoelectric interactions and consequently of attenuation with further increase in energy above the K-edge. Understanding this concept is essential for understanding the behavior of elements on spectral CT.

For example, iodine has a K-edge of 33.2 keV. As such, one would expect that a drop in VMI energy away from the SECT equivalent 70 or 65 keV VMIs would result in an increase in iodine attenuation. This relationship is well demonstrated on spectral Hounsfield unit attenuation curves obtained by ROI analysis, which is a quantitative graphic correlate of attenuation seen on the VMIs. In **Fig. 2**, the spectral Hounsfield unit attenuation curves of 3 different concentration iodine solutions within a phantom are shown. Note the marked increase in attenuation at lower energies, with the highest attenuation at 40 keV, the energy closest to the K-edge of iodine. The error bars in this case represent the SD that can be used to estimate image noise, another important parameter

to be considered. As one would expect, with most DECT systems, there is greater image noise at lower VMI energies, representing a tradeoff between iodine attenuation and noise. Increasing VMI energy, on the other hand, reduces noise but also reduces iodine attenuation. **Fig. 3** shows image examples of the same process for different energy VMIs reconstructed from a DECT scan of a patient with head and neck cancer. An increase in image noise on low-energy VMIs is seen with most currently used DECT systems. However, the exception to this is the layered or sandwich detector-based system with which low-energy VMIs may be obtained without an increase in image noise (**Fig. 4**).

Weighted average images

Another reconstruction routinely obtained when using dual-source CT scanners is the weighted average image (WA) (**Fig. 5**). WA images represent a linear blend of the low- and high-energy acquisitions and are the default reconstructions generated by most dual-source DECT systems, although with some of the newer platforms other types of reconstructions such as VMIs can also be generated automatically. Typically, a linear blend consisting of 30% of the low- and 70% of the high-energy acquisitions are considered equivalent to the standard 120-kVp SECT acquisition and generated for routine clinical interpretation (see **Fig. 5**).[6,12,27,28] However, just like with VMIs, the proportion of the low- and high-energy data that are blended as well as the way they are blended (eg, linear vs nonlinear) can be altered to accentuate different material or tissue characteristics of potential interest.[28,29] For example, altered blending using a higher proportion of the low-energy acquisition would have a similar effect to lowering the VMI energy.

Basis material decomposition, labeling, and maps

Basis material decomposition Depending on the energy (VMI) or blending ratio (WA), VMIs and WA images can resemble images generated using conventional SECT scanning that radiologists are familiar with and comfortable looking at routinely (see **Figs. 1**, **3–5**). For VMIs approaching either end of the spectrum, the images may have much higher contrast (as well as noise) in the low-energy range or lower enhancement and soft tissue contrast in the high energy range, but the basic anatomic information and image "structure" are otherwise the same (see **Fig. 3**). However, in addition to VMIs and WA images, DECT scan data can also be used to create other types of images based on BMD.

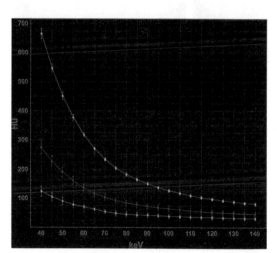

Fig. 2. Strong spectral properties of iodine in CT contrast agents. Spectral Hounsfield unit attenuation curves derived from ROI analysis of iodine solutions at 3 different concentrations, imaged within a phantom, are shown. Note the progressive and marked increase in attenuation at lower energies approaching the K-edge of iodine (33.2 keV). For example, note the higher attenuation at 40 keV compared with conventional SECT equivalent VMI energies at 65 or 70 keV. However, there is a tradeoff, with increasing image noise at lower energies, as represented by the error bars depicting SD of attenuation within the ROI evaluated. The scan was acquired with a fast kilovolt peak switching scanner.

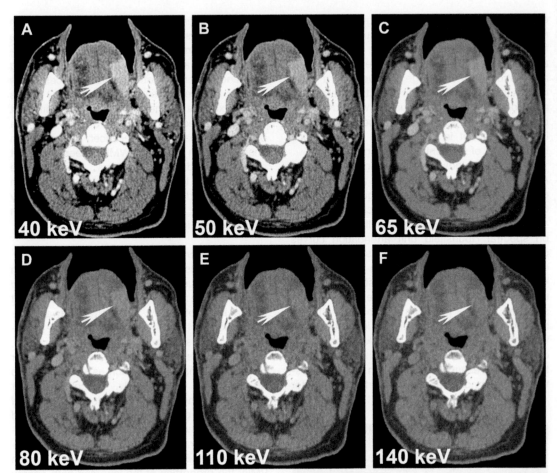

Fig. 3. Examples of VMIs at different energies reconstructed from a contrast-enhanced neck CT of a patient with a left oral tongue cancer (*arrow*). VMIs of the same scan/slice are shown at 40 (*A*), 50 (*B*), 65 (*C*), 80 (*D*), 110 (*E*), and 140 (*F*) keV. In order to emphasize the differences between different VMI energies, all images were displayed using the same window-level setting. Note how enhancing tissues such as the tumor (*arrow*) or vessels have increased attenuation with decreasing VMI energy, with the highest attenuation on the 40 keV VMI (*A*). However, there is a tradeoff as image noise increases with increasing conspicuity of enhancing tissue at lower energies, and this tradeoff is expected with most of the currently used DECT systems, as described in the text. Conversely, at high energies, the lower noise is accompanied by lower attenuation and contrast of enhancing tissues. The scan was acquired with a fast kilovolt peak switching scanner.

DECT BMD is based on the fact that the x-ray attenuation of any material is a linear combination of Compton scatter attenuation and photoelectric attenuation. Strictly speaking, Rayleigh scatter is a third, smaller attenuation mechanism, but for practical purposes, that effect can be ignored here. The energy dependence of these 2 effects can be assumed to be fixed across all materials, but their relative contribution to the overall attenuation changes for different materials. As a result, Compton scatter and the photoelectric effect can form a *material basis pair* in which all materials can be expressed. Photoelectric attenuation has a very strong dependence on energy, and Compton scatter has a weaker dependence on energy, so actual materials have an energy dependence

that is somewhere between the 2. **Fig. 6** shows qualitatively how the x-ray attenuation of different materials (blood, iodine, bone) is fundamentally made up of a combination of Compton scatter and photoelectric absorption.

With DECT scanners, it is more common to express materials in a different material basis pair that is more related to human tissues. One of the most common basis pairs is the combination of water and iodine, as illustrated in **Fig. 6**A. Water and iodine each have their own energy dependence of their attenuation. Water attenuation is close to blood within vessels (blue dot). The attenuation in water is dominated by Compton scatter but also includes some photoelectric effect. Iodine, on the other hand, has a much higher

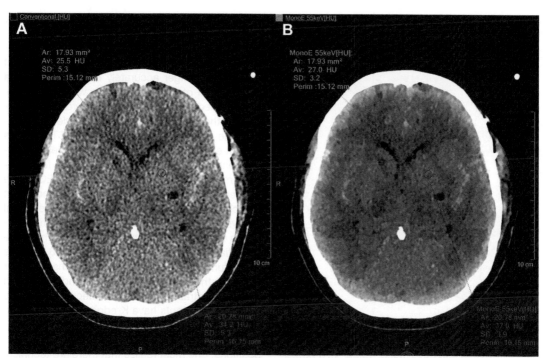

Fig. 4. Example of low-energy VMIs obtained using a layered or sandwich detector system. (*A*) Conventional SECT equivalent and (*B*) 55-keV VMI are shown. With these systems, lower-energy VMIs may be reconstructed without increased image noise. As the ROI analysis shows, the SD, representative of image noise, is actually lower on the 55 keV image compared with the conventional CT image. (*Courtesy of* Professor, David Maintz, MD, The Institute for Diagnostic and Interventional Radiology, Uniklinik, Cologne, Germany; and Philips Healthcare; with permission.)

contribution of the photoelectric effect and hence has a stronger energy dependence. Using water-iodine as the material basis pair, every material is represented as a linear combination of water and iodine, as reflected in **Fig. 6**A by the water density axis and the iodine density axis. For instance, water (and blood) would by definition be 100% water and 0 mg/mL iodine. A mixture of iodine and blood (pink dot) would be 100% water and a certain concentration of iodine. All other materials can be expressed as another weighted combination of water and iodine. The dashed lines represent how each material is mapped in this BMD coordinate system. This does not mean that they physically consist of water and iodine, but it means that their x-ray attenuation is the same as a specific combination of the x-ray attenuations of water and iodine.

These basis material images can be very useful for characterization of materials by cross-correlating their attenuation properties. For instance, a region that is bright or has high intensity on the iodine map but not on the water map is likely to be iodine-containing blood (ie, iodine within the perfused blood volume/vasculature). On the other hand, a region that is bright in both maps is probably bone or calcified tissue. All tissues (eg, muscle,

adipose, cysts) have their own distinct pattern in a given basis material pair. However, it is important to be aware that the basis material images should NOT be interpreted as the physical distribution of pure water and pure iodine.

Multimaterial decomposition and material labeling As alluded to earlier, in principle, DECT only provides 2 independent measurements and is best suited for material decomposition of 2 constituent elements. They are not a reflection of all materials present in the body but truly a decomposition into 2 (somewhat arbitrary) basis pairs. However, DECT has also been used to accurately characterize 3 or more materials occurring in the body. In order to distinguish 3 or more materials based on current DECT scanners providing 2 sets of data, significant assumptions have to be made. One method is assumption of constant volume or mass, and another is a semiempirical method to estimate the effective density in the absence of volume conservation. Both of these approaches have limitations, and for multimaterial decomposition to be effective, the materials under investigation should have sufficiently different spectral characteristics to allow for reasonable discrimination.

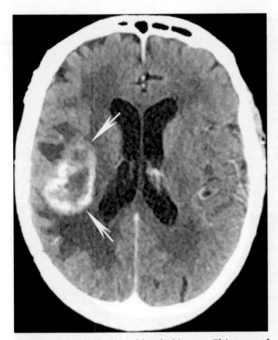

Fig. 5. Example of WA or blended image. This type of reconstruction is obtained when using dual-source CT scanners. Axial head CT obtained after administration of contrast is shown in a patient with an intracranial tumor (*arrows*). A linear blend consisting of 30% of the low- and 70% of the high-energy acquisitions is typically considered equivalent to the standard 120-kVp SECT acquisition. The scan was acquired with a dual-source scanner.

Fig. 6B illustrates how a given voxel (represented here by the white dot) can be expressed as a combination of the true physical material, based on the triangle it is located in. In this case, the white dot falls on the line connecting blood and iodine solution. Hence, this voxel represented by the white dot has zero bone content but contains iodine, although at a lower concentration than the pink dot. Based on this approach, DECT data can also be used for material labeling, or classification of materials into predefined groups.[30] Examples of this application include urinary stone characterization for distinction of uric acid versus nonuric acid stones in abdominal imaging[31,32] or identification of uric acid in crystal arthropathies.[33] The examples provided so far are a few among a list of potential combinations for material decomposition and labeling. As long as there are sufficient differences in the spectral properties of the materials of interest, there is potential for discrimination using DECT. **Fig. 6C, D** illustrates how the same materials would be interpreted in VMI images. Each material is now projected on a respective VMI axis, with the corresponding tradeoffs between contrast and noise discussed earlier.

When materials have an attenuation discontinuity due to a K-edge somewhere in the range of the useful x-ray energy spectrum, their energy dependence actually becomes fundamentally different and can no longer accurately be expressed as a combination of 2 basis materials without K-edge, as explained above; in this case, a third basis material with the appropriate K-edge is needed to represent the position of that K-edge. DECT systems cannot exactly distinguish 3 or more linearly independent basis functions (or conversely, for accurate material decomposition using DECT, the imaged materials should be linearly dependent on the chosen basis materials). Advanced spectral CT systems under development with 3 or more energies such as photon counting scanners have the potential for accurate discrimination of 3 or more basis functions and allow K-edge imaging. For instance, they may allow to image and distinguish multiple contrast agents simultaneously, provided the contrast agents have K-edges that distinguish them from each other.

When performing 2 or multiple material decompositions, one must realize that there are technical limitations to this type of analysis. For example, depending on the material pair, there can be overlap in their spectral characteristics. X-ray measurement noise also impacts the basis material images, which introduces errors in the analysis and may result in overestimation or underestimation of a material of interest or oversubtraction or undersubtraction of a reference material basis pair. Another factor that must be considered is that in vivo, there is a mix of tissues and elements, and not a pure solution or pure theoretic conditions on which the different approaches and algorithms are based. These additional, unpredictable factors can influence the maps and may affect the accuracy for detection or estimation of the concentration of a material of interest. Therefore, although material decomposition maps can be powerful tools in providing estimation of content of certain materials, especially those with strong spectral properties, one must be aware of the potential limitations of this type of analysis.

Virtual unenhanced or virtual noncontrast images and iodine maps One of the most promising applications of DECT is to virtually suppress iodine content to visualize what parts of the images were enhanced due to iodine and what they would look like without iodine or, alternatively, create maps reflecting distribution of iodine in tissues. Similar approaches have been proposed to suppress other tissues such as bone or calcium. There are essentially 3 ways to create images with virtually suppressed iodine.

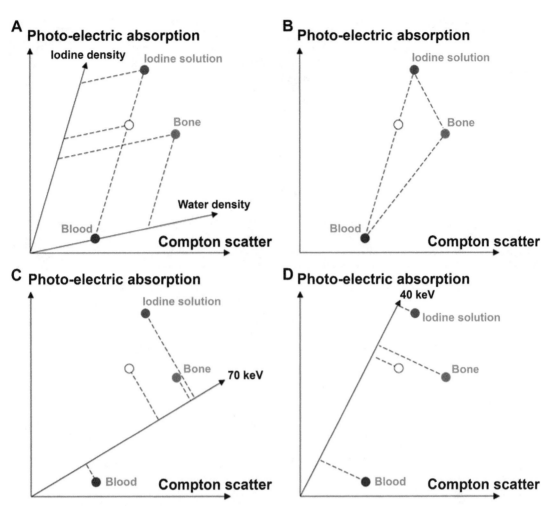

Fig. 6. BMD. All tissue attenuations are fundamentally a combination of Compton scatter and photoelectric absorption (ignoring the small contribution from Rayleigh scatter). Different representations are obtained by projecting these fundamental attenuation properties onto different spaces. Graphs illustrating the principles and approach for (*A*) water-iodine basis-material decomposition, (*B*) multimaterial decomposition, and (*C, D*) virtual monochromatic imaging at 70 keV and 40 keV are shown. Please refer to the text for additional details and explanations. (*Courtesy of* Reza Forghani, MD, PhD, Montreal, Quebec, Canada and Bruno De Man, PhD, Niskayuna, NY)

The first way is to use VMIs at a relatively high kiloelectron volt, where the iodine attenuation is substantially more suppressed than other tissues because of a substantial reduction in photoelectric interactions at energies further away from the iodine K-edge. An example of this can be seen in **Fig. 3**, with progressive suppression of iodine attenuation with increasing VMI energies.

The second way is by looking at the water images after a water-iodine BMD (**Fig. 7**). By definition, the iodine should be captured in the iodine map, and hence, the water map should represent blood without iodine. However, other tissues are also transformed into a water-iodine combination, and hence, this water image is not the same as a regular CT image without iodine. Conversely, for estimation

of iodine content using a fast kilovolt peak switching technique, iodine-water material decomposition maps can be created (see **Fig. 7**), and similar maps can also be created with other DECT systems (**Fig. 8**). These maps represent the iodine content and distribution within tissues. They can be used to estimate the iodine concentration within a tissue and evaluate its distribution for different applications such as assessment of enhancing tumor[34] or determination of perfused tissue blood volume (or blood pool imaging) (see **Figs. 7** and **8**; **Fig. 9**).[35] Water is used as the reference for multiple reasons: it is the most common constituent of the human body; there is significant spectral contrast between iodine and water that enables excellent separation of these 2 materials; and finally, because its CT

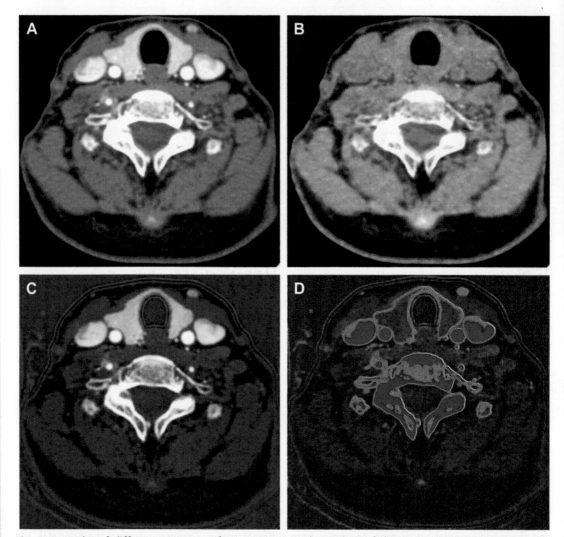

Fig. 7. Examples of different BMD maps from a contrast-enhanced CT of the neck. (*A*) 65 keV VMI (typically considered equivalent to SECT), (*B*) water-iodine BMD map (one type of virtual unenhanced image), and (*C, D*) iodine-water BMD maps displayed in gray scale or color are shown. Note the suppression of iodine in the vessels and thyroid gland on the virtual unenhanced image (*B*). The iodine-water maps represent the iodine distribution and relative iodine content in different tissues (for example higher intensity in the carotid arteries compared with the internal jugular veins). ROI analysis of iodine-water maps can provide an estimate of iodine concentration within a tissue. The scan was acquired with a fast kilovolt peak switching scanner.

number remains relatively constant with respect to change in x-ray energy.

The third and most accurate way is to generate true virtual unenhanced or virtual noncontrast images by performing multimaterial decomposition, characterizing the actual material content for each voxel and replacing the iodine by blood. The resulting image is a VMI (typically at 70 keV), where the iodine has been virtually removed and all other tissues are unchanged.

Commonly performed representations include maps estimating iodine content, iodine subtraction (or virtual unenhanced images), calcium or bone

subtraction, or a combination of the above in order to address an increasing number of clinical scenarios of interest. The earliest investigations and proposed applications of virtual unenhanced images were in body imaging, but there are also potential applications for the use of virtual unenhanced images in neuroradiology and head and neck imaging, including differentiation of intracranial hemorrhage from iodinated contrast material[36] or the evaluation of sialolithiasis, as discussed in detail in other articles in this issue.

Other than the reconstructions discussed so far, DECT enables additional quantitative analysis and

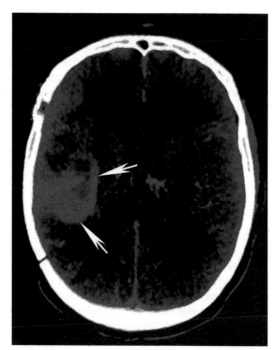

Fig. 8. Example of iodine map of the brain from the same patient as shown in **Fig. 5**. Note increased intensity in the area of the enhancing tumor (*arrows*). The scan was acquired with a dual-source scanner.

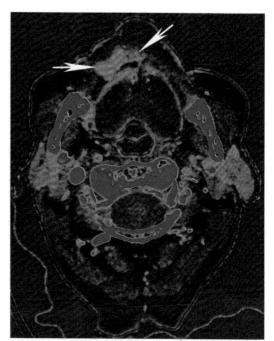

Fig. 9. Example of iodine-water material decomposition map from a contrast-enhanced CT of the neck from a patient with buccal invasion by tumor (*arrows*). The iodine (or iodine-water) maps represent the iodine distribution and relative iodine content in different tissues (for example note the higher "signal" in the tumor compared to surrounding tissues). ROI analysis of iodine-water maps can provide an estimate of iodine concentration within a tissue. The scan was acquired with a fast kilovolt peak switching scanner.

reconstructions. Spectral Hounsfield unit ROI analysis may be used to quantitatively evaluate spectral characteristics of an area or lesion of interest (see **Fig. 2**). Histograms or plots may be created for the evaluation of the effective Z and distribution in an area of interest. Several additional analyses may also be performed on the rich quantitative data from spectral CT[22,37] scans that are discussed in greater detail in a separate article on advanced tissue characterization using DECT in this issue.

Workflow and Other Practical Considerations

As discussed earlier, except for the layered detector DECT scanner, scans must be performed in DECT mode prospectively. However, once acquired in DECT mode, spectral analysis and material characterization can be performed retrospectively as long as the main spectral data set is stored (keeping only a specific reconstructed VMI dataset, WA image, or material decomposition map is not sufficient to allow full retrospective spectral analysis). DECT implementation in clinical practice has workflow implications, at the level of both the technologist and the radiologist. It is also noteworthy that currently the postprocessing software that enables advanced DECT spectral analysis is proprietary and

vendor specific. The authors are not aware of a vendor-neutral independent platform that offers the full spectral analytical and reconstruction capabilities for DECT scans at this time; this is important to consider when planning acquisition of a DECT system, especially for vendors that may not include the full software capabilities as part of their basic or standard package.

One way to facilitate and help integration of DECT into routine clinical workflow is to generate specific sets of useful reconstructions for a given study at the CT console and send to the picture archiving and communication system (PACS) so they are immediately available for review. This is a model some of the authors have previously proposed for evaluation of neck CTs of patients with head and neck cancer[3,4,23,24] and is also discussed in greater detail in separate articles on DECT evaluation of head and neck squamous cell carcinoma and DECT workflow. The advantage of this approach is that the reconstructions are readily available for use. The disadvantage is that by itself, without the capability to do additional postprocessing, the radiologist is limited to preselected reconstructions. Depending on the vendor, certain reconstructions such as material decomposition maps are also not always optimal in terms of use and manipulation when sent to PACS (in contrast to direct use on an advanced workstation), representing another limitation. Even then, this type of approach can ease workflow for most cases, and the radiologist has the option to use an advanced workstation or advanced integrated software for cases where additional analysis or reconstructions are required.

For fast kilovolt peak switching scanners, it is possible to reconstruct VMIs at different energies or limited material decomposition maps at the CT console and send them to PACS (although the range of VMIs that can be generated will vary depending on the model and software version). Some consoles also can generate different energy VMIs automatically, further helping workflow. If additional advanced image analysis or reconstructions are needed, these can be performed on a stand-alone dedicated image processing workstation. Currently, the primary suite of tools for advanced DECT analysis is integrated into the advanced workstation for these systems. However, "thin client" models are available so that DECT software running on a specialized server can be remotely accessed from the PACS workstation. The vendors are continuously pushing to primary reads on the PACS workstation for clinical ease of use.

For dual-source scanners, traditionally the default reconstructions have been blended or WA images that were generated at the CT console and then sent to PACS. However, with some of the newer dual-source systems or the recently introduced TwinBeam CT systems, VMIs or some material decomposition maps can be programmed to be created automatically and sent to the PACS. If not preprogrammed, these reconstructions can also be made retrospectively at the CT console, as long as the original study data are not erased. Advanced spectral CT analysis or generation of different reconstructions is also possible at the radiologist or other workstation using advanced software that may be integrated with the PACS using a thin client application running on any remote workstation, including the PACS. By virtue of these software-based simplifications, it may no longer be necessary to move to a separate dedicated workstation that is physically different from the PACS used for routine radiologic reading. The same software can also be used to perform more advanced spectral analyses or generate material decomposition maps.

Layered detector systems also enable preprogramming for the automatic generation of different DECT reconstructions that are then sent to PACS. In addition, these systems come with software that can be integrated with the PACS or with the radiologist workstation for direct spectral analysis and image manipulation. Increasingly, different systems enable a more seamless flow, which is important for widespread and routine use of DECT in the clinical setting. Workflow implications and challenges of DECT are also discussed in a separate article in this issue, focusing on a single-institution implementation of routine DECT neck scanning.

SUMMARY

DECT is an exciting and evolving technology that has the potential to change the traditional approach to the use of CT in the clinical setting, providing a new layer of information that was previously unavailable. It has the potential to be expanded to elemental or molecular composition analysis far beyond conventional SECT scanning. In this article, the second part of a 2-part review, essential and practical information on the main types of image reconstructions produced by these scanners was reviewed. In addition, important practical considerations on implementation of DECT scanning into routine clinical practice were discussed, ranging from image quality and radiation dose to issues related to workflow-friendly implementation. Familiarity with the topics discussed is essential for any radiologist or group planning to incorporate DECT into their clinical practice, including the types of reconstructions that are expected, reconstructions used for routine interpretation, and those for more advanced analysis.

There are increasing reports of different applications of DECT for the evaluation of brain or head and neck abnormalities, and these are reviewed in multiple articles in this issue. The number of commercially available DECT systems and those deployed in clinical practice is also steadily increasing. As such, there is a great potential for integration of this exciting technology into routine clinical practice. However, there are also competing pressures and barriers; these include increasing scan volumes and at times declining reimbursements for some scans. Although a key determinant of routine use of the technology will obviously be improvements in diagnostic performance and added value for scan interpretation, practical factors, including user-friendly and seamless workflow integration, should not be ignored. The latter is also likely to have a great impact on the use of this technology and integration into routine clinical practice. It is likely that if successfully implemented in a workflow-friendly manner, this technology will play an increasing and important role in neuroradiology and head and neck imaging and will ultimately help further improve the diagnostic evaluation of our patients.

REFERENCES

1. Matsumoto K, Jinzaki M, Tanami Y, et al. Virtual monochromatic spectral imaging with fast kilovoltage switching: improved image quality as compared with that obtained with conventional 120-kVp CT. Radiology 2011;259(1):257–62.
2. Pomerantz SR, Kamalian S, Zhang D, et al. Virtual monochromatic reconstruction of dual-energy unenhanced head CT at 65-75 keV maximizes image quality compared with conventional polychromatic CT. Radiology 2013;266(1):318–25.
3. Forghani R, Levental M, Gupta R, et al. Different spectral hounsfield unit curve and high-energy virtual monochromatic image characteristics of squamous cell carcinoma compared with nonossified thyroid cartilage. AJNR Am J Neuroradiol 2015; 36(6):1194–200.
4. Lam S, Gupta R, Levental M, et al. Optimal virtual monochromatic images for evaluation of normal tissues and head and neck cancer using dual-energy CT. AJNR Am J Neuroradiol 2015;36(8): 1518–24.
5. Forghani R, Kelly H, Yu E, et al. Low-energy virtual monochromatic dual-energy computed tomography images for the evaluation of head and neck squamous cell carcinoma: a study of tumor visibility compared with single-energy computed tomography and user acceptance. J Comput Assist Tomogr 2017. [Epub ahead of print].
6. Wichmann JL, Noske EM, Kraft J, et al. Virtual monoenergetic dual-energy computed tomography: optimization of kiloelectron volt settings in head and neck cancer. Invest Radiol 2014;49(11):735–41.
7. Chesler DA, Riederer SJ, Pelc NJ. Noise due to photon counting statistics in computed X-ray tomography. J Comput Assist Tomogr 1977;1(1):64–74.
8. Riederer SJ, Pelc NJ, Chesler DA. The noise power spectrum in computed X-ray tomography. Phys Med Biol 1978;23(3):446–54.
9. Li B, Avinash GB, Hsieh J. Resolution and noise trade-off analysis for volumetric CT. Med Phys 2007;34(10):3732–8.
10. Ho LM, Yoshizumi TT, Hurwitz LM, et al. Dual energy versus single energy MDCT: measurement of radiation dose using adult abdominal imaging protocols. Acad Radiol 2009;16(11):1400–7.
11. Schenzle JC, Sommer WH, Neumaier K, et al. Dual energy CT of the chest: how about the dose? Invest Radiol 2010;45(6):347–53.
12. Tawfik AM, Kerl JM, Razek AA, et al. Image quality and radiation dose of dual-energy CT of the head and neck compared with a standard 120-kVp acquisition. AJNR Am J Neuroradiol 2011;32(11):1994–9.
13. Li B, Yadava G, Hsieh J. Quantification of head and body CTDI(VOL) of dual-energy x-ray CT with fast-kVp switching. Med Phys 2011;38(5):2595–601.
14. Kamiya K, Kunimatsu A, Mori H, et al. Preliminary report on virtual monochromatic spectral imaging with fast kVp switching dual energy head CT: comparable image quality to that of 120-kVp CT without increasing the radiation dose. Jpn J Radiol 2013; 31(4):293–8.
15. Hwang WD, Mossa-Basha M, Andre JB, et al. Qualitative comparison of noncontrast head dual-energy computed tomography using rapid voltage switching technique and conventional computed tomography. J Comput Assist Tomogr 2016;40(2):320–5.
16. Hoang JK, Reiman RE, Nguyen GB, et al. Lifetime attributable risk of cancer from radiation exposure during parathyroid imaging: comparison of 4D CT and parathyroid scintigraphy. AJR Am J Roentgenol 2015;204(5):W579–85.
17. Siegel JA, Welsh JS. Does imaging technology cause cancer? Debunking the linear no-threshold model of radiation carcinogenesis. Technol Cancer Res Treat 2016;15(2):249–56.
18. Tanaka R, Hayashi T, Ike M, et al. Reduction of dark-band-like metal artifacts caused by dental implant bodies using hypothetical monoenergetic imaging after dual-energy computed tomography. Oral Surg Oral Med Oral Pathol Oral Radiol 2013;115(6): 833–8.
19. Pinho DF, Kulkarni NM, Krishnaraj A, et al. Initial experience with single-source dual-energy CT abdominal angiography and comparison with single-energy CT angiography: image quality, enhancement, diagnosis and radiation dose. Eur Radiol 2013;23(2):351–9.
20. Patel BN, Thomas JV, Lockhart ME, et al. Single-source dual-energy spectral multidetector CT of pancreatic adenocarcinoma: optimization of energy level viewing significantly increases lesion contrast. Clin Radiol 2013;68(2):148–54.
21. Srinivasan A, Hoeffner E, Ibrahim M, et al. Utility of dual-energy CT virtual keV monochromatic series for the assessment of spinal transpedicular hardware-bone interface. AJR Am J Roentgenol 2013;201(4):878–83.
22. Srinivasan A, Parker RA, Manjunathan A, et al. Differentiation of benign and malignant neck pathologies: preliminary experience using spectral computed tomography. J Comput Assist Tomogr 2013;37(5): 666–72.
23. Forghani R. Advanced dual-energy CT for head and neck cancer imaging. Expert Rev Anticancer Ther 2015;15(12):1489–501.

24. Lam S, Gupta R, Kelly H, et al. Multiparametric evaluation of head and neck squamous cell carcinoma using a single-source dual-energy CT with fast kVp switching: state of the art. Cancers (Basel) 2015;7(4):2201–16.

25. Stolzmann P, Winklhofer S, Schwendener N, et al. Monoenergetic computed tomography reconstructions reduce beam hardening artifacts from dental restorations. Forensic Sci Med Pathol 2013;9(3):327–32.

26. Albrecht MH, Scholtz JE, Kraft J, et al. Assessment of an advanced monoenergetic reconstruction technique in dual-energy computed tomography of head and neck cancer. Eur Radiol 2015;25(8):2493–501.

27. Graser A, Johnson TR, Hecht EM, et al. Dual-energy CT in patients suspected of having renal masses: can virtual nonenhanced images replace true nonenhanced images? Radiology 2009;252(2):433–40.

28. Tawfik AM, Kerl JM, Bauer RW, et al. Dual-energy CT of head and neck cancer: average weighting of low- and high-voltage acquisitions to improve lesion delineation and image quality-initial clinical experience. Invest Radiol 2012;47(5):306–11.

29. Scholtz JE, Husers K, Kaup M, et al. Non-linear image blending improves visualization of head and neck primary squamous cell carcinoma compared to linear blending in dual-energy CT. Clin Radiol 2015;70(2):168–75.

30. Krauss B, Schmidt B, Flohr TG. Dual source CT. In: Johnson T, Fink C, Schönberg SO, et al, editors. Dual energy CT in clinical practice. Berlin: Springer-Verlag Berlin Heidelberg; 2011. p. 10–20.

31. Primak AN, Fletcher JG, Vrtiska TJ, et al. Noninvasive differentiation of uric acid versus non-uric acid kidney stones using dual-energy CT. Acad Radiol 2007;14(12):1441–7.

32. Boll DT, Patil NA, Paulson EK, et al. Renal stone assessment with dual-energy multidetector CT and advanced postprocessing techniques: improved characterization of renal stone composition–pilot study. Radiology 2009;250(3):813–20.

33. Glazebrook KN, Guimaraes LS, Murthy NS, et al. Identification of intraarticular and periarticular uric acid crystals with dual-energy CT: initial evaluation. Radiology 2011;261(2):516–24.

34. Kuno H, Onaya H, Iwata R, et al. Evaluation of cartilage invasion by laryngeal and hypopharyngeal squamous cell carcinoma with dual-energy CT. Radiology 2012;265(2):488–96.

35. McCollough CH, Leng S, Yu L, et al. Dual- and multi-energy CT: principles, technical approaches, and clinical applications. Radiology 2015;276(3):637–53.

36. Gupta R, Phan CM, Leidecker C, et al. Evaluation of dual-energy CT for differentiating intracerebral hemorrhage from iodinated contrast material staining. Radiology 2010;257(1):205–11.

37. Forghani R, Roskies M, Liu X, et al. Dual-energy CT characteristics of parathyroid adenomas on 25-and 55-second 4D-CT acquisitions: preliminary experience. J Comput Assist Tomogr 2016;40(5):806–14.

Dual-Energy Computed Tomographic Applications for Differentiation of Intracranial Hemorrhage, Calcium, and Iodine

CrossMark

Ranliang Hu, MD[a],*, Atul Padole, MD[b], Rajiv Gupta, MD, PhD[b]

KEYWORDS

- Dual-energy CT • Intracranial hemorrhage • Calcification • Iodine staining • Iodine map
- Calcium overlay maps • Material decomposition • Virtual non-contrast images

KEY POINTS

- Dual-energy computed tomography (CT) uses the energy-dependent attenuation of different elements to allow decomposition of materials on a voxel-by-voxel basis.
- Dual-energy CT (DECT) material decomposition can accurately differentiate between calcification and hemorrhage for any indeterminate hyperdensity in the brain.
- In patients who have previously received intra-arterial or intravenous iodinated contrast, DECT can differentiate intracranial hemorrhage from contrast.

INTRODUCTION

Computed tomography (CT) remains an important tool in neuroimaging despite the advent and popularity of MR imaging, due in part to its wide availability, rapid acquisition, and high spatial resolution. Limited ability to differentiate materials with similar x-ray attenuation is an important limitation of this modality, whereby images are typically acquired using a single peak kilovoltage (kVp) that produces a polychromatic spectrum. Dual-energy CT (DECT) offers the ability to exploit the energy-dependent attenuation of different elements to allow decomposition of materials on a voxel-by-voxel basis. Emerging applications of this powerful technique in neurologic imaging include differentiation of intracranial calcification versus hemorrhage, postprocedure iodine staining versus hemorrhagic transformation, and bland versus tumoral hemorrhage, among others.

MATERIAL DECOMPOSITION PRINCIPLES

Attenuation of radiographs used in diagnostic imaging is dependent on 2 major interactions: the photoelectric effect and Compton scattering. The photoelectric effect is highly dependent on the atomic number (Z) of the element and energy of the x-ray beam (E) and dominates at lower energies with a spike of photon absorption near the

The authors report no relevant disclosures.
[a] Department of Radiology and Imaging Sciences, Emory University, 1364 Clifton Road Northeast, Suite BG20, Atlanta, GA 30322, USA; [b] Department of Radiology, Massachusetts General Hospital, 55 Fruit Street, Boston, MA 02114, USA
* Corresponding author.
E-mail address: Ranliang.Hu@emory.edu

Neuroimag Clin N Am 27 (2017) 401–409
http://dx.doi.org/10.1016/j.nic.2017.03.004
1052-5149/17/

K-edge. Compton scattering, on the other hand, is dependent on electron density and has little energy dependence. The CT attenuation value used in clinical imaging relies on a combination of these 2 interactions and is therefore a function of the atomic number and electron density of the material being measured as well as the energy spectrum of the x-ray beam used for measurement.

Conventional CT uses a single peak voltage (kVp) and thus performs a measurement with a single energy spectrum, while DECT enables measurements using 2 different energy spectra. Measurement using a single spectrum does not allow the differentiation or decomposition of materials, because the attenuation coefficient is not unique to a material but is dependent on the energy of the x-ray beam and concentration of each material. For example, a lower concentration of a higher Z material (ie, iodine) may have the same attenuation as higher concentration of a lower Z material (ie, calcium) at a given energy. However, measurement at 2 different energies may be able to distinguish between these 2 materials because their total attenuation (which is a sum of their photoelectric and Compton scattering components) will not be the same at both energies.

DECT exploits the energy-dependent attenuation differences of elements to allow the decomposition of a mixture of materials in each voxel. The most widely available systems use 2 distinct energy spectra, using either a single source that rapidly switches between 2 energy levels, typically 80 and 140 kVp (GSI; GE Healthcare, Waukesha, WI, USA), or 2 orthogonally oriented imaging chains each operated at a different peak voltage, either 80 and 140 kVp (SOMATOM Flash; Siemens, Forchheim, Germany) or 80 and 150 kVp (SOMATOM Force; Siemens). Other implementations include a multilayer detector system (IQon Spectral CT; Philips, Andover, MA, USA) that allows detection of low and high energy at different layers, and photon-counting systems under development that allow separation of incident radiograph into multiple energy bins.

The attenuation coefficient of a mixture of materials can be modeled as a combination of photoelectric effect and Compton scattering, or as the linear combination of attenuation coefficient of individual basis materials (excluding the k-edges). The latter method is of interest in material decomposition because it allows for the calculation of the concentrations of the 2 known materials in a voxel, using available data on energy-dependent mass attenuation coefficient of standard materials. Two-material decomposition assumes the presence of only 2 basis materials, and models other constituents

as a combination of the 2. Two-material decomposition is the most straightforward implementation and is practical when decomposition of 2 materials is the question of clinical interest (eg, iodine vs hemorrhage). Two-material decomposition algorithm can be performed before reconstruction using projection data or after reconstruction of 2 sets of different energy images. Three-material composition algorithm allows the determination of the mass fraction of 3 known materials based on assumption of conservation of mass.[1] Detailed description of dual-energy principles and methods can be found in separate articles in this issue as well as a recent review by McCollough and colleagues.[2]

DUAL-ENERGY COMPUTED TOMOGRAPHIC IMAGE POSTPROCESSING

Commercial software is available from each of the major DECT vendors that allows for postprocessing of images and analysis. Software packages differ in their implementation and terminology, but in general, vendor-specific workstations are used for postprocessing, qualitative analysis, and construction of material-specific images sent to PACS for clinical interpretation. In addition to material-specific images, a mixed image using a combination of high- and low-energy data is often created to simulate a conventional CT image performed at 120 kVp. Each material has a characteristic ratio of attenuation at high and low energies, and a threshold often referred to as the dual-energy ratio or iodine ratio can be specified in the postprocessing workflow to achieve the best separation of 2 materials. In 2-material decomposition, pairs of basis material images can be generated, each displaying the distribution of one of the specified materials (eg, water-calcium, water-iodine, calcium-iodine). The pixels attributable to a specific material are sometimes color coded and displayed as material-specific images (ie, calcium-overlay, iodine-overlay), removed from the image to produce subtraction images (ie, virtual noncalcium, virtual noncontrast), or superimposed on conventional images in a sliding scale.

DIFFERENTIATION OF HEMORRHAGE AND CALCIFICATION

Intracranial hemorrhage and calcification can both appear hyperdense on conventional polychromatic CT and can have overlapping attenuation coefficients depending on their respective concentrations. Although the 2 can usually be differentiated based on clinical history, location, morphology, and density characteristics, diagnostic dilemmas

Table 1
Diagnostic algorithm to differentiate between calcification and hemorrhage

Material	Polychromatic CT	Calcium Overlay or Calcium Density	Virtual Noncalcium or Water Density
Calcium	Hyperdense	Hyperdense	Isodense
Hemorrhage	Hyperdense	Isodense	Hyperdense
Calcium and hemorrhage	Hyperdense	Hyperdense	Hyperdense

sometimes occur and necessitate further workup with follow-up imaging or MR imaging. In a recent study of emergency department patients, 9% of brain intraparenchymal hyperdensities were indeterminate on polychromatic head CT, and DECT decomposition was 99% accurate in differentiating between hemorrhage and calcification.[3]

A practical diagnostic algorithm to differentiate between calcification and hemorrhage is presented in **Table 1**. Using a dual-energy calcium and water decomposition, material with energy-dependent attenuation compatible with calcium would be mapped on the calcium overlay image and not on virtual noncalcium image, whereas material similar to water (ie, blood) would be mapped on the virtual noncalcium image and not on the calcium overlay image. This diagnostic algorithm is useful when the 2 main differential considerations are hemorrhage versus calcification, such as in a patient presenting with headache who has a CT demonstrating focal hyperdensity in the pons that could represent hypertensive hemorrhage or calcification (**Fig. 1**). In this case, the hyperdensity mapped to the calcium overlay

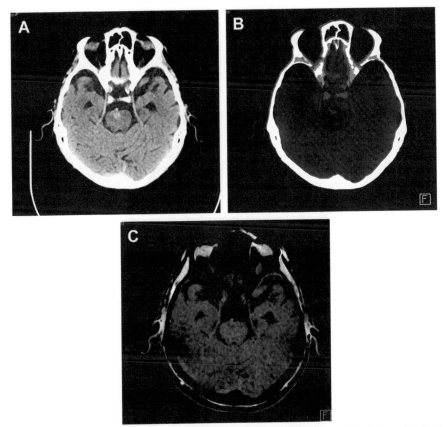

Fig. 1. DECT in a patient presenting with headache demonstrates indeterminate focal hyperdensity in the pons on simulated 120-kVp image (*A*). Material decomposition maps the hyperdensity onto the calcium overlay image (*B*) but not the virtual noncalcium image (*C*). Based on the presence of calcium, this was a cavernous malformation rather than a hypertensive hemorrhage. Although both entities commonly occur in this location, DECT could distinguish the 2 based on energy-dependent attenuation.

image and a follow-up MR imaging confirmed the presence of a cavernous malformation with mineralization and an adjacent developmental venous malformation (not shown). In a future clinical scenario such as this, dual-energy decomposition could enable rapid triage of the patient to the appropriate level of care and eliminate the need for intensive monitoring and follow-up imaging.

Fig. 2 demonstrates the case of a patient with known glioma who presented with seizure, and CT demonstrated a new focal hyperdensity in the region of the tumor, measuring 62 HU. It was unclear whether the surrounding hypodensity represented edema or tumor, and the focal hyperdensity was interpreted as possible acute hemorrhage, which prompted urgent neurosurgical consultation and escalation of care. DECT decomposition demonstrates that the hyperdensity maps entirely to the calcium overlay image, and a follow-up CT performed several months later confirmed increased density of the focus compatible with

calcification. This case reminds us that even if a lesion is new and has Hounsfield values similar to blood, it can still be a focus of calcification that is evolving and not reached its maximal concentration.

It should be noted that this simple diagnostic algorithm is based on the assumption that the 2 possible contributions to attenuation are calcium and hemorrhage, and additional sources of attenuation such as high-density tumor or iodine are not taken into account. The diagnostic approach should always take the relevant clinical scenario into consideration, and sometimes further imaging and postprocessing of dual-energy datasets are necessary. Fig. 3 demonstrates a case where a new hyperdensity in a treated metastasis was initially interpreted as calcification, but on dual-energy decomposition, the density mapped to the virtual noncalcium image. The possibilities in this case are hemorrhage versus hyperdense tumor. MR imaging showed an enhancing

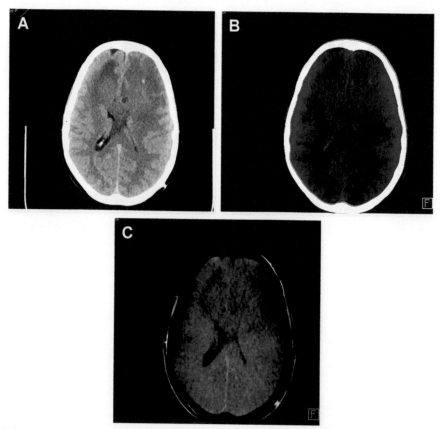

Fig. 2. DECT in a patient with known left frontal glioma demonstrates an indeterminate focal hyperdensity in the tumor on simulated 120-kVp image (A), which could either represent tumoral hemorrhage or calcification. Material decomposition maps the hyperdensity onto the calcium overlay image (B) but not the virtual noncalcium image (C). A follow-up conventional CT several weeks later demonstrated increased mineralization of the focus of question, compatible with calcification (not shown).

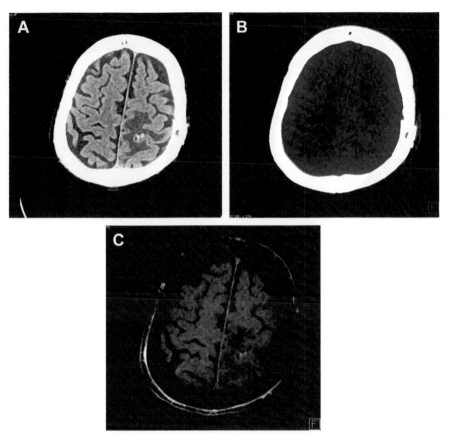

Fig. 3. DECT in a patient with treated cerebral metastasis demonstrates hyperdensity within a left frontal lesion on simulated 120-kVp image (*A*) that was initially interpreted as dystrophic calcification. The hyperdense components of the lesion do not map to the calcium overlay image (*B*) and instead appear on the virtual noncalcium image (*C*), which excludes calcification and leaves the possibility of blood versus hyperdense tumor.

metastasis with superimposed hemorrhage, and a follow-up CT demonstrated resolution of the density compatible with expected evolution of blood. In this case, the utility of dual-energy material decomposition would be its ability to exclude treatment-related calcification and prompt further workup.

PITFALLS OF MATERIAL DECOMPOSITION IN THE PRESENCE OF ARTIFACT

Beam-hardening artifact is commonly encountered in neurologic imaging, such as due to dense bone in the skull base, dental amalgam, or hardware implants. This artifact poses a challenge for dual-energy material decomposition because low-energy radiographs are absorbed by the high-density material and the actual measured energy spectrum is altered, leading to distortions in material decomposition images. DECT has been effectively used to reduce beam-hardening artifact by harnessing the additional information obtained from 2

separate acquisitions, one at a higher energy than routine conventional CT (140 or 150 kVp). Corrections can be applied in the projection space in geometrically consistent acquisitions (ie, fast kVP switching), which has theoretic advantages, but actual results vary due to imperfect calibrations. Material decomposition in the image space is theoretically more prone to beam-hardening artifact, and caution must be used to review all images and not just the material-selective images. A case where extensive beam hardening artifact from metal hardware masks a focus of hemorrhage on the virtual noncalcium image is illustrated in **Fig. 4**.

DIFFERENTIATION OF IODINE AND HEMORRHAGE

Acute hemorrhage and lower concentrations of iodine can have overlapping density on conventional CT and can be difficult to differentiate in cases when they can coexist in the same compartment. Intracranial hemorrhage may be

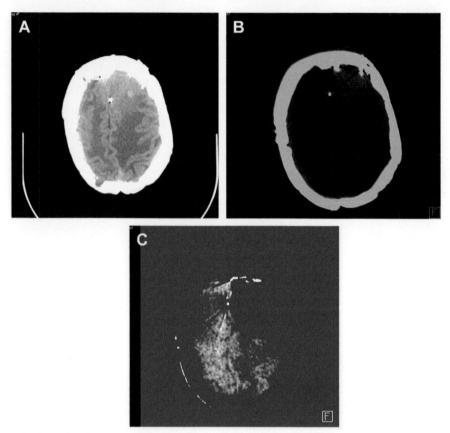

Fig. 4. Extensive beam hardening artifact related to metallic implants from prior craniotomy degrades simulated 120-kVp image (*A*) but a focus of intraparenchymal hemorrhage in the left frontal lobe is still discernible. Material decomposition falsely classifies the region of artifact as calcification (*B*) and subtracts it from the virtual noncalcium images (*C*).

differentiated from iodinated contrast material using iodine-water material decomposition in a similar fashion as the one used for calcium-hemorrhage (**Table 2**). The clinical utility of this technique was demonstrated in acute stroke patients who underwent head CT after intra-arterial thrombolysis, where DECT was shown to reliably differentiate between hemorrhagic conversion and contrast staining of the infarct territory.[4,5] An example of hemorrhagic conversion of stroke that occurred during arterial intervention is shown in **Fig. 5**, where

both extravasated iodinated contrast and hemorrhage are clearly shown in the infarct bed and adjacent lateral ventricle. In less clinically obvious cases, accurate exclusion of hemorrhage in a patient who had just undergone intra-arterial thrombolysis would be important for clinical management.

DECT material decomposition has also been shown to be useful in differentiation between tumoral versus bland hemorrhage in patients presenting with unknown cause of intraparenchymal

Table 2
Diagnostic algorithm to differentiate between iodine and hemorrhage

Material	Polychromatic CT	Iodine Overlay or Iodine Density	Virtual Noncontrast or Water Density
Iodine	Hyperdense	Hyperdense	Isodense
Hemorrhage	Hyperdense	Isodense	Hyperdense
Iodine and hemorrhage	Hyperdense	Hyperdense	Hyperdense

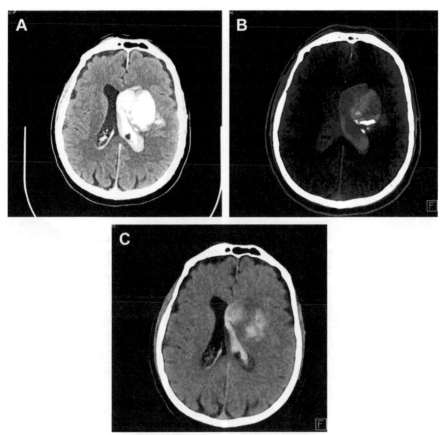

Fig. 5. DECT in a patient who underwent mechanical thrombectomy for left middle cerebral artery stroke demonstrates hemorrhage in the left basal ganglia and corona radiata with intraventricular extension on simulated 120-kVp image (*A*). Material decomposition maps some of the density to iodine overlay (*B*) and others to virtual noniodine image (*C*), representing a combination of extravasated contrast and hemorrhage.

hemorrhage, by detecting tumoral enhancement in hyperdense hemorrhage on contrast-enhanced CT.[6] Other investigators have shown that DECT material decomposition improves sensitivity for detection of contrast extravasation (spot sign) in intraparenchymal hematoma on CT angiography.[7] **Fig. 6** shows a case of a patient presenting for noncontrast head CT after receiving intravenous iodinated contrast for a chest CT performed to evaluate for pulmonary embolism. A hyperdense lesion was identified and not readily discernible as hemorrhage or enhancement from prior intravenous contrast administration. The patient underwent a contrast-enhanced DECT, with material decomposition images clearly demonstrating an enhancing component posteriorly and a hemorrhagic component anteriorly. This lesion was a hemorrhagic tumor, and the confirmation of hemorrhage was instrumental in management of anticoagulation for this patient, who was also diagnosed with pulmonary embolism.

SUMMARY

DECT is a powerful technique that uses the energy-dependent attenuation of materials to distinguish between 2 materials of similar attenuation and determine the concentration of 2 or more known materials within a voxel. Application of this powerful technique has been explored extensively in body and musculoskeletal imaging, such as characterizing renal stone composition, differentiating a hyperdense renal cyst from enhancement, detection of pulmonary embolism, and others. Emerging application in neurologic imaging includes metal artifact reduction, characterization of carotid artery plaque, bone subtraction CT angiography, and others.

This review focused on the role of DECT in differentiating between hyperdense materials commonly encountered in neurologic imaging: hemorrhage, calcium, and iodine. Studies show that DECT is useful in differentiating between

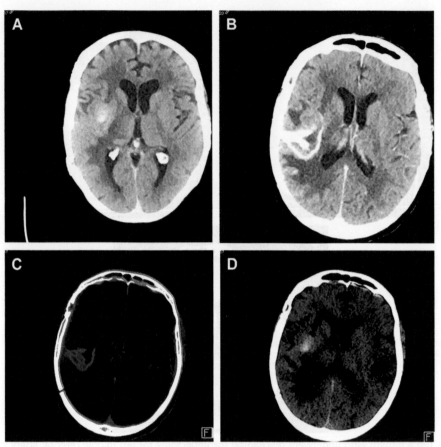

Fig. 6. Routine noncontrast head acquired after a contrast-enhanced chest CT demonstrates hyperdensity in a known right frontal mass that could represent residual contrast or hemorrhage (*A*). DECT performed after administration of second dose of contrast demonstrates enhancement around the periphery of the mass on simulated 120-kVp image (*B*). Material decomposition accurately maps iodinated contrast enhancement onto the iodine overlay image (*C*), whereas tumoral hemorrhage maps onto the virtual noniodine image (*D*).

hemorrhage and calcification in indeterminate intracranial lesions in the emergency department population and in differentiating between iodine staining and hemorrhage after intra-arterial stroke treatment. The advantage of this technique is that it relies on the intrinsic physical properties of the radiograph interaction with materials and is highly reproducible and generalizable to other applications where characterization of hyperdense materials is important.

It is important to recognize the basic assumptions underlying the material decomposition algorithm and always review material-selective images alongside conventional or simulated conventional CT, much like the way different MR imaging sequences are reviewed together in a complementary manner. Material decomposition is very good at separating materials of very different Z numbers, such as calcium and iodine versus water. In practical terms, hemorrhage can

be assumed to behave more like water in its radiograph interaction and thus can be distinguished from calcium and iodine. Other materials, such as hyperdense tumor and other mineralization types, can be erroneously classified as either water or calcium/iodine based on 2-material decomposition, and judgment must be used to determine whether this is relevant in a specific clinical context and if further workup is needed.

Material-selective images may also suffer from increased noise propagated by the material decomposition algorithm, limiting its effectiveness in characterizing small or inconspicuous lesions. Beam hardening artifact can theoretically be corrected in the projection space in some circumstances, but the effectiveness of correction techniques is variable and caution must be used in recognizing misclassification of materials due to artifact. Different scanner manufacturers have developed different approaches in scanner configuration and postprocession algorithms, and further work is being done to improve current techniques and in development of newer techniques such as photon-counting scanners. As the technology matures, DECT material decomposition holds much promise in becoming an important tool in our imaging armamentarium.

REFERENCES

1. Liu X, Yu L, Primak AN, et al. Quantitative imaging of element composition and mass fraction using dual-energy CT: three-material decomposition. Med Phys 2009;36:1602–8.

2. McCollough CH, Leng S, Yu L, et al. Dual- and multi-energy CT: principles, technical approaches, and clinical applications. Radiology 2015;276:637–53.

3. Hu R, Daftari Besheli L, Young J, et al. Dual-energy head CT enables accurate distinction of intraparenchymal hemorrhage from calcification in emergency department patients. Radiology 2016;280:177–83.

4. Gupta R, Phan CM, Leidecker C, et al. Evaluation of dual-energy CT for differentiating intracerebral hemorrhage from iodinated contrast material staining 1. Radiology 2010;257:205–11.

5. Phan CM, Yoo AJ, Hirsch JA, et al. Differentiation of hemorrhage from iodinated contrast in different intracranial compartments using dual-energy head CT. AJNR Am J Neuroradiol 2012;33:1088–94.

6. Kim SJ, Lim HK, Lee HY, et al. Dual-energy CT in the evaluation of intracerebral hemorrhage of unknown origin: differentiation between tumor bleeding and pure hemorrhage. AJNR Am J Neuroradiol 2012;33:865–72.

7. Watanabe Y, Tsukabe A, Kunitomi Y, et al. Dual-energy CT for detection of contrast enhancement or leakage within high-density haematomas in patients with intracranial haemorrhage. Neuroradiology 2014;56:291–5.

Miscellaneous and Emerging Applications of Dual-Energy Computed Tomography for the Evaluation of Intracranial Pathology

Hirofumi Kuno, MD, PhD[a,b],*, Kotaro Sekiya, DDS, PhD[b],
Margaret N. Chapman, MD[a], Osamu Sakai, MD, PhD[a,c,d]

KEYWORDS

- Dual-energy CT • Virtual monochromatic image • Bone removal • Bone subtraction image
- Iodine distribution map • Effective atomic number • Basis material analysis

KEY POINTS

- Dual-energy computed tomography (CT) has the potential to improve detection of abnormalities and increase diagnostic confidence in the evaluation of a variety of neurologic conditions.
- Virtual monochromatic imaging (VMI) can be used as an additional tool to help differentiate materials and may be useful to determine optimal VMI energy level for visualization of brain lesions.
- Three-material decomposition techniques can be readily performed to create calcium maps, virtual noncalcium images, and iodine distribution maps.
- Iodine distribution maps potentially provide additional "contrast resolution" to the standard contrast-enhanced CT images for skull base lesions and intracranial extension of extracranial tumors.
- Bone removal or subtraction images can be used for identifying small or subtle intracranial abnormalities that lie adjacent to osseous structures.

INTRODUCTION

Since the introduction of clinical dual-energy computed tomography (CT) scanners in 2006, the ability of dual-energy CT to differentiate materials of different effective atomic numbers (Z_{eff}) has made several new clinically relevant CT applications possible.[1,2] There is increasing evidence to support the advantages of dual-energy CT in evaluating intracranial abnormalities. One of the significant advantages in neuroradiology is to differentiate hemorrhage, calcium, and iodine. Using this 3-material decomposition algorithm, dual-energy CT has proven to be very helpful in differentiating contrast-related hyperdensity from acute intracranial hemorrhage.[3–7] Dual-energy CT

[a] Department of Radiology, Boston Medical Center, Boston University School of Medicine, FGH Building, 3rd Floor, 820 Harrison Avenue, Boston, MA 02118, USA; [b] Department of Diagnostic Radiology, National Cancer Center Hospital East, 6-5-1, Kashiwanoha, Kashiwa, Chiba 277-8577, Japan; [c] Department of Otolaryngology–Head and Neck Surgery, Boston Medical Center, Boston University School of Medicine, FGH Building, 3rd Floor, 820 Harrison Avenue, Boston, MA 02118, USA; [d] Department of Radiation Oncology, Boston Medical Center, Boston University School of Medicine, FGH Building, 3rd Floor, 820 Harrison Avenue, Boston, MA 02118, USA
* Corresponding author. Department of Diagnostic Radiology, National Cancer Center Hospital East, 6-5-1, Kashiwanoha, Kashiwa, Chiba 277-8577, Japan.
E-mail address: hkuno@east.ncc.go.jp

Neuroimag Clin N Am 27 (2017) 411–427
http://dx.doi.org/10.1016/j.nic.2017.03.005
1052-5149/17/© 2017 Elsevier Inc. All rights reserved.

applications have provided a significant impact in neurovascular imaging, such as automated bone and plaque removal for CT angiography. Bone removal, material characterization, and monochromatic reconstructions can be achieved with one scan and improve detection of aneurysms, vascular malformations, and iodine enhancement.[8–13] Therefore, dual-energy CT may provide significant added value, particularly in the emergency department setting.[14]

Other clinically useful applications to evaluate intracranial abnormalities have also been developed in addition to those mentioned above. This article reviews the virtual monochromatic imaging (VMI) applications of dual-energy CT, particularly material decomposition algorithms to improve lesion conspicuity, define lesion-normal tissue interface using different reconstruction techniques, and discuss miscellaneous emerging applications of dual-energy CT for neuroimaging, with an emphasis on their potential clinical utility.

TECHNICAL CONSIDERATION FOR DUAL-ENERGY COMPUTED TOMOGRAPHY

In practice, 2 CT images taken at different tube voltages, typically 80 and 140 kV, are sufficient to classify many tissues. Processing dual-energy data to generate material selective or virtual monochromatic images can be performed either in the raw data space or in the image data space. Then, low-energy and high-energy images are reconstructed as a first step, and the dual-energy processing is applied to these images. Raw data-based evaluation is often considered superior to image data-based evaluation, because image-based methods are thought to be limited by beam-hardening problems, although further validation studies are needed. In this article, the discussion is limited to 2 types of dual-energy CT: 2-rotation kilovolt-milliampere switching system with a 320-detector CT scanner (Aquilion ONE Vision; Toshiba Medical Systems Corp, Tokyo, Japan) and 128-slice dual-source dual-energy CT (SOMATOM Definition Flash; Siemens Healthcare, Forchheim, Germany).

VIRTUAL MONOCHROMATIC IMAGING

CT exposures, including dual-energy mode acquisitions, consist of photons within a broad spectrum of energies (polychromatic). The data from the 2 polychromatic exposures of a dual-energy scan can be reconstructed into a single data set that reflects the properties of a scan with a monochromatic x-ray beam, which is called "virtual monochromatic or monoenergetic imaging." VMI represents one of the most widely applicable attributes of dual-energy CT and has the potential to optimize the image quality of unenhanced and enhanced CT.[15] As in polychromatic CT, with increasing tube voltage, the signal-to-noise ratio (SNR) increases, whereas tissue contrast decreases. Lowering the tube voltage will increase the contrast-to-noise ratio (CNR), whereas the SNR decreases. Monochromatic images with dual-energy CT may be able to provide the best balanced CNR and SNR images for a specific target in one scanning process.

Currently available algorithms allow reconstruction of virtual monochromatic images far beyond the range of mean kilovolt levels available with current CT technology (35–190 keV in steps of 1 keV). The CT number (attenuation value) of a region of interest (ROI) is displayed as a function of the kiloelectron volt and leads to material-specific curves on a Cartesian graph (Fig. 1). Target ROIs composed of materials with high atomic number, such as calcium and tissues containing an iodinated contrast agent, will show a significant increase in the CT number at lower kiloelectron volt (see Fig. 1). On the other hand, target ROIs containing materials with low atomic number will show only small variations in the CT number as a function of the kiloelectron volt (see Fig. 1). Unlike the other materials, the CT number of fat will decrease with decreasing kiloelectron volts. In several clinical studies, investigators have tried to characterize lesions by their specific curves in the CT number versus kiloelectron volt diagram.[16,17]

Optimal Virtual Monochromatic Imaging Energy Level for Noncontrast Brain Imaging

Several studies have been performed to determine the best VMI energy levels, which provide the best CNR and SNR, for unenhanced head CT. Pomerantz and colleagues[18] demonstrated that maximal brain parenchymal image quality in dual-energy unenhanced head CT with dual-energy rapid 80 to 140 peak kilovolt (kVp) switching mode occurs in the 65- to 70-keV range, and the maximum SNR and CNR for the supratentorial gray and white matter was at 65 keV, with significant improvement of image quality measurement compared with conventional 120-kV head CT images (corrected improvement ratios in the range of 17%–46%). For posterior fossa evaluation, a 75-keV VMI reconstruction had the lowest posterior fossa artifact index and a 50% reduction in posterior fossa artifact index compared with the conventional 120-kV head CT images (Fig. 2).[18] Hwang and colleagues[19] demonstrated that optimal monochromatic energy levels in evaluating

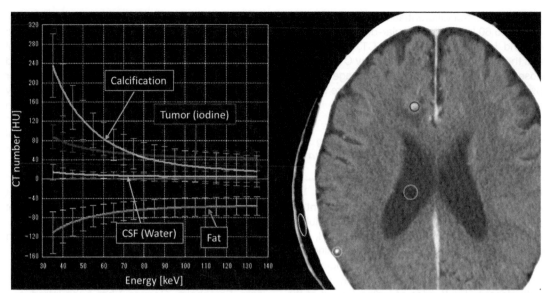

Fig. 1. The CT number of an ROI is displayed as a function of the kiloelectron volt and leads to material specific curves. Brain calcification (*green*) and enhancing tumor (*pink*) demonstrate a significant increase in CT number at lower kiloelectron volts. On the other hand, the cerebrospinal fluid (*blue*) showed only small variations in CT number as a function of the kiloelectron volt. The CT number of fat (*yellow*) decreased with decreasing kiloelectron volt.

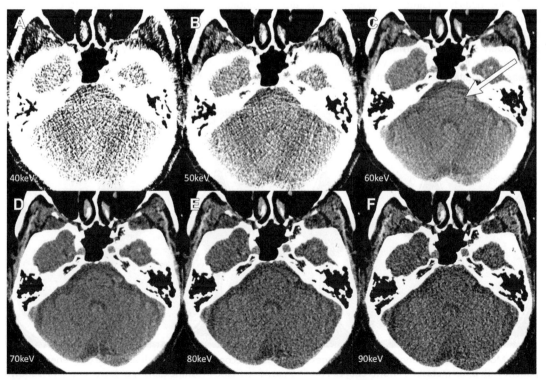

Fig. 2. Dual-energy unenhanced head CT at the posterior fossa level. Monochromatic images (*A–F*) at 40, 50, 60, 70, 80, and 90 keV show a progressive reduction in the severity of posterior fossa beam-hardening artifact (*arrow*) at the expense of reduced soft tissue contrast.

gray–white matter differentiation were 50 to 55 keV and 50 to 60 keV, using regular-dose dual-energy CT and low-dose dual-energy CT, respectively, and they suggested that dual-energy CT may offer dose savings with acceptable image quality, particularly in those patients who require multiple repeat head CT.

Optimal Virtual Monochromatic Imaging Energy Level for Contrast-Enhanced Brain Imaging (Best Contrast-to-Noise Ratio)

For contrast-enhanced CT, the optimal VMI energy levels may be objective dependent. In general, the low-energy VMI may be useful for improvement of lesion enhancement, CNR, subjective overall image quality, and tumor delineation for malignancies.[20,21] Enhancing tumors have increased attenuation on lower-kiloelectron volt VMI, closer to the K-edge of iodine,[2] albeit at the expense of other factors such as increased image noise (Fig. 3). Several studies have shown that optimal VMI has an advantage in head and neck oncology imaging.[20–24] Therefore, it might be useful to determine the optimal VMI energy level (best CNR) for visualization of brain lesions.

CNR is a quantitative parameter with even greater clinical significance. Images with higher CNR are usually desired because lesions are more readily detectable when they appear in higher contrast than the background normal tissue. Such quantitative image evaluations have been widely investigated in various organs and disease conditions. A recent application has

been further developed that can automatically identify the optimal VMI energy level (Best CNR; Toshiba Medical Systems Corp, Tokyo, Japan) based on 2 different target ROIs (base ROI and contrast ROI) (Figs. 4 and 5). For example, for assessment of a brain tumor, the best VMI energy level may be different for the purpose of each assessment; that is, tumor versus brain tissue (improved tumor boundary delineation) and normal brain tissue versus brain edema (assessment of brain edema) (see Fig. 5). An optimal monochromatic image set is automatically selected for obtaining the best VMI energy level for each target lesion corresponding to the objective or target of interest for each patient, until the best image quality and contrast for an individual scan is reached (see Fig. 5).

Another novel monoenergetic algorithm (syngo.CT DE Monoenergetic Plus; Siemens Healthcare, Forchheim, Germany) has been introduced with the goal to improve the image quality of monoenergetic (monochromatic) data sets at low-kiloelectron volt levels (40 keV) by substantially reducing the image noise using an advanced image-based algorithm.[25,26] Using this algorithm, a spatial, frequency-based recombination is performed to combine the high signal at lower energies and the superior noise properties at medium to high energies in order to create VMIs with an optimal balance of signal/contrast and noise at the target kiloelectron volt.[25,26] The low kiloelectron volt VMIs may also allow reduction of intravenous contrast material volume while maintaining adequate detection of parenchymal

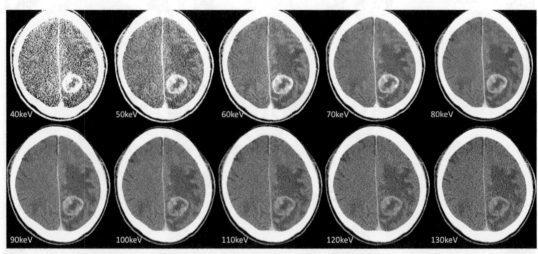

Fig. 3. Monoenergetic (monochromatic) images (40–130 keV) reconstructed from dual-source dual-energy CT in a patient with brain metastases from renal cell carcinoma. An increase in iodine density at lower energies is shown, although this is at the expense of increased image noise. At higher energies, the brain edema is better appreciated, whereas the iodine attenuation decreases. CNR is higher at lower energies, whereas SNR increases with higher energies. All images are displayed using the same window-level settings.

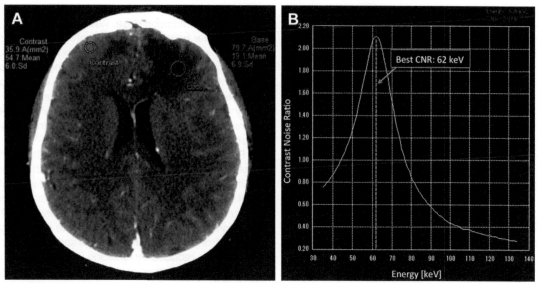

Fig. 4. Selecting the best CNR for the assessment of brain edema with *Best CNR* application in a patient with a history of brain necrosis after chemoradiation for recurrent nasal carcinoma. Axial contrast-enhanced CT (*A*) demonstrates the ROI in an edematous area (Base ROI) and cerebral cortex (Contrast ROI). The CNR curve (*B*) shows the optimal monochromatic energy of 62 keV for the best CNR.

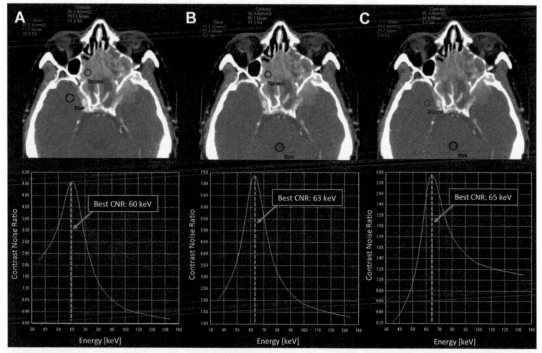

Fig. 5. The *Best CNR* of 3 different objective ROIs for optimal VMI energy level in a patient with olfactory neuroblastoma (Kadish stage C). (*A*) ROI set on the tumor and brain tissue for tumor boundary delineation (60 keV for the best CNR). (*B*) ROI set on the tumor and cerebrospinal fluid for increasing attenuation difference between tumor and secondary sinusitis (63 keV for the best CNR). (*C*) ROI set on the cerebrospinal fluid and brain tissue for detecting brain edema (65 keV for the best CNR).

enhancement and image quality. The reduction of intravenous contrast material volume has the potential to improve patient safety, particularly in patients with impaired renal function, and may impact examination protocols and reduce cost. However, these methods are time consuming and currently can only be done at a dedicated workstation. A more practical approach is to reconstruct predetermined image data set or data sets, including those with the best CNR VMI energy level, and send it to the PACS at the time of CT acquisition so that it is readily available at the time of interpretation.

Artifact Reduction

In patients with intracranial metal, such as aneurysm clips, coils, stents, and foreign bodies (shrapnel, bullet fragments), CT and MR imaging are often challenging. The presence of metal can severely degrade CT image quality because of summative artifacts including beam hardening, photon starvation, and photon scattering. With a single-energy CT, increasing the kVp reduces beam-hardening artifacts, however, at the expense of increased radiation dose. With dual-energy CT, on the other hand, virtual monochromatic images can be generated at high predicted energy levels, substantially reducing beam-hardening artifacts from metallic structures and significantly improving image quality.[27–30] These high monochromatic energy level images may improve interpretation of intracranial lesions in patients with intracranial metallic devices (Figs. 6 and 7).

Shinohara and colleagues[31] demonstrated that fast-kilovolt switching dual-energy CT with metal artifact reduction software (MARS) reduces metal artifact of platinum coils, resulting in favorable vessel visualization around the coil mass on CT angiography after embolization.[32] With increasing kiloelectron volt, the SNR increased and metallic artifacts were reduced by reducing beam-hardening artifacts. Reduction of metal artifact achieved by high-monochromatic energy images partly depends on the amount and type of metal, because VMI cannot correct for photon starvation and scattering if there are inadequate data at the low kilovolt setting to perform dual-energy postprocessing. In

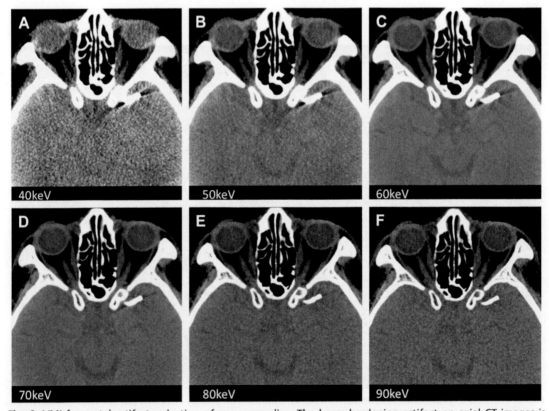

Fig. 6. VMI for metal artifact reduction of aneurysm clips. The beam-hardening artifact on axial CT images is partially reduced with VMI. The artifact is greater on the 40-keV (A), 50-keV (B), and 60-keV (C) virtual monochromatic CT images than on the corresponding 70-keV (D), 80-keV (E), and 90-keV images (F). The reduced artifact on the high-kiloelectron volt images may enable improved visibility of the adjacent intracranial tissue.

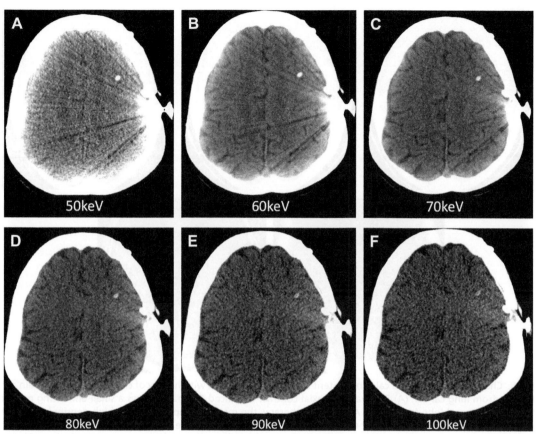

Fig. 7. VMI for metal artifact reduction of extracranial metal. The beam-hardening artifact on axial CT images is partially reduced with VMI. The artifact is greater on the 40-keV (*A*), 50-keV (*B*), and 60-keV (*C*) virtual monochromatic CT images than on the corresponding 70-keV (*D*), 80-keV (*E*), and 90-keV images (*F*). The reduced artifact on the high-kiloelectron volt images may enable improved visibility of the adjacent intracranial tissue.

addition, the high monochromatic energy values needed to reduce beam-hardening artifacts result in a decrease in iodine attenuation and consequently contrast enhancement, a tradeoff between artifact reduction and lesion visualization.[14] Recently, additional metal artifact reduction postprocessing, such as MARS, has been applied to improve overall image quality and increase diagnostic confidence in the assessment of soft tissues near and far from the metallic implants,[33] although potential new artifacts may be created by MARS reconstructions because of systematic errors near and far from the metallic implant. Further studies are needed to validate the ability of virtual monochromatic images to reduce metal artifacts and how they compare to other methods developed for single-energy CT with MARS.

MATERIAL SEPARATION USING DUAL-ENERGY COMPUTED TOMOGRAPHY

One of the most versatile techniques made possible by dual-energy CT is material separation.

Different vendors have adopted different algorithms for material decomposition with dual-energy CT. With a dual-source dual-energy CT (SOMATOM Definition Flash; Siemens Healthcare, Forchheim, Germany), a 3-material decomposition (default set: iodine, soft tissue, and fat) algorithm has been developed to process the data in the image-data space. With a 2-rotation kilovolt-milliampere switching system with a 320-detector CT scanner (Aquilion ONE Vision; Toshiba Medical Systems Corp), a material decomposition algorithm has been developed to process the data in the raw data space.

Differentiation Between Iodine-Enhanced Tumor and Calcification

For conventional single-energy CT images, iodine and calcium may be difficult to distinguish, as both are hyperattenuating. Material decomposition with dual-energy CT can be used to characterize such hyperattenuating material as calcium or iodine. Multiple studies have investigated the

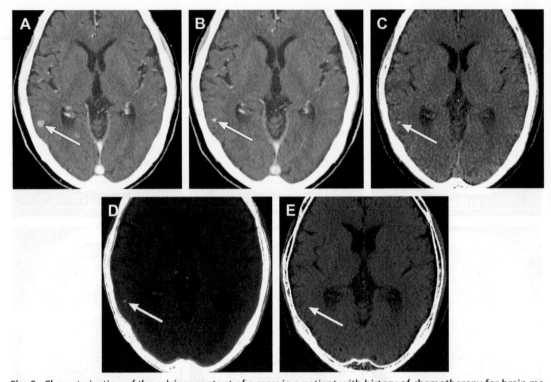

Fig. 8. Characterization of the calcium content of a mass in a patient with history of chemotherapy for brain metastases from lung cancer. (*A*) Pretreatment axial contrast-enhanced CT image shows a small enhancing mass in the right temporal lobe (*arrow*). (*B*) After chemotherapy, the metastasis appeared as a high-density lesion with decreasing size (*arrow*). The high density within the lesion remains visible on the VNC image (*C*). The lesion is therefore shown to be calcium rather than residual enhancing tumor, because it appears as a bright focus (*arrow*) on the axial calcium overlay map (*D*) and is completely absent (*arrow*) on the axial VNCa image (*E*).

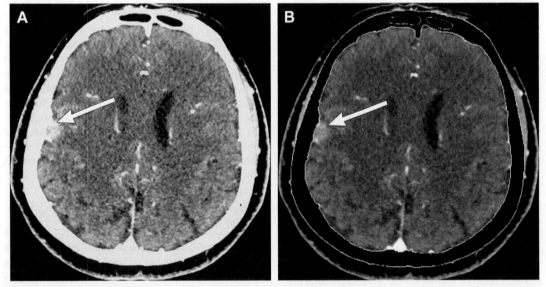

Fig. 9. Improved visibility of extra-axial masses using bone removal. An enhancing mass (*arrow*) overlying the right frontal convexity was incidentally detected on axial CT images obtained without (*A*) and with (*B*) bone removal. The dural-based mass is more evident on the bone-subtraction image.

utility of dual-energy CT to visually detect iodine and calcium using virtual noncontrast (VNC) and virtual noncalcium (VNCa) images.[3,4,6] Calcium and iodine exhibit very different x-ray absorption at low and high kilovolt settings. As a result, 3-material decomposition techniques can be readily performed to create VNCa images. These VNC and VNCa images may be helpful in characterizing high-attenuating foci in brain parenchyma encountered in the emergency department setting as acute hemorrhage or calcification that would otherwise have similar attenuation values on single-energy CT.[3–7,14,34] This 3-material decomposition method may also be used to identify calcium within intracranial lesions (vs enhancement or hemorrhage). This decomposition method may be useful for assessment of treatment response, or identification of iodine-containing, enhancing lesions that may indicate residual or recurrent tumor and require further close follow-up (**Fig. 8**).[35]

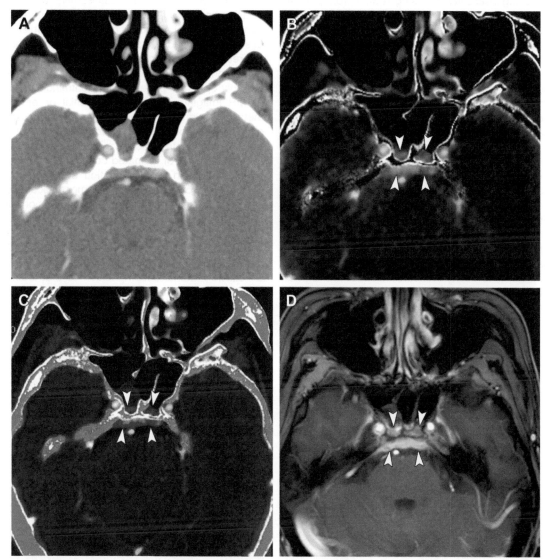

Fig. 10. An 82-year-old man who presented with sudden double vision 2 years after completion of CRT for nasopharyngeal carcinoma. An enhancing lesion along the clivus in the prepontine cistern was incidentally detected on axial CT images obtained without (*A*) or with (*B*) dual-energy bone subtraction and on the iodine overlay image (*C*). The mass extended into the sphenoid sinus (*arrowheads*) and was more clearly seen on the bone subtraction (*B*) and iodine overlay images (*C*). Corresponding slice on a contrast-enhanced fat-saturated T1-weighted image also demonstrates the mass (*D*).

Bone Removal or Bone Subtraction Imaging

Various methods have been used to remove bone to facilitate interpretation of the cerebral vasculature. Semiautomatic segmentation with threshold-based software using density differences of structures has been widely used. Disadvantages of this method include possible subtraction artifacts when the Hounsfield unit (HU) of vessels, calcified plaque, and bone are similar. Depending on the system used, dual-energy CT bone removal methods based on 3-material decomposition may have a significant benefit of being insensitive to misregistration from patient motion, and they are not susceptible to partial subtraction of the vessel lumen, which is often seen with threshold-based or region-growing bone subtraction methods. In addition, with dual-energy CT, it is possible to hide or highlight calcified plaque (plaque removal). Therefore, dual-energy CT bone removal method is a powerful tool for evaluation of the intracranial vessels in CT angiography[8–13] and CT venography.[36]

In addition to enabling vessel visualization, bone removal or subtraction images (subtracting the VNC CT from the contrast-enhanced CT generated by dual-energy CT) can be used for identifying small or subtle intracranial abnormalities that lie adjacent to osseous structures. In CT imaging of soft tissues near the base of the skull, the thick layers of bone preferentially absorb the radiographs from CT, sometimes creating imaging artifacts that impair the ability to clearly delineate lesions in this region. Dual-energy CT bone removal/subtracted images may be helpful for detecting small lesions near the skull base, improving conspicuity of small extra-axial tumors (**Fig. 9**) and tumor invasion into the skull base (**Fig. 10**).[14]

Iodine Distribution Map

The literature on dual-energy CT in brain tumor imaging is limited because MR imaging, rather than CT, is usually the modality of choice for tumor imaging. Even then, CT still plays an important role in evaluating skull base involvement and intracranial extension of extracranial malignancies. CT is excellent for the evaluation of bone detail and complements MR imaging for assessment of bone invasion, in particular for the evaluation of cortical bone invasion. CT also does not have the problems of susceptibility artifact seen with MR imaging that can result in image degradation and preclude accurate diagnostic evaluation. In addition, CT may be the only option in patients with contraindications to MR imaging, such as intracranial or orbital metallic foreign bodies and pacemaker devices, or patients who cannot tolerate MR imaging because of claustrophobia.[37,38]

Administration of iodinated contrast agents improves detection and delineation of tumors on CT because of differences in tumor vascularity and enhancement patterns compared with normal soft tissues. However, even on contrast-enhanced CT scans, tumor can have similar attenuation to certain normal tissues, and differentiating the 2 can often be challenging (**Fig. 11**). Dual-energy CT allows material decomposition so that iodine can be differentiated from soft tissue and can potentially provide additional further "contrast

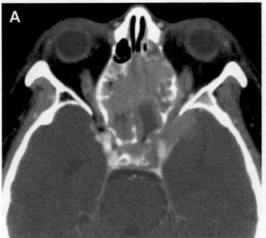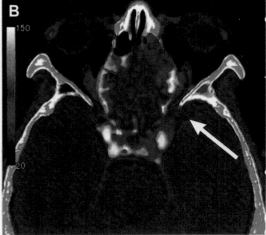

Fig. 11. Iodine overlay image for intracranial extension of olfactory neuroblastoma (same patient as **Fig. 5**). Axial contrast-enhanced CT image (*A*) and iodine overlay image (*B*) show an invasive mass extending into the intracranial space with cavernous sinus invasion. Note improved delineation of tumor extension and margins on the iodine overlay image (*B, arrow*) compared with the standard CT image.

resolution" to the standard contrast-enhanced CT images (**Figs. 10–13**). Recent applications have shown several ways to improve the contrast resolution (see **Fig. 12**). One method is iodine overlay images, which are generated using 3-material decomposition algorithms with dual-energy CT. Iodine overlay images can highlight the area of tumor enhancement as different-colored pixels, because iodine images use a color gradient to display quantitative iodine content within various tissues. Several studies have shown that iodine overlay images have an advantage in head and neck oncology imaging.[39–41] In neuroradiology, the color-coded map is thought to increase visual lesion detection for skull base lesions and intracranial extension of extracranial tumors (see **Figs. 10–13**). Because color is superimposed on original CT images, the details of complex anatomy of the skull base are preserved (see **Fig. 13**). Enhancing tumor may be differentiated from other

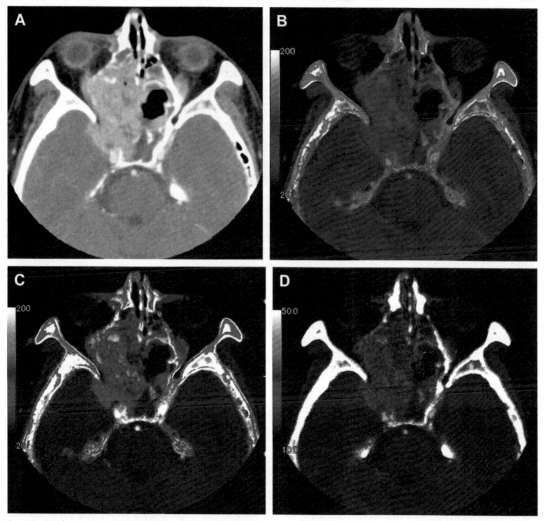

Fig. 12. Dual-energy CT applications for improving contrast resolution using iodine overlay images with several different approaches. Axial contrast-enhanced image (120 kV) (*A*) and iodine overlay images generated by high-kiloelectron volt base (75 keV) (*B*), low-kiloelectron volt base (58 keV) (*C*), and energy subtraction (60–65 keV) in a patient with sphenoid sinus squamous cell carcinoma with intracranial extension. High-kiloelectron volt base iodine overlay image (*B*) has less image noise than the low-kiloelectron volt base (*C*), yet iodine attenuation also decreases. On the other hand, the enhancing tumor has increased attenuation on lower-kiloelectron volt base (*C*), closer to the K-edge of iodine, albeit at the expense of other factors such as increased image noise. The energy subtraction (in this case, 60–65 keV) algorithm can also be used to generate iodine overlay images (*D*), but it is also possible to enhance other materials, which have large changes in attenuation when imaged at 2 different x-ray energy spectra.

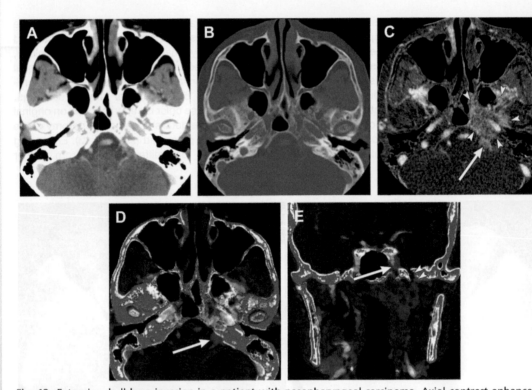

Fig. 13. Extensive skull base invasion in a patient with nasopharyngeal carcinoma. Axial contrast-enhanced CT does not show extensive destruction of the skull base (*A*: soft tissue window; *B*: bone window). DSA-like bone subtracted image (*C*) shows remarkable skull base invasion (*arrowheads*) with intracranial extension (*arrow*). Axial iodine overlay image (*D*) also demonstrates the intracranial extension more clearly (*arrow*). Coronal iodine overlay image (*E*) shows invasion into the left cavernous sinus (*arrow*), and perineural spread via V3 into the foramen ovale (*arrowheads*).

nonenhancing or non-iodine-containing tissue such as the brain, even if the CT attenuation values are similar (see **Fig. 11**). This technique improves pretreatment target delineation, which is very important for optimal treatment planning and favorable therapeutic outcomes.

Imaging Assessment of Tumor Extent into the Bone Marrow Space

It is still challenging to assess tumor extent in the bone marrow using dual-energy CT. There are several reports in the literature of the use of unenhanced dual-energy CT for the diagnosis of bone marrow edema in patients with bone fractures[42,43] and for detection of bone marrow involvement in patients with multiple myeloma.[44] However, if the material decomposition algorithm is applied to bone marrow on contrast-enhanced CT, dual-energy CT cannot separate the constituent materials of bone and iodinated contrast and will misclassify them because bone and iodine share a similar high tissue density. The separating iodinate contrast from bone would require 4- (or more) material decomposition with use of x-ray energy absorption data from at least 3 distinct x-ray energy bins. As a result, with current dual-energy CT acquisitions and iodine 3-material decomposition postprocessing, calcium (bone) remains visible on both the iodine map and the VNC image.

As a way to supplement such shortcomings of dual-energy CT, additional methods could include subtracting the unenhanced CT from the contrast-enhanced CT using subtraction software (SURESubtraction application; Toshiba Medical Systems, Tokyo, Japan), used recently in musculoskeletal applications.[45,46] Teixeira and colleagues[45] demonstrated that CT with digital subtraction angiography (DSA)-like bone subtraction imaging using wide-area detector CT showed high performance for the visual identification of bone marrow enhancement adjacent to lytic bone lesions. These data can also be technically obtained by a single-energy CT system, but the low-kiloelectron volt image performed with dual-energy CT is advantageous for improved detection of iodine distribution in the bone marrow as well as soft tissue (see **Fig. 13**).

Bone subtraction images allow calcification and bone removal (both cortical and trabecular) without affecting the visualization of contrast enhancement. This technique enables identification of contrast enhancement on CT in a nonlytic bone background and may be useful for the diagnosis of bone marrow invasion with or without erosive changes in cortical bone (see **Fig. 13**; **Fig. 14**). For this DSA-like bone subtraction procedure, the mask volume scan (a nonenhanced volume scan, 5–7 seconds after start of contrast injection) and the postcontrast volume scan (60 seconds after start of contrast injection) are acquired using dual-energy mode with fixation of the patient's head to the bed of CT. Skull base registration and subtraction is actually one of the simplest algorithms, although slight movement of the neck can result in spatial mismatch of the skeleton between the precontrast and postcontrast scans. Conventional volume scanning using wide-area detector CT can reduce this mismatch, because the wide coverage provided by the 160-mm-wide detector enables scanning of the head in one rotation, eliminating the need for helical scanning and for moving the patient bed, which can eliminate the moment of inertia or helical artifact radically. Furthermore, an additional bone subtraction algorithm can be used that uses a

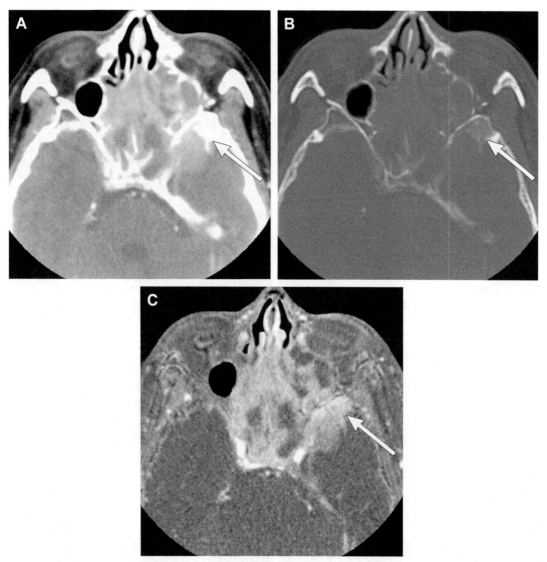

Fig. 14. Skull base invasion of olfactory neuroblastoma (same patient as **Figs. 5** and **11**). Contrast-enhanced CT images (*A*: soft tissue window; *B*: bone window) show ill-defined lytic and sclerotic foci in the sphenoid bone (*arrow*). The DSA-like bone subtraction image (*C*) clearly shows enhancement of the bone marrow (*arrow*).

high-resolution deformable registration algorithm to ensure accurate subtraction of skeletal structures and calcified lesion.[45-48]

EMERGING APPLICATIONS OF DUAL-ENERGY COMPUTED TOMOGRAPHY: FUTURE DEVELOPMENTS AND CHALLENGES

Recently, dual-energy CT postprocessing techniques with raw data-based analysis have been used to create a real-time interactive display of VMI, the Z_{eff}, and electron density, which can be readily displayed on an advanced workstation (**Fig. 15**). Z_{eff} and the characteristics of the spectral HU curves may help to distinguish different lesions and have been investigated in many clinical settings, including classification of benign and malignant thyroid nodules[17] and differentiation between benign and malignant abnormalities for patients with palpable masses in the neck.[16] However, research regarding the value of spectral curve and Z_{eff} remain limited in oncologic or other neuroimaging applications. Recent phantom studies have shown that Z_{eff} and electron density can be potentially calculated and displayed with high accuracy using raw data-based dual-energy CT,[49] which may help to improve accuracy in radiotherapy treatment planning.[49,50] Another potential application using raw data-based dual-energy imaging is the use of basis material analysis (Toshiba Medical Systems, Tokyo,

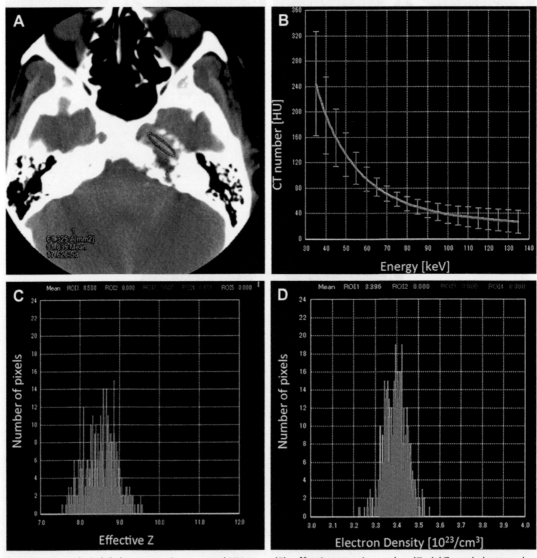

Fig. 15. ROI analysis (*A*) demonstrating spectral HU curve (*B*), effective atomic number (Z_{eff}) (*C*), and electron density (*D*) in a patient with chordoma.

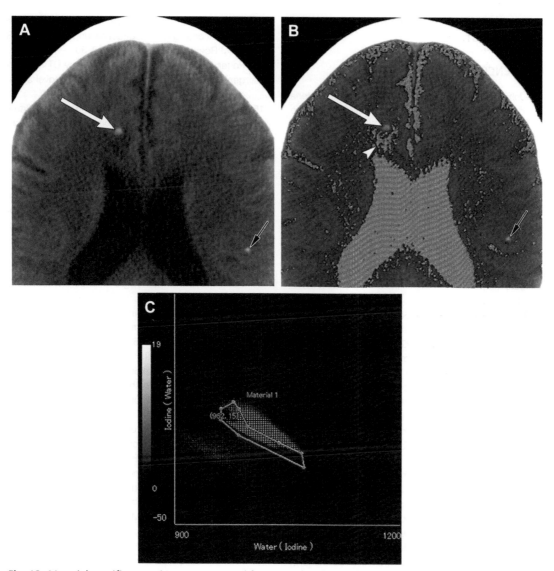

Fig. 16. Material-specific water images generated from raw data-based dual-energy CT analysis in a patient with small brain metastases from lung cancer. Axial contrast-enhanced CT (*A*) demonstrated 2 small parenchymal metastases (*white arrow* and *black arrow*). The water images (*B*) showed edematous area (*arrowhead*) surrounding the right-sided lesion (*white arrow*), as represented by the yellow pixels, but none surrounding the left lesion (*black arrow*). The water image was generated by basis material analysis (ROI placed in cerebral spinal fluid) (*C*).

Japan) for generation of water maps (using ROIs within cerebral spinal fluid). These maps have the potential to improve detection of brain edema, which can be challenging on CT (**Fig. 16**).

SUMMARY

With rising clinical interest and widely available scanner technology, it is likely that dual-energy CT will increasingly be incorporated into the clinical routine as radiologists further integrate this technology into their daily practice. Various postprocessing software for dual-energy CT, although vendor dependent, are available, enable additional analysis, and provide effective tools for more accurate interpretation of clinical images. Preliminary studies have shown their additional benefits in a wide range of neurologic applications that were discussed in detail in this review, although further validation of their diagnostic value in a broader range of diseases is still needed.

ACKNOWLEDGMENTS

The authors greatly appreciate the participation of So Tsushima, MSc, Toshiba Medical Systems

Corporation, Tokyo, Japan, for technical advice on dual-energy CT.

REFERENCES

1. Johnson TR, Krauss B, Sedlmair M, et al. Material differentiation by dual energy CT: initial experience. Eur Radiol 2007;17(6):1510–7.
2. McCollough CH, Leng S, Yu L, et al. Dual- and multi-energy CT: principles, technical approaches, and clinical applications. Radiology 2015;276(3):637–53.
3. Gupta R, Phan CM, Leidecker C, et al. Evaluation of dual-energy CT for differentiating intracerebral hemorrhage from iodinated contrast material staining. Radiology 2010;257(1):205–11.
4. Kim SJ, Lim HK, Lee HY, et al. Dual-energy CT in the evaluation of intracerebral hemorrhage of unknown origin: differentiation between tumor bleeding and pure hemorrhage. AJNR Am J Neuroradiol 2012; 33(5):865–72.
5. Postma AA, Hofman PA, Stadler AA, et al. Dual-energy CT of the brain and intracranial vessels. AJR Am J Roentgenol 2012;199(5 Suppl):S26–33.
6. Hu R, Daftari Besheli L, Young J, et al. Dual-energy head ct enables accurate distinction of intraparenchymal hemorrhage from calcification in emergency department patients. Radiology 2016;280(1):177–83.
7. Payabvash S, Khan AA, Qureshi MH, et al. Detection of intraparenchymal hemorrhage after endovascular therapy in patients with acute ischemic stroke using immediate postprocedural flat-panel computed tomography scan. J Neuroimaging 2016;26(2):213–8.
8. Morhard D, Fink C, Graser A, et al. Cervical and cranial computed tomographic angiography with automated bone removal: dual energy computed tomography versus standard computed tomography. Invest Radiol 2009;44(5):293–7.
9. Watanabe Y, Uotani K, Nakazawa T, et al. Dual-energy direct bone removal CT angiography for evaluation of intracranial aneurysm or stenosis: comparison with conventional digital subtraction angiography. Eur Radiol 2009;19(4):1019–24.
10. Brockmann C, Scharf J, Nolte IS, et al. Dual-energy CT after peri-interventional subarachnoid haemorrhage: a feasibility study. Clin Neuroradiol 2010; 20(4):231–5.
11. Buerke B, Puesken M, Wittkamp G, et al. Bone subtraction CTA for transcranial arteries: intra-individual comparison with standard CTA without bone subtraction and TOF-MRA. Clin Radiol 2010;65(6):440–6.
12. Muhlenbruch G, Das M, Mommertz G, et al. Comparison of dual-source CT angiography and MR angiography in preoperative evaluation of intra- and extracranial vessels: a pilot study. Eur Radiol 2010;20(2):469–76.
13. Zhang LJ, Wu SY, Niu JB, et al. Dual-energy CT angiography in the evaluation of intracranial aneurysms: image quality, radiation dose, and comparison with 3D rotational digital subtraction angiography. AJR Am J Roentgenol 2010;194(1):23–30.
14. Potter CA, Sodickson AD. Dual-energy CT in emergency neuroimaging: added value and novel applications. Radiographics 2016;36(7):2186–98.
15. Matsumoto K, Jinzaki M, Tanami Y, et al. Virtual monochromatic spectral imaging with fast kilovoltage switching: improved image quality as compared with that obtained with conventional 120-kVp CT. Radiology 2011;259(1):257–62.
16. Srinivasan A, Parker RA, Manjunathan A, et al. Differentiation of benign and malignant neck pathologies: preliminary experience using spectral computed tomography. J Comput Assist Tomogr 2013;37(5): 666–72.
17. Li M, Zheng X, Li J, et al. Dual-energy computed tomography imaging of thyroid nodule specimens: comparison with pathologic findings. Invest Radiol 2012;47(1):58–64.
18. Pomerantz SR, Kamalian S, Zhang D, et al. Virtual monochromatic reconstruction of dual-energy unenhanced head CT at 65–75 keV maximizes image quality compared with conventional polychromatic CT. Radiology 2013;266(1):318–25.
19. Hwang WD, Mossa-Basha M, Andre JB, et al. Qualitative comparison of noncontrast head dual-energy computed tomography using rapid voltage switching technique and conventional computed tomography. J Comput Assist Tomogr 2016;40(2):320–5.
20. Albrecht MH, Scholtz JE, Kraft J, et al. Assessment of an advanced monoenergetic reconstruction technique in dual-energy computed tomography of head and neck cancer. Eur Radiol 2015;25(8):2493–501.
21. Wichmann JL, Noske EM, Kraft J, et al. Virtual monoenergetic dual-energy computed tomography: optimization of kiloelectron volt settings in head and neck cancer. Invest Radiol 2014;49(11):735–41.
22. Tawfik AM, Kerl JM, Bauer RW, et al. Dual-energy CT of head and neck cancer: average weighting of low- and high-voltage acquisitions to improve lesion delineation and image quality-initial clinical experience. Invest Radiol 2012;47(5):306–11.
23. Lam S, Gupta R, Kelly H, et al. Multiparametric evaluation of head and neck squamous cell carcinoma using a single-source dual-energy CT with fast kVp switching: state of the art. Cancers (Basel) 2015; 7(4):2201–16.
24. Lam S, Gupta R, Levental M, et al. Optimal virtual monochromatic images for evaluation of normal tissues and head and neck cancer using dual-energy CT. AJNR Am J Neuroradiol 2015;36(8):1518–24.
25. Grant KL, Flohr TG, Krauss B, et al. Assessment of an advanced image-based technique to calculate virtual monoenergetic computed tomographic images from a dual-energy examination to improve contrast-to-noise ratio in examinations using

iodinated contrast media. Invest Radiol 2014;49(9): 586–92.

26. Lell MM, Jost G, Korporaal JG, et al. Optimizing contrast media injection protocols in state-of-the art computed tomographic angiography. Invest Radiol 2015;50(3):161–7.

27. Wang Y, Qian B, Li B, et al. Metal artifacts reduction using monochromatic images from spectral CT: evaluation of pedicle screws in patients with scoliosis. Eur J Radiol 2013;82(8):e360–6.

28. Meinel FG, Bischoff B, Zhang Q, et al. Metal artifact reduction by dual-energy computed tomography using energetic extrapolation: a systematically optimized protocol. Invest Radiol 2012;47(7):406–14.

29. Pessis E, Campagna R, Sverzut JM, et al. Virtual monochromatic spectral imaging with fast kilovoltage switching: reduction of metal artifacts at CT. Radiographics 2013;33(2):573–83.

30. Srinivasan A, Hoeffner E, Ibrahim M, et al. Utility of dual-energy CT virtual keV monochromatic series for the assessment of spinal transpedicular hardware-bone interface. AJR Am J Roentgenol 2013;201(4):878–83.

31. Shinohara Y, Sakamoto M, Iwata N, et al. Usefulness of monochromatic imaging with metal artifact reduction software for computed tomography angiography after intracranial aneurysm coil embolization. Acta Radiol 2014;55(8):1015–23.

32. Jia Y, Zhang J, Fan J, et al. Gemstone spectral imaging reduced artefacts from metal coils or clips after treatment of cerebral aneurysms: a retrospective study of 35 patients. Br J Radiol 2015;88(1055): 20150222.

33. Pessis E, Sverzut JM, Campagna R, et al. Reduction of metal artifact with dual-energy CT: virtual monospectral imaging with fast kilovoltage switching and metal artifact reduction software. Semin Musculoskelet Radiol 2015;19(5):446–55.

34. Postma AA, Das M, Stadler AA, et al. Dual-energy CT: what the neuroradiologist should know. Curr Radiol Rep 2015;3(5):1–16.

35. Inomata M, Hayashi R, Kambara K, et al. Miliary brain metastasis presenting with calcification in a patient with lung cancer: a case report. J Med Case Rep 2012;6(1):279.

36. Seo H, Choi DS, Shin HS, et al. Bone subtraction 3D CT venography for the evaluation of cerebral veins and venous sinuses: imaging techniques, normal variations, and pathologic findings. AJR Am J Roentgenol 2014;202(2):W169–75.

37. Kuno H, Jara H, Buch K, et al. Global and regional brain assessment with quantitative MR imaging in patients with prior exposure to linear gadolinium-based contrast agents. Radiology 2017;283(1):195–204.

38. Kanda T, Ishii K, Kawaguchi H, et al. High signal intensity in the dentate nucleus and globus pallidus on unenhanced T1-weighted MR images: relationship with increasing cumulative dose of a gadolinium-based contrast material. Radiology 2014;270(3): 834–41.

39. Kuno H, Onaya H, Iwata R, et al. Evaluation of cartilage invasion by laryngeal and hypopharyngeal squamous cell carcinoma with dual-energy CT. Radiology 2012;265(2):488–96.

40. Kuno H, Onaya H, Fujii S, et al. Primary staging of laryngeal and hypopharyngeal cancer: CT, MR imaging and dual-energy CT. Eur J Radiol 2014; 83(1):e23–35.

41. Ginat DT, Mayich M, Daftari-Besheli L, et al. Clinical applications of dual-energy CT in head and neck imaging. Eur Arch Otorhinolaryngol 2016;273(3): 547–53.

42. Pache G, Krauss B, Strohm P, et al. Dual-energy CT virtual noncalcium technique: detecting posttraumatic bone marrow lesions—feasibility study. Radiology 2010;256(2):617.

43. Kaup M, Wichmann JL, Scholtz JE, et al. Dual-energy CT-based display of bone marrow edema in osteoporotic vertebral compression fractures: impact on diagnostic accuracy of radiologists with varying levels of experience in correlation to MR imaging. Radiology 2016;280(2): 510–9.

44. Thomas C, Schabel C, Krauss B, et al. Dual-energy CT: virtual calcium subtraction for assessment of bone marrow involvement of the spine in multiple myeloma. AJR Am J Roentgenol 2015;204(3): W324–31.

45. Teixeira PAG, Hossu G, Lecocq S, et al. Bone marrow edema pattern identification in patients with lytic bone lesions using digital subtraction angiography–like bone subtraction on large-area detector computed tomography. Invest Radiol 2014;49(3):156–64.

46. Teixeira PAG, Gervaise A, Louis M, et al. Musculoskeletal wide detector CT: principles, techniques and applications in clinical practice and research. Eur J Radiol 2015;84(5):892–900.

47. Fujiwara H, Momoshima S, Akiyama T, et al. Whole-brain CT digital subtraction angiography of cerebral dural arteriovenous fistula using 320-detector row CT. Neuroradiology 2013;55(7):837–43.

48. Luo Z, Wang D, Sun X, et al. Comparison of the accuracy of subtraction CT angiography performed on 320-detector row volume CT with conventional CT angiography for diagnosis of intracranial aneurysms. Eur J Radiol 2012;81(1):118–22.

49. Tatsugami F, Higaki T, Kiguchi M, et al. Measurement of electron density and effective atomic number by dual-energy scan using a 320-detector computed tomography scanner with raw data-based analysis: a phantom study. J Comput Assist Tomogr 2014;38(6):824–7.

50. van Elmpt W, Landry G, Das M, et al. Dual energy CT in radiotherapy: current applications and future outlook. Radiother Oncol 2016;119(1):137–44.

Dual-Energy Computed Tomography Angiography of the Head and Neck and Related Applications

Shahmir Kamalian, MD[a,*], Michael H. Lev, MD, FAHA[a],
Stuart R. Pomerantz, MD[b]

KEYWORDS

- Dual-energy CT • Neurovascular • Bone-removal • Virtual non-contrast • Virtual monochromatic
- "Spot-sign"

KEY POINTS

- Neurovascular dual-energy CT applications include automated bone removal, creation of virtual noncontrast, noncalcium, and monochromatic images, and metallic artifact reduction.
- Automated bone removal reduces interpretation time and potentially increases accuracy by improved depiction of neurovascular structures and abnormalities.
- Virtual noncontrast and iodine overlay images improve depiction of "spot sign" as a marker of active bleeding and to predict hematoma expansion and patient prognosis.
- Low keV virtual monochromatic images can be used to improve iodinated contrast attenuation and/ or reduce contrast dose.
- High-keV virtual monochromatic images and other DECT-based metal artifact techniques can significantly reduce image degradation from aneurysm clips and coils.

INTRODUCTION

Dual-energy computed tomography (DECT) technology has become increasingly available on the high-end computed tomography (CT) platforms most common at large medical centers and teaching institutions with the potential for much wider adoption given its proposed capacity to improve CT diagnosis. For neuroimaging, the advantages of DECT lie in greater tissue characterization and differentiation than conventional CT, more akin to the capabilities of MR imaging in advanced neurodiagnostics. For neurovascular indications, increased accuracy, efficiency, and diagnostic confidence can be achieved, especially in the acute setting where CT remains the preferred imaging method or in patients with contraindications to MR imaging.

DECT tissue characterization is based on predictable attenuation differences of various materials when exposed to 2 different energy x-ray spectra and is discussed in detail in the first 2 articles in this issue (see Reza Forghani and colleagues' article, "Dual Energy CT: Physical Principles, Approaches to Scanning, Usage, and Implementation - Part 1"; and Reza Forghani and colleagues' article, "Dual Energy CT: Physical

Conflicts of Interest: None (S. Kamalian, S.R. Pomerantz). Consultant for Takeda Pharm, GE Healthcare, Medy-Match, and D-Pharm (M.H. Lev).
[a] Division of Emergency Radiology, Department of Radiology, Massachusetts General Hospital, 55 Fruit Street, Blake SB Room 29A, Boston, MA 02114, USA; [b] Division of Neuroradiology, Department of Radiology, Massachusetts General Hospital, 55 Fruit Street, Gray 2, Room 273A, Boston, MA 02114, USA
* Corresponding author.
E-mail address: skamalian@mgh.harvard.edu

Neuroimag Clin N Am 27 (2017) 429–443
http://dx.doi.org/10.1016/j.nic.2017.04.009
1052-5149/17/© 2017 Elsevier Inc. All rights reserved.

Principles, Approaches to Scanning, Usage, and Implementation - Part 2" in this issue). If using a dual-source DECT system, mixed or blended images are created from weighted averages of the high- and low- peak kilovoltage (kVp) image data to simulate traditional single-source CT images. However, the changes in tissue attenuation between these 2 datasets can be mathematically correlated to expected characteristic changes of constituent basis materials such as iodine, calcium, and water. The degree to which the expected characteristic attenuation differences for the basis materials are observed when mathematically comparing the high- and low-energy data sets enables an estimation of the relative percentage of the various basis materials on a voxel-wise basis. This material decomposition can then be used to create material-selective or tissue-weighted image reconstructions such as bone- or calcium-subtracted images, iodine overlay, and virtual noncontrast (VNC) images. Virtual monochromatic (monoenergetic) images can also be derived from this material decomposition. By reconstructing images reflecting the lower or higher energies within the polychromatic x-ray spectra used for CT acquisition, accentuation of iodine contrast enhancement or reduction of metallic artifact from aneurysm coils or clips can be achieved, respectively. This article provides an illustrative overview of the key applications of DECT technique for neurovascular imaging and their clinical utility.

FUNDAMENTAL PRINCIPLES OF DUAL-ENERGY COMPUTED TOMOGRAPHY ACQUISITION, MATERIAL CHARACTERIZATION, AND POSTPROCESSING
Dual-Energy Computed Tomography Acquisition and Material Characterization

The various commercially available DECT scanners and different methods for acquiring images are discussed in detail in the first 2 articles of this issue and will not be reviewed here. A detailed discussion of DECT principles and material characterization can also be found in the first 2 articles in this issue, but will be briefly reviewed here (see Reza Forghani and colleagues' article, "Dual Energy CT: Physical Principles, Approaches to Scanning, Usage, and Implementation - Part 1"; and Reza Forghani and colleagues' article, "Dual Energy CT: Physical Principles, Approaches to Scanning, Usage, and Implementation - Part 2" in this issue). Tissue characterization in both conventional and DECT is based on the differential x-ray photon attenuation from the various materials that are encountered during medical scanning, including different soft tissues, fluids, and

bone, as well as exogenous materials such as metal and contrast agents. In the energy range used in medical imaging, x-ray attenuation is attributable primarily to photoelectric absorption (PEA) and photon scatter (Compton effect). The likelihood of PEA depends on an element's K-edge, atomic number, and the incident photon energy. The K-edge is the binding energy of the atom's innermost electron shell. At energies slightly above the K-edge of an element, the probability of PE absorption is sharply increased. Therefore, at energies just above the K-edge, there is a sharp increase in attenuation followed by a rapid decline with increases in energy away from the K-edge. Furthermore, PEA is proportional to the cube of the atomic number (Z^3) and inversely proportional to the cube of the incident photon energy ($1/E^3$). Therefore, elements with a higher Z have a much higher likelihood of PEA, which can be exploited using DECT approaches.

Compton effect is the decrease in energy of an incident photon scattered by its interaction with outer shell electrons of a particular atomic material. The likelihood of this event is proportional to the number of outer shell electrons, which relates both to electron density of the given element and to the physical density of the overall material. The likelihood of the Compton effect does not change with the atomic number and shows little energy dependence, in contrast to PEA.

In DECT, attenuation data are gathered from materials exposed to 2 different polychromatic x-ray beams, enabling evaluation and characterization of the energy-dependent attenuation characteristics of different materials and tissues. In general, the elements constituting most soft tissues in the body, such as hydrogen, carbon, oxygen, and nitrogen, have low atomic numbers and typically demonstrate little energy-dependent changes in their attenuation. Elements with higher atomic numbers such as iodine, on the other hand, demonstrate significant energy dependency of their attenuation that can be exploited using DECT approaches.

Dual-Energy Computed Tomography Postprocessing

The imaging datasets acquired by DECT can be used to calculate effective atomic numbers, for 2- or 3-material decomposition, and to create virtual monochromatic images. The postprocessing tools and different DECT reconstructions are discussed in detail in multiple accompanying articles in this issue but are briefly reviewed here as well.

Calculation of effective atomic number
When dealing with materials composed of more than one element, a useful tool is to calculate an

effective atomic number. In conventional single-energy computed tomography (SECT), images are displayed in Hounsfield units, which are based on the attenuation coefficients of the various materials. The attenuation coefficient is a function of 2 fundamental parameters of a material: its effective atomic number and electron density. In DECT, data expressed in Hounsfield units can be converted into the effective atomic number and the electron density. The ability to determine the effective atomic number of individual voxels with reasonable accuracy is one of the advantages of DECT.[1–3]

Material decomposition
DECT material decomposition relies on the fact that the x-ray attenuation of a material can be represented as a linear combination of attenuation secondary to Compton scatter and the photoelectric effect. As a result, Compton scatter and the photoelectric effect can form a material basis pair in which all materials can be expressed, although with DECT scanners, it is more common to express materials in a different material basis pair that is more related to human tissues, for example, a combination of water and iodine. When evaluating material decomposition maps, it is important to keep in mind that material characterization on these maps is performed by cross-correlating their attenuation properties with reference materials. Therefore, although these could be used to generate maps demonstrating the distribution and estimated concentration of a material of interest, they should not be interpreted as the physical distribution of a pure solution such as pure water or pure iodine.

The DECT material decomposition approach can be very powerful and may be used to distinguish 2 presumed materials from each other in ways not possible with conventional single-energy CT. For example, a standard CT at 120 kVp may show similar Hounsfield unit numbers for a mixture of iodine with brain tissue and a mixture of hemorrhage with brain tissue on postcontrast images, but at lower kVp closer to the iodine K-edge, the attenuation of the iodine with brain tissue shows a much higher increase in Hounsfield number than the mixture of hemorrhage and brain tissue, which can be used to distinguish iodine from hemorrhage. The same method is used for bone subtraction based on characterization of each voxel as behaving more like a mixture of iodine with blood or calcium with bone marrow at 2 x-ray energy levels. Each voxel is characterized as falling above or below a separation line slope. The voxels characterized as containing predominantly calcium are replaced with a very lower number in order to better evaluate adjacent structures.[4] Other maps

commonly used in neuroradiology or head and neck imaging include iodine overlay maps, VNC images, or virtual calcium or noncalcium images. For a more detailed discussion of the material decomposition process, including different approaches (eg, 2 vs 3 material decomposition), the reader is referred to the first 2 articles in this issue (see Reza Forghani and colleagues' article, "Dual Energy CT: Physical Principles, Approaches to Scanning, Usage, and Implementation - Part 1"; and Reza Forghani and colleagues' article, "Dual Energy CT: Physical Principles, Approaches to Scanning, Usage, and Implementation - Part 2" in this issue).

Virtual monochromatic image reconstruction
The attenuation values recorded in the high- and low-energy polychromatic datasets (measured in kVp) acquired from dual-energy scanning can be used to simulate the expected attenuation values, which would be recorded if a monochromatic x-ray beam at a given hypothetical energy value (measured in kiloelectronvolts [keV]) was used for scanning.[5] Postprocessing of DECT angiography data allows reconstruction of virtual monoenergetic images at the arbitrary energy levels ranging from 40 keV to 190 keV (or higher for some DECT systems).[6,7] As the monochromatic energy level is reduced closer to their K-edge, the attenuation of the materials with higher effective atomic numbers increases much greater than the attenuation of the material with lower effective atomic numbers. Therefore, materials with high effective atomic numbers such as iodine and calcium demonstrate higher densities in Hounsfield units, whereas materials with low effective atomic numbers such as water and soft tissues remain relatively flat.[4] In general, at higher monoenergetic levels, images are less noisy, but there is also decreased iodine attenuation and soft tissue contrast. Conversely, at lower monoenergetic levels, there is increased soft tissue contrast but also greater image noise (**Fig. 1A–C**).

DUAL-ENERGY COMPUTED TOMOGRAPHY BONE AND CALCIUM REMOVAL FOR NEUROVASCULAR COMPUTED TOMOGRAPHY ANGIOGRAPHY

Bone and calcified atheromatous plaques can obscure arterial and venous anatomy on CT angiographic images, especially when maximal intensity projection (MIP) and volume rendering images are used.

Before DECT, various methods were being used to generate bone- or calcium-subtracted images for optimal depiction of the vessel lumen and to facilitate interpretation of complex vascular anatomy.[8–18] These methods include the following

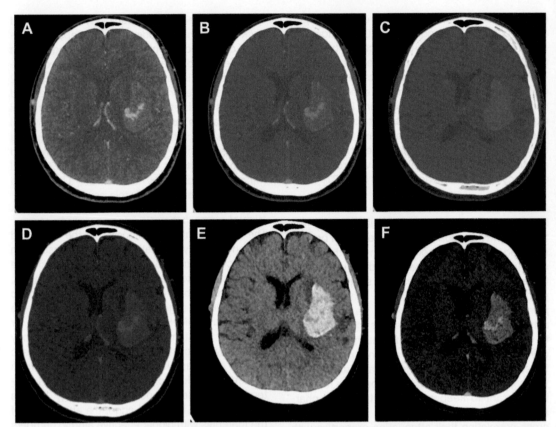

Fig. 1. (*A–C*) Virtual 40-, 60-, and 190-keV monoenergetic images; (*D*) weighted-average image of the high- and low-kVp datasets; (*E*) VNC image; and (*F*) iodine overlay image. CT images demonstrate an intraparenchymal hematoma within the left basal ganglia and insula with active extravasation of iodinated contrast. The iodine (vessels and contrast extravasation within the hemorrhage) is better depicted at lower virtual monoenergetic levels (40 and 60 keV; *A* and *B*) than the weighted-average image (*D*). At higher virtual monoenergetic levels, the attenuation of iodine decreases. Note, for example, that the reconstructed virtual 190-keV monoenergetic image (*C*) appears similar to an unenhanced study. The iodinated contrast is successfully subtracted on the VNC image (*E*). In addition, the iodine map can be used as iodine overlay on the weighted-average dual-energy images (*F*) to differentiate iodine from dense hemorrhage.

approaches and their limitations: (1) Manual segmentation of bones and vessels, which is labor-intensive and operator-dependent; (2) Threshold-based semiautomatic segmentation, which is prone to subtraction artifacts when the density of contrast material in the vessels is similar to the adjacent calcium and bone; and (3) Digital subtraction of non-contrast CT from the computed tomography angiography (CTA) images, which is susceptible to motion artifact and misregistration between the 2 acquisitions and increases the radiation dose.[8–10]

DECT-based techniques for bone and calcium removal are effective in revealing underlying vascular anatomy without the time costs of manual segmentation, motion artifacts (different image sets are created from the same acquisition avoiding problems with misregistration of multiple phase acquisitions), and increased radiation dose of the previously listed techniques (**Fig. 2**).

In addition, material decomposition enables discrimination of atheromatous calcium and intraluminal contrast, which can have similar attenuation on SECT images.[11–14,19]

Aneurysm Detection and Morphologic Visualization

Bone-subtraction DECT angiography is a highly accurate test for aneurysm detection compared with digital subtraction angiography (DSA) and facilitates visualization of the morphology of aneurysms at the skull base (**Fig. 3**).[15,16,20] Watanabe and colleagues[15] demonstrated that bone-removed DE-CTA is superior to conventional CTA in visualization of aneurysms near the skull base and calcified aneurysms compared with the gold-standard DSA. Zhang and colleagues[16,20] demonstrated that DE-CTA has a lower radiation

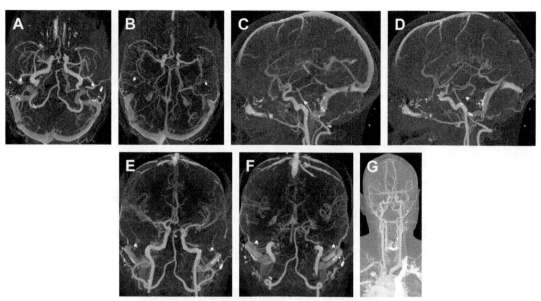

Fig. 2. The intracranial arteries and veins are well depicted and evaluated with these 6 axial, coronal, and sagittal 7-cm-thick MIP reconstructions after bone removal. (*A, B*) Axial MIP; (*C*) sagittal MIP through the right hemisphere; (*D*) sagittal MIP through the left hemisphere; (*E, F*) coronal MIP. A representative image from automatic bone-subtraction rotational MIP (*G*) depicts all the major head and neck arteries in a single view.

dose compared with DSA and facilitates evaluation of surgically treated aneurysms by reducing the metallic artifact from the aneurysm clips using postprocessing techniques (discussed in the following sections).

Evaluation of Atherosclerotic Arterial Stenosis

Carotid CTA has become an important test in the evaluation of atherosclerotic carotid stenosis as a major ischemic risk factor, helping to decide between different treatment strategies, such as medical therapy, carotid endarterectomy, or stent placement. This assessment can be challenging in the presence of heavily calcified atherosclerotic plaques, which can appear isodense to the immediately adjacent residual contrast-enhanced lumen. DE-CTA techniques based on calcium material decomposition have been shown to be beneficial in this setting.[21–24] DE-CTA postprocessing techniques can be used to either highlight or remove calcified plaques,[13,14] potentially affording better visualization of the residual lumen and more accurate quantitative measures for stenosis grading.[25] Virtual monochromatic CTA reconstructions can further increase the accuracy of stenosis assessment, although care must be taken as the choice of energy level can change the apparent size of the calcified plaque by improving or exaggerating a "blooming" effect (**Fig. 4**).[22,26]

Bone removal is another DE-CTA technique that can be used to improve neurovascular CTA

interpretation. Overlying bone can obscure vascular anatomy, especially on volume-rendered and MIP reformatted views. DE-CTA bone removal techniques can thus reduce interpretation time and increase efficiency compared with standard CT angiography.[8,12] In addition, bone subtraction may facilitate detection of other subtle intracranial abnormalities that may otherwise be obscured by the adjacent bone such an as acute subdural hematoma. A potential pitfall of both calcium and bone removal techniques is overestimation of the stenosis. In places where the vessels closely abut or are surrounded by bone, such as at the skull base and in the paraclinoid regions, bone-removal DE-CTA can result in artifactual defects in the vessels (**Fig. 5**).[8,15,18] Correlation of apparent defects, especially in these regions, to source CTA images is a critical element of DE-CTA interpretation workflow.[24]

Computed Tomography Venography

By delaying the time of acquisition after intravenous injection, CTA techniques can be used for evaluation of the superficial and deep venous drainage systems. CT venography is an important technique for identifying acute cortical vein and dural venous sinus thrombosis, for preoperative assessment of the degree of tumoral encasement and venous patency in lesions along the calvarium and skull base (such as meningiomas), and for evaluating chronic venoocclusive disease. As the dural venous sinuses and cortical veins course directly adjacent

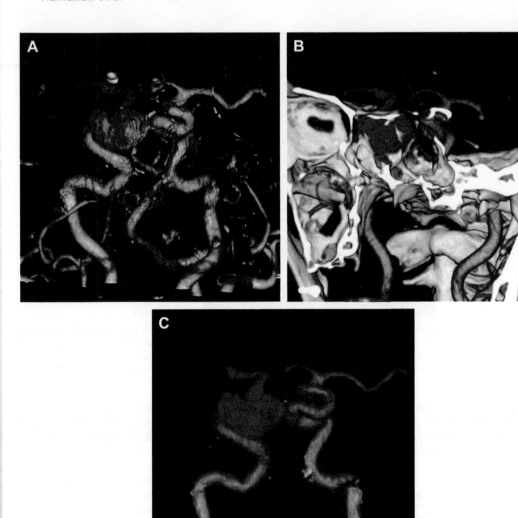

Fig. 3. Automatic bone-subtraction DECT 3D volume rendering (*A*) provides adequate visualization of the morphology of aneurysms at the skull base compared with 3D volume rendering without bone removal (*B*) and labor-intensive manual or semi-automatic bone subtraction (*C*).

to the skull, conventional 3-dimensional (3D) venographic postprocessing techniques are more challenging and time consuming than visualizing the arterial branches of the circle of Willis in arterial-phase CTA evaluations. DE-CTA bone removal techniques provide a fast and robust tool for display of the normal venous anatomy and any potential abnormality (see **Fig. 2**).[27,28]

CLINICAL USE OF VIRTUAL MONOCHROMATIC IMAGES

Virtual monochromatic images can be used to accentuate iodine contrast with a potential to decrease contrast material dose and to decrease artifact from metal implants. Multiple specialized clinical applications of different energy virtual monochromatic image are discussed in accompanying articles in this issue. The authors briefly review applications of these reconstructions focusing on vascular imaging.

Accentuation of Iodine Contrast Enhancement

The K-edge of iodine is 33.2 keV, and therefore, monoenergetic images at lower energies than those considered equivalent to a 120-kVp single-energy CT acquisition, approaching the iodine

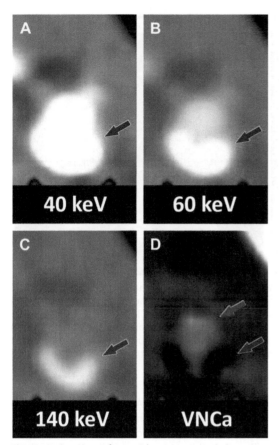

Fig. 4. Estimation of carotid artery stenosis is a common problem in the presence of dense atherosclerotic plaques on the conventional CT imaging and virtual monochromatic energy reconstructions in DECT (A–C). Material decomposition with calcium removal (D, VNCa) can offer a more accurate estimation of carotid stenosis (D). Blue arrows show the calcified plaque. The red arrow shows a reasonable diagnostic depiction of the contrast material in the residual vessel lumen. (*Courtesy of* Dr Shervin Kamalian, Boston, MA.)

K-edge, can increase iodine attenuation and therefore improve visibility of vascular opacification.[29–32] Therefore, DECT approaches can potentially lower the dose of contrast needed for sufficient vascular delineation[30,33] or even generate vessel images from delayed postcontrast images. The caveat is that at lower monoenergetic levels the noise also increases. At least one study has suggested that the optimal monoenergetic level for vessel visualization in head and neck CT angiography is 60 keV due to a tradeoff between vessel opacification and image noise.[29] However, the noise level can vary depending on the vendor and postprocessing techniques used and the contrast-to-noise ratio will also partly depend on the absolute opacification (or iodine content) within a vessel. Last, newer postprocessing techniques are under development that decrease image noise at the lower energy virtual monoenergetic images (see **Fig. 1**A, B).[34] Therefore, the optimal monoenergetic energy level will likely vary depending on vendor and the algorithm used for data postprocessing[4] and the type of examination performed. Overall, accentuation of iodinated contrast enhancement in combination with better postprocessing techniques provides an opportunity for contrast material dose reduction. Contrast dose reduction is especially important in patients with renal insufficiency or in patients receiving multiple contrast injections over a short time period.[35–37]

Metal Artifact Reduction

Approximately 20% of CT studies are at least partially degraded by beam hardening artifact from metallic materials.[38] Beam hardening artifact is seen with polychromatic x-ray beams and is caused by materials with high effective atomic numbers, such as metallic implants, high concentrations of iodine, or dense bone.[39] As the polychromatic x-ray beam passes through these materials, low-energy x-ray photons are absorbed more readily and the proportion of the high-energy photons increases (higher energy x-ray beam or hardened beam). The reconstruction algorithms are based on the presumed similarity of the x-ray beams entering and exiting the patient. As the hardened beam passes through the remaining soft tissues with little attenuation, a dark line is seen on the reconstructed image.[39]

The use of monoenergetic imaging at higher energy levels reduces beam-hardening artifacts and improves the delineation of metal implants, such as aneurysm coils or clips, or spine fixation hardware (**Fig. 6**).[40–44] However, there is a limitation to this process, and inadequate data due to photon starvation in the presence of large amount of materials with very high atomic numbers cannot be entirely corrected with virtual monochromatic imaging.[4]

CTA assessment and surveillance after aneurysm coiling or clipping may benefit from this technique. Use of monoenergetic imaging in DE-CTA with or without additional metal artifact reduction software can potentially improve vessel visualization near aneurysm coils and clips.[40,42] However, a potential limitation of the higher keV monochromatic images is reduction in the attenuation of contrast enhancement from iodine,[4,40,45] and the optimal monoenergetic energy level and contrast material dose are yet to be determined. Artifact reduction using DECT is discussed in a separate article in this issue.

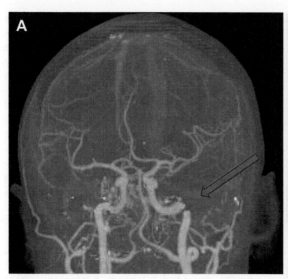
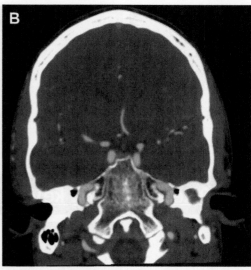

Fig. 5. A potential pitfall of bone removal techniques in places where the vessels are surrounded by bone, such as at the skull base, is artifactual defects in the vessels. A representative image from automatic bone-subtraction rotational MIP (*A*) demonstrates a defect in the proximal petrous segment of the left internal carotid artery (*blue arrow*). This vessel was in fact widely patent, with the artifactual defect created by the misregistration of the contrast within the vessel lumen as bone in the bone removal technique. Coronal reconstruction from CTA source image (*B*) demonstrates normal appearance of the petrous segment of the left internal carotid artery (ICA).

ICA–PLAQUE EVALUATION: CA++ PLAQUE REMOVAL, IMPROVING RESIDUAL LUMINAL MEASUREMENT ACCURACY, AND REDUCING BLOOMING FROM CONTRAST AND CA++

Current clinical algorithms for treatment of carotid stenosis are largely based on the degree of narrowing (in addition to other clinical factors). However, such algorithms do not take into account the characteristics of the atherosclerotic plaque, which can have a significant impact on the risk for future stroke. Atherosclerotic carotid plaques are composed of a lipid-rich necrotic core, a fibrous cap/covering tissue, and occasionally calcifications and intraplaque hemorrhage. A thin fibrous cap, a large lipid-rich core, intraplaque hemorrhage, and vasa vasorum enhancement have been identified as markers of plaque vulnerability and higher risk of future strokes.[46–49] Large amounts of fibrous tissue and calcified components are considered markers of plaque stability.[46–49] Hence, assessment of plaque vulnerability can potentially guide treatment.

Although the ability of conventional SECT to visualize and evaluate vulnerable plaque is somewhat controversial, some studies suggested that the plaques with large lipid-rich necrotic core and intraplaque hemorrhage can be identified based on CT attenuation values (Hounsfield unit).[50–52] A few recent studies demonstrated that DECT allows for assessment of the different carotid plaque components with a higher accuracy compared with

conventional SECT.[53,54] Another recent study suggested that effective atomic number (Z) maps can differentiate vulnerable from stable carotid plaques with reasonable accuracy.[55] In that study, vulnerable carotid plaques had lower effective Z numbers compared with stable plaques with an area under the curve of 0.88 and a cutoff effective Z value of 7.9.[55] Potentially, DE-CTA with calcium removal may facilitate visualization of vasa vasorum enhancement and intraplaque hemorrhage, which can be obscured by plaque calcification.

ROLE OF VIRTUAL NONCONTRAST IMAGING IN INTRACRANIAL HEMORRHAGE

Material decomposition allows for virtual extraction of iodine and creation of VNC imaging and iodine maps, which are useful in various neuroradiologic indications.

Hemorrhage versus Leaked Iodine

A serious complication after endovascular thrombolysis for treatment of acute ischemic stroke is hemorrhagic conversion, which can be seen in up to 15% of patients.[56–59] A common finding in these patients after angiography is contrast material staining due to breakdown of the blood-brain barrier. It is often difficult to differentiate contrast staining from acute hemorrhage with conventional SECT due to similar Hounsfield numbers and overlap in attenuation,

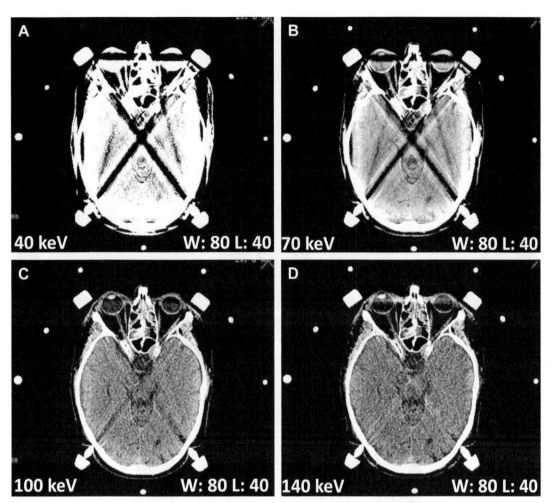

Fig. 6. Virtual monochromatic images created from axial noncontrast DECT acquired in a patient in a stereotactic head fixation device at 40 keV (*A*), 70 keV (*B*), 100 keV (*C*), and 140 keV (*D*) demonstrate a decrease in beam hardening and streak artifacts with an increase in virtual monoenergetic level.

which can lead to a delay in antithrombotic therapy.[60–62] VNC imaging, used in conjunction with the standard CT equivalent reconstructions, is particularly useful in distinguishing hemorrhagic conversion from contrast material staining after endovascular thrombolysis in patients with acute ischemic stroke.[63–66] The reported accuracy of DECT in differentiation of hemorrhage from contrast staining ranges from 87% to 100% (**Fig. 7**).[4,63,66,67]

A potential pitfall is the presence of both calcium and contrast staining after endovascular thrombolysis (such as basal ganglia calcifications) because calcium remains visible on VNC images similar to blood products and may be misclassified as hemorrhage.[67] In the same way, contrast staining remains visible on virtual noncalcium (VNCa) images similar to the blood products and may be misclassified as hemorrhage. In these situations, correlation with older comparison studies or VNCa images from noncontrast DECT (if obtained before the endovascular thrombolysis) is helpful for making the distinction.

DECT is also a potentially valuable tool in discrimination and subtraction of blood and iodine mixed within the subarachnoid spaces for detection of rebleeding during and after endovascular treatment of patients with aneurysmal subarachnoid hemorrhage.[17] In addition, the iodine map can be used as iodine overlay on the weighted-average dual-energy images, which can potentially serve as perfusion-weighted imaging.

Intracranial Hemorrhage: Detection of Spot Sign or Underlying Lesion

Active extravasation of contrast within a parenchymal hemorrhage on CT angiography ("spot sign") is an imaging marker of active bleeding,

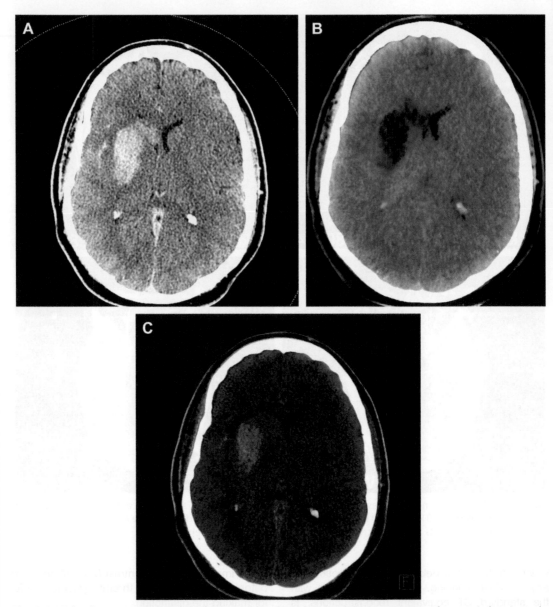

Fig. 7. Weighted-average image of the high- and low-kVp datasets (*A*) in a patient with acute ischemic stroke after endovascular thrombectomy shows subarachnoid hyperdensity in the Sylvian fissure and a hyperdense parenchymal focus in the right lentiform nucleus and caudate head. The VNC (*B*) and iodine overlay (*C*) images demonstrate that these finding represent contrast staining rather than subarachnoid and intraparenchymal hemorrhage.

and an independent predictor of hematoma expansion and poor prognosis.[68–74] The CT angiography spot sign represents contrast material extravasation on arterial phase and/or delayed images not present on the precontrast images.[75–77] VNC images in conjunction with iodine overlay maps derived from DECT angiography can identify leaked iodine and facilitate detection of a spot sign, particularly within heterogenous hematomas with areas of dense blood products (see **Fig.** 1D–F;

Fig. 8).[78] The use of VNC images also has the potential to decrease the radiation dose in comparison to multiphase conventional SECT techniques, which typically use noncontrast, angiographic, and delayed phase images.

Up to 30% of intracranial hemorrhages are due to underlying neoplastic lesions or vascular malformations.[79] However, such lesions can be obscured in the acute setting by a large parenchymal hematoma. Similar to the spot sign, VNC

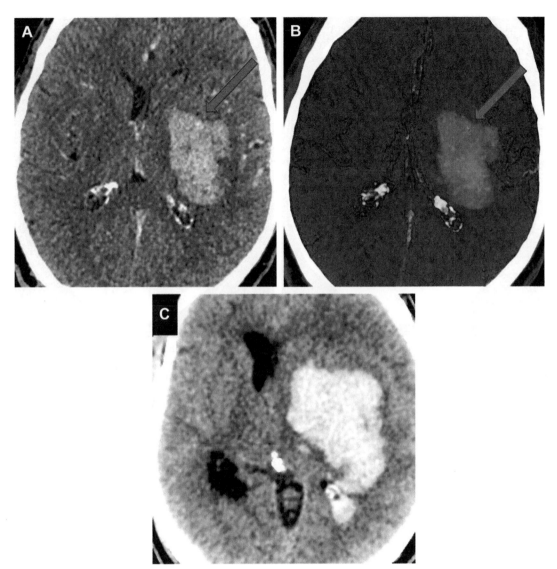

Fig. 8. Delayed CTA source image (*A*) demonstrates a subtle active extravasation of contrast (spot sign), which is difficult to detect (*blue arrow*). The iodine overlay image (*B*) facilitates detection of the spot sign (*blue arrow*). Follow-up noncontrast CT image (*C*) after a few hours demonstrates interval increase in size of the hematoma.

images in conjunction with iodine overlay maps have been shown to be superior to conventional CT angiography or weighted-average dual-energy images for the detection of underlying neoplastic or vascular causes of hemorrhage.[80] DECT can potentially play an important role in detection of an underlying neoplasm in the acute and subacute phases,[80] leading to earlier diagnosis (**Fig. 9**).

Opportunity for Radiation Dose Reduction: Reality?

VNC images can be created by the removal of iodine with no additional radiation exposure, which closely mimics the noncontrast image obtained from single-energy CT. Hence, at least in theory, noncontrast CT

and CTA could be replaced by a single acquisition of DECT angiography images and reconstruction of VNC images. Although the VNC images are noisier and not as visually appealing as a separately acquired noncontrast dataset, they are of sufficient diagnostic quality for detection of intracranial hemorrhages.[81,82] Hence, by omitting the noncontrast CT radiation dose can be reduced.

LIMITATIONS

The limitations in use of DECT angiography include hardware and software costs, and workflow inefficiencies related to added time required for postprocessing, without compensatory increases

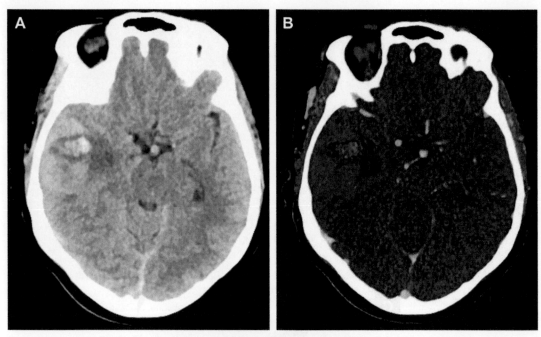

Fig. 9. Noncontrast CT (*A*) demonstrates a parenchymal hemorrhage in the right temporal lobe. The iodine overlay map (*B*) from the contrast-enhanced DE-CTA demonstrates absence of intravenous contrast. However, the image depicts thick irregular peripheral enhancement, suggesting an underlying lesion. Subsequently, the patient was diagnosed with glioblastoma.

in reimbursement. Workflow inefficiencies are of particular concern in the acute setting, when rapid diagnosis is critical for timely patient management. Newer DECT systems at least partly address these challenges by enabling automatic generation of many of the specialized DECT reconstructions at the CT technologist console, which in turn can be sent to PACS and will be available for review without additional radiologist postprocessing. Systems enabling advanced DECT manipulations directly from PACS will also facilitate the use of this technology and help increase adoption in the clinical setting. Ultimately, if DECT is proven to have significant added value, modifications in reimbursement that take into account the additional time requirements for processing and interpretation would be desirable to promote its use.

SUMMARY

DECT angiography is emerging as an invaluable problem-solving tool in clinical practice that offers a diverse and expanding range of applications in detection and diagnosis of different cerebrovascular diseases.

REFERENCES

1. Goodsitt MM, Christodoulou EG, Larson SC. Accuracies of the synthesized monochromatic CT numbers and effective atomic numbers obtained with a rapid kVp switching dual energy CT scanner. Med Phys 2011;38:2222–32.
2. Landry G, Seco J, Gaudreault M, et al. Deriving effective atomic numbers from DECT based on a parameterization of the ratio of high and low linear attenuation coefficients. Phys Med Biol 2013;58:6851–66.
3. Landry G, Reniers B, Granton PV, et al. Extracting atomic numbers and electron densities from a dual source dual energy CT scanner: experiments and a simulation model. Radiother Oncol 2011;100: 375–9.
4. Potter CA, Sodickson AD. Dual-energy CT in emergency neuroimaging: added value and novel applications. Radiographics 2016;36:2186–98.
5. Yu L, Leng S, McCollough CH. Dual-energy CT-based monochromatic imaging. AJR Am J Roentgenol 2012;199:S9–15.
6. Kuchenbecker S, Faby S, Sawall S, et al. Dual energy CT: how well can pseudo-monochromatic imaging reduce metal artifacts? Med Phys 2015;42:1023–36.
7. Tsunoo T, Torikoshi M, Ohno Y, et al. Measurement of electron density in dual-energy x-ray CT with monochromatic x rays and evaluation of its accuracy. Med Phys 2008;35:4924–32.
8. Morhard D, Fink C, Becker C, et al. Value of automatic bone subtraction in cranial CT angiography: comparison of bone-subtracted vs. standard CT angiography in 100 patients. Eur Radiol 2008;18:974–82.

9. Lell MM, Ruehm SG, Kramer M, et al. Cranial computed tomography angiography with automated bone subtraction: a feasibility study. Invest Radiol 2009;44:38–43.

10. Romijn M, Gratama van Andel HA, van Walderveen MA, et al. Diagnostic accuracy of CT angiography with matched mask bone elimination for detection of intracranial aneurysms: comparison with digital subtraction angiography and 3D rotational angiography. AJNR Am J Neuroradiol 2008;29:134–9.

11. Hegde A, Chan LL, Tan L, et al. Dual energy CT and its use in neuroangiography. Ann Acad Med Singapore 2009;38:817–20.

12. Morhard D, Fink C, Graser A, et al. Cervical and cranial computed tomographic angiography with automated bone removal: dual energy computed tomography versus standard computed tomography. Invest Radiol 2009;44:293–7.

13. Ma R, Liu C, Deng K, et al. Cerebral artery evaluation of dual energy CT angiography with dual source CT. Chin Med J (Engl) 2010;123:1139–44.

14. Muhlenbruch G, Das M, Mommertz G, et al. Comparison of dual-source CT angiography and mr angiography in preoperative evaluation of intra- and extracranial vessels: a pilot study. Eur Radiol 2010; 20:469–76.

15. Watanabe Y, Uotani K, Nakazawa T, et al. Dual-energy direct bone removal CT angiography for evaluation of intracranial aneurysm or stenosis: comparison with conventional digital subtraction angiography. Eur Radiol 2009;19:1019–24.

16. Zhang LJ, Wu SY, Niu JB, et al. Dual-energy CT angiography in the evaluation of intracranial aneurysms: image quality, radiation dose, and comparison with 3D rotational digital subtraction angiography. AJR Am J Roentgenol 2010;194:23–30.

17. Brockmann C, Scharf J, Nolte IS, et al. Dual-energy CT after peri-interventional subarachnoid haemorrhage: a feasibility study. Clin Neuroradiol 2010;20:231–5.

18. Buerke B, Puesken M, Wittkamp G, et al. Bone subtraction CTA for transcranial arteries: intra-individual comparison with standard CTA without bone subtraction and TOF-MRA. Clin Radiol 2010;65:440–6.

19. Deng K, Liu C, Ma R, et al. Clinical evaluation of dual-energy bone removal in CT angiography of the head and neck: comparison with conventional bone-subtraction CT angiography. Clin Radiol 2009;64:534–41.

20. Zhang LJ, Wu SY, Poon CS, et al. Automatic bone removal dual-energy CT angiography for the evaluation of intracranial aneurysms. J Comput Assist Tomogr 2010;34:816–24.

21. Uotani K, Watanabe Y, Higashi M, et al. Dual-energy CT head bone and hard plaque removal for quantification of calcified carotid stenosis: utility and comparison with digital subtraction angiography. Eur Radiol 2009;19:2060–5.

22. Mannelli L, Mitsumori LM, Ferguson M, et al. Changes in measured size of atherosclerotic plaque calcifications in dual-energy CT of ex vivo carotid endarterectomy specimens: effect of monochromatic kev image reconstructions. Eur Radiol 2013;23:367–74.

23. Watanabe Y, Nakazawa T, Higashi M, et al. Assessment of calcified carotid plaque volume: comparison of contrast-enhanced dual-energy CT angiography and native single-energy CT. AJR Am J Roentgenol 2011;196:W796–9.

24. Thomas C, Korn A, Ketelsen D, et al. Automatic lumen segmentation in calcified plaques: dual-energy CT versus standard reconstructions in comparison with digital subtraction angiography. AJR Am J Roentgenol 2010;194:1590–5.

25. Postma AA, Das M, Stadler AA, et al. Dual-energy CT: what the neuroradiologist should know. Curr Radiol Rep 2015;3:16.

26. Mannelli L, MacDonald L, Mancini M, et al. Dual energy computed tomography quantification of carotid plaques calcification: comparison between monochromatic and polychromatic energies with pathology correlation. Eur Radiol 2015;25:1238–46.

27. Gratama van Andel HA, van Boven LJ, van Walderveen MA, et al. Interobserver variability in the detection of cerebral venous thrombosis using CT venography with matched mask bone elimination. Clin Neurol Neurosurg 2009;111:717–23.

28. Majoie CB, van Straten M, Venema HW, et al. Multisection CT venography of the dural sinuses and cerebral veins by using matched mask bone elimination. AJNR Am J Neuroradiol 2004;25:787–91.

29. Schneider D, Apfaltrer P, Sudarski S, et al. Optimization of kiloelectron volt settings in cerebral and cervical dual-energy CT angiography determined with virtual monoenergetic imaging. Acad Radiol 2014; 21:431–6.

30. Cho ES, Chung TS, Oh DK, et al. Cerebral computed tomography angiography using a low tube voltage (80 kVp) and a moderate concentration of iodine contrast material: a quantitative and qualitative comparison with conventional computed tomography angiography. Invest Radiol 2012;47:142–7.

31. Apfaltrer P, Sudarski S, Schneider D, et al. Value of monoenergetic low-kV dual energy CT datasets for improved image quality of CT pulmonary angiography. Eur J Radiol 2014;83:322–8.

32. Sudarski S, Apfaltrer P, Nance JW Jr, et al. Optimization of keV-settings in abdominal and lower extremity dual-source dual-energy CT angiography determined with virtual monoenergetic imaging. Eur J Radiol 2013;82:e574–81.

33. Bahner ML, Bengel A, Brix G, et al. Improved vascular opacification in cerebral computed tomography angiography with 80 kVp. Invest Radiol 2005;40:229–34.

34. Albrecht MH, Scholtz JE, Kraft J, et al. Assessment of an advanced monoenergetic reconstruction

technique in dual-energy computed tomography of head and neck cancer. Eur Radiol 2015;25:2493–501.

35. Delesalle MA, Pontana F, Duhamel A, et al. Spectral optimization of chest CT angiography with reduced iodine load: experience in 80 patients evaluated with dual-source, dual-energy CT. Radiology 2013; 267:256–66.

36. Yuan R, Shuman WP, Earls JP, et al. Reduced iodine load at CT pulmonary angiography with dual-energy monochromatic imaging: comparison with standard CT pulmonary angiography–a prospective randomized trial. Radiology 2012;262:290–7.

37. Agrawal MD, Oliveira GR, Kalva SP, et al. Prospective comparison of reduced-iodine-dose virtual monochromatic imaging dataset from dual-energy CT angiography with standard-iodine-dose single-energy CT angiography for abdominal aortic aneurysm. AJR Am J Roentgenol 2016;207: W125–32.

38. Boas FE, Fleischmann D. Evaluation of two iterative techniques for reducing metal artifacts in computed tomography. Radiology 2011;259:894–902.

39. Park HS, Hwang D, Seo JK. Metal artifact reduction for polychromatic x-ray CT based on a beam-hardening corrector. IEEE Trans Med Imaging 2016;35:480–7.

40. Shinohara Y, Sakamoto M, Iwata N, et al. Usefulness of monochromatic imaging with metal artifact reduction software for computed tomography angiography after intracranial aneurysm coil embolization. Acta Radiol 2014;55:1015–23.

41. Guggenberger R, Winklhofer S, Osterhoff G, et al. Metallic artefact reduction with monoenergetic dual-energy CT: systematic ex vivo evaluation of posterior spinal fusion implants from various vendors and different spine levels. Eur Radiol 2012;22:2357–64.

42. Jia Y, Zhang J, Fan J, et al. Gemstone spectral imaging reduced artefacts from metal coils or clips after treatment of cerebral aneurysms: a retrospective study of 35 patients. Br J Radiol 2015;88:20150222.

43. Grams AE, Sender J, Moritz R, et al. Dual energy CT myelography after lumbar osteosynthesis. Rofo 2014;186:670–4.

44. Srinivasan A, Hoeffner E, Ibrahim M, et al. Utility of dual-energy CT virtual keV monochromatic series for the assessment of spinal transpedicular hardware-bone interface. AJR Am J Roentgenol 2013;201:878–83.

45. Lambert JW, Edic PM, FitzGerald PF, et al. Complementary contrast media for metal artifact reduction in dual-energy computed tomography. J Med Imaging (Bellingham) 2015;2:033503.

46. Lovett JK, Gallagher PJ, Hands LJ, et al. Histological correlates of carotid plaque surface morphology on lumen contrast imaging. Circulation 2004;110:2190–7.

47. Ballotta E, Da Giau G, Renon L. Carotid plaque gross morphology and clinical presentation: a prospective study of 457 carotid artery specimens. J Surg Res 2000;89:78–84.

48. Kamalian S, Kamalian S, Pomerantz SR, et al. Role of cardiac and extracranial vascular CT in the evaluation/management of cerebral ischemia and stroke. Emerg Radiol 2013;20:417–28.

49. Hsu CC, Kwan GN, Singh D, et al. Principles and clinical application of dual-energy computed tomography in the evaluation of cerebrovascular disease. J Clin Imaging Sci 2016;6:27.

50. de Weert TT, Ouhlous M, Meijering E, et al. In vivo characterization and quantification of atherosclerotic carotid plaque components with multidetector computed tomography and histopathological correlation. Arterioscler Thromb Vasc Biol 2006;26:2366–72.

51. Wintermark M, Jawadi SS, Rapp JH, et al. High-resolution CT imaging of carotid artery atherosclerotic plaques. AJNR Am J Neuroradiol 2008;29:875–82.

52. Saba L, Anzidei M, Marincola BC, et al. Imaging of the carotid artery vulnerable plaque. Cardiovasc Intervent Radiol 2014;37:572–85.

53. Obaid DR, Calvert PA, Gopalan D, et al. Dual-energy computed tomography imaging to determine atherosclerotic plaque composition: a prospective study with tissue validation. J Cardiovasc Comput Tomogr 2014;8:230–7.

54. Das M, Braunschweig T, Muhlenbruch G, et al. Carotid plaque analysis: comparison of dual-source computed tomography (CT) findings and histopathological correlation. Eur J Vasc Endovasc Surg 2009;38:14–9.

55. Shinohara Y, Sakamoto M, Kuya K, et al. Assessment of carotid plaque composition using fast-kV switching dual-energy CT with gemstone detector: comparison with extracorporeal and virtual histology-intravascular ultrasound. Neuroradiology 2015;57:889–95.

56. Mokin M, Kan P, Kass-Hout T, et al. Intracerebral hemorrhage secondary to intravenous and endovascular intraarterial revascularization therapies in acute ischemic stroke: an update on risk factors, predictors, and management. Neurosurg Focus 2012;32:E2.

57. Fiorelli M, Bastianello S, von Kummer R, et al. Hemorrhagic transformation within 36 hours of a cerebral infarct: relationships with early clinical deterioration and 3-month outcome in the European Cooperative Acute Stroke Study I (ECASS I) cohort. Stroke 1999;30:2280–4.

58. Jang YM, Lee DH, Kim HS, et al. The fate of high-density lesions on the non-contrast CT obtained immediately after intra-arterial thrombolysis in ischemic stroke patients. Korean J Radiol 2006;7:221–8.

59. Nakano S, Iseda T, Kawano H, et al. Parenchymal hyperdensity on computed tomography after intra-arterial reperfusion therapy for acute middle cerebral artery occlusion: incidence and clinical significance. Stroke 2001;32:2042–8.

60. Macdougall NJ, McVerry F, Baird S, et al. Iodinated contrast media and cerebral hemorrhage after intravenous thrombolysis. Stroke 2011;42:2170–4.

61. Kim JT, Heo SH, Cho BH, et al. Hyperdensity on noncontrast CT immediately after intra-arterial revascularization. J Neurol 2012;259:936–43.

62. Payabvash S, Qureshi MH, Khan SM, et al. Differentiating intraparenchymal hemorrhage from contrast extravasation on post-procedural noncontrast CT scan in acute ischemic stroke patients undergoing endovascular treatment. Neuroradiology 2014;56:737–44.

63. Gupta R, Phan CM, Leidecker C, et al. Evaluation of dual-energy CT for differentiating intracerebral hemorrhage from iodinated contrast material staining. Radiology 2010;257:205–11.

64. Phan CM, Yoo AJ, Hirsch JA, et al. Differentiation of hemorrhage from iodinated contrast in different intracranial compartments using dual-energy head CT. AJNR Am J Neuroradiol 2012;33:1088–94.

65. Morhard D, Ertl L, Gerdsmeier-Petz W, et al. Dual-energy CT immediately after endovascular stroke intervention: prognostic implications. Cardiovasc Intervent Radiol 2014;37:1171–8.

66. Tijssen MP, Hofman PA, Stadler AA, et al. The role of dual energy CT in differentiating between brain haemorrhage and contrast medium after mechanical revascularisation in acute ischaemic stroke. Eur Radiol 2014;24:834–40.

67. Dinkel J, Khalilzadeh O, Phan CM, et al. Technical limitations of dual-energy CT in neuroradiology: 30-month institutional experience and review of literature. J Neurointerv Surg 2015;7:596–602.

68. Brouwers HB, Greenberg SM. Hematoma expansion following acute intracerebral hemorrhage. Cerebrovasc Dis 2013;35:195–201.

69. Huynh TJ, Aviv RI, Dowlatshahi D, et al. Validation of the 9-point and 24-point hematoma expansion prediction scores and derivation of the predict a/b scores. Stroke 2015;46:3105–10.

70. Sun SJ, Gao PY, Sui BB, et al. "Dynamic spot sign" on CT perfusion source images predicts haematoma expansion in acute intracerebral haemorrhage. Eur Radiol 2013;23:1846–54.

71. Wada R, Aviv RI, Fox AJ, et al. CT angiography "spot sign" predicts hematoma expansion in acute intracerebral hemorrhage. Stroke 2007;38:1257–62.

72. Del Giudice A, D'Amico D, Sobesky J, et al. Accuracy of the spot sign on computed tomography angiography as a predictor of haematoma enlargement after acute spontaneous intracerebral haemorrhage: a systematic review. Cerebrovasc Dis 2014;37:268–76.

73. Park SY, Kong MH, Kim JH, et al. Role of 'spot sign' on CT angiography to predict hematoma expansion in spontaneous intracerebral hemorrhage. J Korean Neurosurg Soc 2010;48:399–405.

74. Hallevi H, Abraham AT, Barreto AD, et al. The spot sign in intracerebral hemorrhage: the importance of looking for contrast extravasation. Cerebrovasc Dis 2010;29:217–20.

75. Hu R, Daftari Besheli L, Young J, et al. Dual-energy head CT enables accurate distinction of intraparenchymal hemorrhage from calcification in emergency department patients. Radiology 2016;280:177–83.

76. Brouwers HB, Goldstein JN, Romero JM, et al. Clinical applications of the computed tomography angiography spot sign in acute intracerebral hemorrhage: a review. Stroke 2012;43:3427–32.

77. Delgado Almandoz JE, Yoo AJ, Stone MJ, et al. Systematic characterization of the computed tomography angiography spot sign in primary intracerebral hemorrhage identifies patients at highest risk for hematoma expansion: the spot sign score. Stroke 2009;40:2994–3000.

78. Watanabe Y, Tsukabe A, Kunitomi Y, et al. Dual-energy CT for detection of contrast enhancement or leakage within high-density haematomas in patients with intracranial haemorrhage. Neuroradiology 2014;56:291–5.

79. Gazzola S, Aviv RI, Gladstone DJ, et al. Vascular and nonvascular mimics of the CT angiography "spot sign" in patients with secondary intracerebral hemorrhage. Stroke 2008;39:1177–83.

80. Kim SJ, Lim HK, Lee HY, et al. Dual-energy CT in the evaluation of intracerebral hemorrhage of unknown origin: differentiation between tumor bleeding and pure hemorrhage. AJNR Am J Neuroradiol 2012;33:865–72.

81. Ferda J, Novak M, Mirka H, et al. The assessment of intracranial bleeding with virtual unenhanced imaging by means of dual-energy CT angiography. Eur Radiol 2009;19:2518–22.

82. Jiang XY, Zhang SH, Xie QZ, et al. Evaluation of virtual noncontrast images obtained from dual-energy CTA for diagnosing subarachnoid hemorrhage. AJNR Am J Neuroradiol 2015;36:855–60.

Applications of Dual-Energy Computed Tomography for the Evaluation of Head and Neck Squamous Cell Carcinoma

Reza Forghani, MD, PhD[a],*, Hillary R. Kelly, MD[b],
Hugh D. Curtin, MD[c]

KEYWORDS

- Dual-energy CT • Head and neck squamous cell carcinoma • Thyroid cartilage invasion
- Lymphadenopathy • Dental artifact • Virtual monochromatic images
- Material decomposition iodine maps • Spectral Hounsfield unit attenuation curves

KEY POINTS

- There is increasing evidence that supplementary DECT reconstructions can improve diagnostic evaluation of head and neck cancer compared with conventional single-energy CT.
- Low-energy virtual monochromatic images or altered blending of weighted average images can improve visualization of tumors and their boundaries.
- High-energy virtual monochromatic images and iodine maps may improve accuracy for evaluation of thyroid cartilage invasion.
- Additional potential DECT applications are emerging for dental artifact reduction and evaluation of lymphadenopathy.
- A multiparametric strategy using a combination of various reconstructed image sets seems to be the optimal DECT approach for head and neck cancer evaluation.

INTRODUCTION

Since its introduction into clinical practice, there have been ongoing technical improvements in dual-energy computed tomography (DECT) systems and an increase in the availability of these scanners. This in turn has led to an increase in the use of DECT in the clinical setting, with emergence of an increasing number of applications in neuroimaging and head and neck imaging. This article reviews DECT applications for the diagnostic evaluation of head and neck cancer, focusing on head and neck squamous cell carcinoma (HNSCC). The evidence for optimal

Disclosures: R. Forghani has acted as a consultant for GE Healthcare and has served as a speaker at lunch and learn sessions titled "Dual-Energy CT Applications in Neuroradiology and Head and Neck Imaging" sponsored by GE Healthcare at the 27th and 28th Annual Meetings of the Eastern Neuroradiological Society in 2015 and 2016 (no personal compensation or travel support for these sessions).
[a] Department of Radiology, Segal Cancer Centre and Lady Davis Institute for Medical Research, Jewish General Hospital, McGill University, Room C-212.1, 3755 Cote Sainte-Catherine Road, Montreal, Quebec H3T 1E2, Canada; [b] Departments of Radiology, Massachusetts General Hospital and Massachusetts Eye and Ear Infirmary, Harvard Medical School, 55 Fruit Street, GRB-273A, Boston, MA 02114, USA; [c] Department of Radiology, Massachusetts Eye and Ear Infirmary, Harvard Medical School, 243 Charles Street, Boston, MA 02114, USA
* Corresponding author.
E-mail address: rforghani@jgh.mcgill.ca

Neuroimag Clin N Am 27 (2017) 445–459
http://dx.doi.org/10.1016/j.nic.2017.04.001

reconstructions for routine evaluation of the neck, visualization of the tumor and its boundaries, and critical structure invasion (eg, invasion of the thyroid cartilage) are reviewed. This is followed by a brief review of other emerging applications that may be relevant for head and neck cancer evaluation, such as dental artifact reduction and evaluation of lymphadenopathy. The article concludes with a summary of current evidence, including potentially useful DECT reconstructions using a multiparametric approach for head and neck cancer evaluation, and areas of interest for future research.

BASIC PRINCIPLES UNDERLYING DUAL-ENERGY COMPUTED TOMOGRAPHY MATERIAL CHARACTERIZATION

The fundamentals underlying DECT, including the technical details of different systems and approaches used, are discussed in detail elsewhere in this issue and are only briefly reviewed here. Attenuation on clinical CT scanning is based on three physical processes. Compton scatter typically accounts for the greatest attenuation. However, the Compton effect is nearly independent of photon energy.[1] The other important physical process accounting for CT attenuation, the photoelectric effect, is strongly energy dependent and key for material characterization using DECT. The third physical process, Rayleigh (or coherent) scatter, accounts for a small percentage of CT attenuation and is generally considered negligible.

The photoelectric effect refers to the ejection of an electron from the innermost shell (K-shell) of an atom by an incident photon.[2] For an electron to be ejected, the incident photon must have a minimum energy, equal to the binding energy of the electron to its shell. In addition, the probability of photoelectric interactions (and therefore the degree of attenuation of the photon beam from this process) is greatest when the incident photon energy is equal to or just higher than the binding energy of a K-shell electron. The energy at which this sharp increase or spike in the attenuation coefficient of photons occurs is represented by the K-edge of a given material or element, followed by a rapid drop in attenuation with further increases in photon energy. Understanding this concept is essential for understanding the behavior of elements with spectral CT.

The other essential concept is that the photoelectric effect is strongly dependent on the atomic number (Z) of the tissue elements, which represents the number of protons within their atomic nucleus.[3,4] The probability of the photoelectric effect is approximately proportional to the third power of the atomic number (Z) of the element.[4] Therefore, elements with a high atomic number (Z) have strong spectral effects, meaning that they demonstrate large differences in attenuation at different photon energies, and are good candidates for evaluation and characterization using DECT. Elements with a small atomic number (Z), however, are not good candidates for characterization based on their energy-dependent (or "spectral") properties because they have small differences in attenuation at different X-ray energies.[4] For example, common elements found in the human body, such as hydrogen (Z = 1), carbon (Z = 6), nitrogen (Z = 7), and oxygen (Z = 8), have low atomic numbers and only small differences between their atomic numbers. These would not be expected to have sufficient energy-dependent differences to enable reliable differentiation based on their spectral properties.[4,5]

However, elements with high atomic numbers and significant differences between their atomic numbers are amenable to spectral characterization using DECT. One that is particularly relevant to CT scanning is iodine, the main constituent of most CT contrast agents used clinically. Iodine has a high atomic number (Z = 53) and strong energy-dependent (spectral) properties (**Fig. 1**) that can be exploited for the evaluation of iodine-containing and/or enhancing structures on DECT. Calcium (Z = 20) is another element found in the human body that has a high atomic number and good spectral properties. If there is sufficient difference in the Z and K-edge of two materials, DECT can be used to separately identify and differentiate between them based on the differences in their attenuation at various energies.

OVERVIEW OF DUAL-ENERGY COMPUTED TOMOGRAPHY RECONSTRUCTIONS AND OPTIMAL RECONSTRUCTIONS FOR ROUTINE EVALUATION OF THE NECK

With DECT, the data from the low- and high-energy acquisitions are combined in a variety of ways to produce images for routine interpretation or advanced material (or tissue) characterization. In broad terms, the most common types of reconstructions generated using DECT are virtual monochromatic images (VMIs), weighted average (WA) or blended images (for acquisitions using dual-source scanners), and material decomposition maps (**Box 1**).[4,6–11] With modern DECT scanners, scans are obtained at an acceptable dose similar to single-energy CT (SECT), while maintaining or even improving image quality.[12–17]

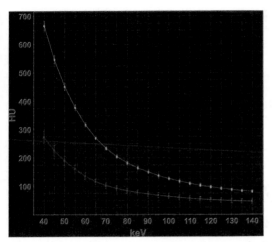

Fig. 1. Energy-dependent/spectral properties of iodine in CT contrast agents. Spectral Hounsfield unit attenuation curves derived from region of interest analysis of two solutions with different concentrations of iodine, imaged within a phantom, are shown. There is a progressive increase in attenuation at lower energies approaching the K-edge of iodine (33.2 keV). For example, note the much higher attenuation at 40 keV compared with conventional single-energy CT equivalent virtual monochromatic image energies at 65 or 70 keV. The trade-off is the increasing image noise at lower energies, as represented by the error bars depicting standard deviation of attenuation within the region of interest evaluated. The scan was acquired with a fast kVp switching scanner.

Therefore, the additional reconstructions, postprocessing, and quantitative capabilities made possible with DECT have the potential to produce clinically useful information beyond what is achievable with SECT, without impacting patient dose.

Box 1

Common DECT reconstructions

- Virtual monochromatic images are images at prescribed or predicted energy levels that are reconstructed using the data from the different energy acquisitions, that is, what the image would look like if the study was acquired with a monochromatic beam at a given energy.

- Weighted average or blended images are reconstructed by blending of data from the low and high energy acquisitions from dual-source scanners.

- Basis material decomposition maps display the estimated distribution and quantity of a material of interest based on its elemental composition and unique spectral characteristics. One example is an iodine map.

Virtual Monochromatic Images

VMIs are reconstructed using sophisticated software and algorithms. With these reconstructions, the data from the different energy acquisitions are combined to generate images at distinct prescribed or predicted energy levels, that is, what the image would look like if the study was acquired with a monochromatic beam at a given energy (**Fig. 2**A, B). Typical VMIs that are generated with current DECT systems range between 40 and 140 keV, but VMIs may be reconstructed at even higher energies with some systems.[18]

Based on data extrapolated from phantom studies and body imaging, the 70-keV VMIs are generally considered equivalent to the standard 120-kVp SECT acquisition and are frequently the default setting for routine reconstructions on some DECT systems, such as fast kVp switching scanners.[16,19,20] In one study, the optimal VMIs for the evaluation of the neck were directly evaluated using a fast kVp switching scanner.[21] This study evaluated the signal-to-noise ratio (SNR) of different tissues and pathologic lesions in the neck as a measure of overall image quality. The SNR was determined using regions of interest (ROIs) in normal muscles, normal glandular tissue, HNSCC, and metastatic lymph nodes. The highest SNR in the soft tissue discrimination range was consistently at 65 keV, closely matched by that of VMIs at 70 or 60 keV.[21]

Similar SNR trends were observed when enhancing tumor in patients with HNSCC was evaluated in a subsequent study with a larger number of patients (60) from two different institutions.[17] In the same study, on subjective evaluation of the neck CTs that included VMI reconstructions at 40, 50, 60, and 65 keV, the 60- and 65-keV VMIs were found to be the most visually appealing and least noisy VMIs, corroborating the quantitative SNR results. Therefore, at least at one of the authors' institutions, 65-keV VMIs are generated for every DECT scan for routine clinical interpretation (see **Fig. 2**A). However, the SNRs for the 70-keV VMIs are close to that of 65-keV VMIs and the 70-keV reconstructions are likely an acceptable alternative (**Box 2**). The 65- or 70-keV VMIs can then be supplemented with VMIs at other energies for specific clinical applications,[9,10,17,18,21–25] as discussed later in this article.

Weighted Average Images

Another type of reconstruction routinely created when using dual-source DECT scanners are the WA or blended images. Typically, a linear blend consisting of 30% of the low and 70% of the high-energy acquisitions is considered equivalent to

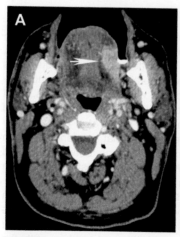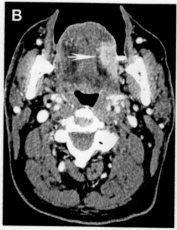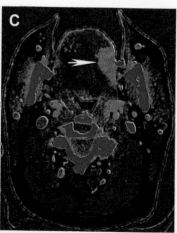

Fig. 2. Examples of different DECT reconstructions are shown from a contrast-enhanced neck CT of a patient with a left oral tongue cancer (*arrow*). (*A*) 65-keV VMI (typically considered equivalent to a 120-kVp single-energy CT acquisition), (*B*) 40-keV VMI, and (*C*) iodine-water map are shown. Note the increase in tumor attenuation and contrast/tumor boundary on the low-energy (40 keV) VMI compared with the 65-keV VMI. The iodine-water map represents the iodine distribution and iodine content in different voxels and is used to estimate iodine concentration within tissues. The scan was acquired with a fast kVp switching scanner.

the standard 120-kVp SECT acquisition and is the default reconstruction generated by many of the earlier versions of these scanners for routine clinical interpretation (see **Box 2**).[13,24,26,27] However, it should be noted that some of the new platforms being introduced also enable automatic reconstruction of VMIs from dual-source scanners. Just as with VMIs, the proportion of the low- and high-energy data that are blended and the ways in which they are blended (eg, linear vs nonlinear) can be altered to accentuate different materials or tissue characteristics of potential clinical interest.[27,28]

Material Decomposition Maps

In SECT, mixtures of various elements or materials can be represented by the same (or similar) HU, in some instances making characterization and differentiation of distinct types of tissues challenging. In DECT, having two measurements of attenuation obtained with two different X-ray spectra allows not only for differentiation of different materials,

but also enables estimation of the quantity or concentration of elements in a material based on the energy-dependent attenuation characteristics of known elements. The ability of DECT to separate (or decompose) a material into its basic elements is known as basis material decomposition.[4,7,11]

The algorithms for material decomposition can mathematically convert attenuation data at the different energies into estimates of the concentrations of two-material pairs of interest that would be necessary to produce the measured attenuation within each voxel, based on their specific energy-dependent attenuation characteristics. Image pairs can then be generated that display the distribution or content of one of the specified materials. For example, two-material decomposition of iodine and water is used to generate "iodine maps," displaying and providing an estimate of the quantity of iodine within each voxel. Iodine maps (**Fig. 2**C) are of particular interest for the evaluation of HNSCC, because they can potentially make enhancing tumor easier to identify and differentiate it from adjacent normal tissues.

DUAL-ENERGY COMPUTED TOMOGRAPHY APPLICATIONS FOR THE EVALUATION OF HEAD AND NECK SQUAMOUS CELL CARCINOMA

In the previous section, the different types of DECT reconstructions and reconstructions typically considered equivalent to the standard 120-kVp acquisition were reviewed (see **Box 2**). These reconstructions are important and in the opinion of the authors, should be generated for every DECT neck scan. However, other DECT reconstructions can provide complementary or supplementary information and may be useful for specific applications, such as increasing tumor visibility, soft tissue contrast, and helping distinguish tumor from nonossified thyroid cartilage.

Differences in iodine attenuation observed at different energies (see **Fig. 1**; **Fig. 3**) are exploited to visually accentuate the differences between materials or tissues of interest, such as tumor and normal adjacent structures.[21,22,29,30] Many supplementary DECT reconstructions can be generated using this concept, potentially improving diagnostic evaluation of HNSCC. In the review of the potential applications that follows, one should keep in mind that most of the published studies in the peer reviewed literature on DECT applications for HNSCC evaluation were performed using either a fast kVp switching scanner or one of the many generations of dual-source CT scanners. Therefore, this review predominantly covers studies based on those two scanner types. Because the fundamental principles underlying DECT are the same, it is likely that the observations from these studies can be extrapolated to other scanner systems in one way or another. However, because there are significant technical differences between different DECT systems, any cross-platform application requires validation and is likely to require some degree of fine tuning to obtain the expected and optimal results.

Tumor Visibility and Soft Tissue Contrast

One of the most fundamental roles of imaging for the evaluation of head and neck cancer is accurate determination of tumor extent. This is essential for appropriate staging of the cancer, which in turn guides the optimal treatment approach. CT scans of the neck performed for the evaluation of patients with head and neck cancer are almost always performed after administration of intravenous iodinated contrast agents, unless contraindicated. Contrast administration improves anatomic discrimination of tumor from normal tissues, including critical vascular structures. Tumor visualization and boundary discrimination on contrast-enhanced CT is primarily based on its differential vascularity and architecture compared with normal tissues. However, tumor attenuation can be similar to muscle, and the boundary between the tumor and surrounding soft tissues may not always be clearly defined.

Several studies have reported that VMIs reconstructed at energies lower than the standard 65- or 70-keV VMI can improve tumor visibility and discrimination of tumor-muscle interface using either a fast kVp switching system or a dual-source system. The basis for these studies is the strong spectral properties of iodine, its K-edge of 33.2 keV, and the differences in energy-dependent attenuation characteristics of different elements or tissues, as discussed previously (see **Figs. 1** and **3**; **Fig. 4**).[17,21,24,25] There

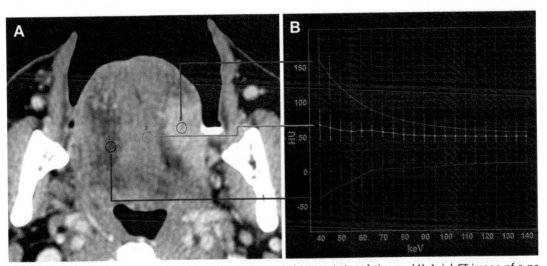

Fig. 3. Example of differential energy-dependent/spectral characteristics of tissues. (*A*) Axial CT image of a patient with a left oral tongue cancer (same patient as in **Fig. 2**) shows ROI analysis of different tissues: tumor (*purple*), normal tongue muscle (*green*), and a more fatty part of the tongue (*blue*). (*B*) Spectral Hounsfield unit attenuation curves from the ROI analysis in *A* are shown. Note the differences in energy-dependent attenuation of the different tissues, with increased separation of the curves at low energies. These differences in tissue attenuation form the basis for the use of low-energy virtual monochromatic images for increasing tumor visibility and improving boundary discrimination.

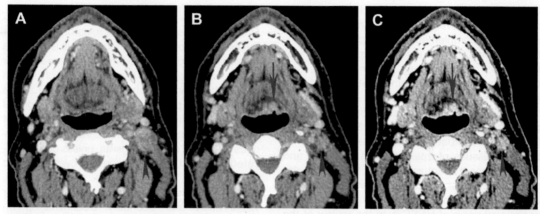

Fig. 4. Use of low-energy VMIs for the evaluation of HNSCC. (*A, B*) 65-keV (typically considered equivalent to a 120-kVp single-energy CT acquisition) and (*C*) 40-keV VMIs are shown from a patient presenting with left level II lymphadenopathy (*arrowhead*). Note the improved visibility of the primary tumor (*arrow*) and its boundary on the 40-keV VMI (*C*) compared with the 65-keV VMI at the same level (*B*). The scan was acquired with a fast kVp switching scanner.

is a substantial and progressive increase in the attenuation of enhancing tumor on VMIs approaching the K-edge of iodine (see **Figs. 2, 3** and **4**). However, lower energy VMIs also have greater image noise, as would be expected for a lower energy "beam," representing a trade-off. Multiple studies have evaluated the potential use of low-energy VMIs and this trade-off for the evaluation of HNSCC.[21,24,25]

In the study discussed previously that evaluated the optimal VMIs for the evaluation of the neck, the optimal VMIs for tumor assessment were also investigated.[21] In addition to the SNR, the investigators compared pooled spectral Hounsfield unit attenuation curves of tumor with that of normal muscle, and calculated the contrast-to-noise ratio (CNR) as a quantitative measure of tumor–soft tissue contrast. Muscle was selected because it is one of the normal soft tissue structures that can have attenuation similar to tumor, occasionally making determination of tumor boundary challenging. Similar to the example in **Fig. 3**, although the average attenuation of tumor and muscle progressively increased on lower-energy VMIs secondary to their iodine content, there was progressive spectral separation between the curves on low-energy VMIs, with the greatest difference in attenuation seen at 40 keV. When the CNR was calculated (to take into account image noise), the greatest CNR was also at 40 keV. The investigators concluded that 40-keV VMIs can improve visualization of HNSCC and tumor boundary compared with the SECT equivalent VMIs at 65 or 70 keV.[21] It was suggested that low-energy VMIs might represent a useful reconstruction to complement the high SNR SECT equivalent 65- or 70-keV VMIs for tumor evaluation.[21]

In a subsequent larger study using data from two institutions (also using a fast kVp switching scanner), similar trends were seen, with the highest attenuation difference between tumor and muscle at 40 keV.[17] The latter study also performed an extensive subjective evaluation, comparing 40-, 50-, 60-, and 65-keV VMIs. Radiologists specialized in head and neck radiology and radiologists without subspecialty expertise in head and neck or neuroradiology performed the subjective evaluation. When surveyed on image quality overall, the radiologists consistently ranked the 60- or 65-keV VMIs the highest and preferred these by far over 50- or 40-keV VMIs. However, when the radiologists were asked specifically regarding tumor conspicuity or boundary visualization, regardless of overall image quality, the 40-keV VMIs were the most frequently selected images.[17] Likewise, when asked to select the one reconstruction most useful for tumor assessment, the 40-keV VMIs were by far the favored reconstructions. This was concordant with the quantitative results and suggested that these could be acceptable for clinical use. It is noteworthy that both studies included cases of primary tumors and recurrent cancers.[17,21] Furthermore, another study also found that 40-keV VMIs (and tumor iodine content on iodine maps) could improve distinction of primary or recurrent tumor from benign posttreatment changes.[31] As such, these results should be applicable to the initial pretreatment scan and posttreatment surveillance studies.

Although the previously mentioned results support the use of low-energy VMIs and favor the 40-keV VMIs for tumor visibility and soft tissue boundary evaluation (see **Figs. 2–4**), not all studies agree on the exact VMI energy considered optimal for tumor evaluation. In one study performed using a dual-source scanner, 40-, 60-, 80-, and 100-keV VMIs were reconstructed and compared with each other, and with standard WA images considered equivalent to SECT.[24] Similar to these studies, tumors were found to have the highest attenuation on 40-keV VMIs. However, the CNR was reported to be highest at 60 keV and the same energy VMIs were found to have the highest subjective overall image quality and provide the best tumor delineation.[24] Only four VMI energies were evaluated in this study and other VMI energies between 40 and 60 keV were not evaluated. The reason for the discrepancy between the two studies is not clear. One possibility is that it is related to technical differences, because different DECT systems were used. However, there were also differences in patient dose between the two studies. Although the scan coverage may not have been the same (which could have contributed to the difference), the former studies using a fast kVp switching scanner reported average CTDIvol of 17.3 mGy or more, whereas the study using a dual-source DECT reported an average CTDIvol of 9.96 mGy. It is possible that the difference in dose could have tipped the balance on the 40-keV VMIs and because the next lowest VMI energy used was at 60 keV, it is not possible to determine whether an energy in between would have represented a more suitable alternative.

A subsequent report also using a dual-source scanner by the same group found that if an advanced form of VMI is reconstructed, the quantitative tumor CNR was actually highest at 40 keV.[25] These advanced monoenergetic reconstructions or "Mono+" VMIs were generated by combining the high signal data at low energies with the superior noise properties at medium energies. However, on subjective evaluation, the 55-keV images were overall preferred on that study.[25] There is no clear explanation for the discrepancy between the objective and subjective analysis on this study.

Although many studies have focused on the use of VMIs to enhance tumor visibility, alterations in WA images using dual-source CT systems can also be made for this purpose. In one study, it was reported that HNSCC was best seen when a blend of 60% of the low-energy spectra and 40% of high-energy spectra are used (instead of the standard 30%–70% blend simulating the standard SECT acquisition).[27] The concept is in some ways similar to using low-energy VMIs, by using a greater portion of the low-energy spectra to improve tumor visualization. Yet another study found that nonlinear blending methods could improve tumor visualization on WA average images.[28]

For obvious practical reasons, most studies evaluating tumor visibility compare different reconstructions of interest to SECT equivalent images derived from the same DECT acquisition, such as the 65- or 70-keV VMIs or the 30% and 70% low/high-energy spectra blending for WA average images.[21,24,25,27,28] It would not be ethically acceptable to perform two separate back to back acquisitions on a patient to provide a true DECT-SECT comparison, and the former approach increases the statistical power of the study because all other variables are controlled for each case (ie, comparison at the different energy reconstructions is made for the same tumor and identical ROIs). The approach of comparing special DECT reconstructions with the SECT equivalent reconstructions generated from the same DECT acquisition is common and sound, given that several studies have independently evaluated the VMIs or WA DECT images that can be used as a substitute for the standard 120-kVp SECT acquisition.[13,16,19,20,26] However, at least one study compared low-energy VMIs directly with SECT acquisitions. This study compared 40-keV VMIs generated from 60 DECT cases with 60 true SECT acquisitions and again found that quantitatively, tumor attenuation and tumor-muscle attenuation difference were significantly higher on 40-keV compared with true SECT images (in addition to SECT equivalent DECT images).[17] This study also did not find a significant difference in the average tumor attenuation on 65- or 70-keV DECT images and true SECT images.[17] These results further support the extrapolation and use of SECT equivalent images acquired from a DECT acquisition as representative of a true SECT acquisition.

Overall, there are multiple independent studies suggesting that low-energy VMIs lower than the usual standard reconstructions at 65 or 70 keV improve tumor visibility and contour delineation (see **Figs. 2** and **4**). There is, however, no absolute consensus on the exact optimal energy for these VMIs, as discussed extensively previously. As is frequently the case in medicine, it is likely that multiple approaches are valid. There is likely some leeway in the exact reconstruction energy used based on the exact technique and acquisition dose, the scanner system used, and radiologist preference. In at least one of the authors' institutions, 40-keV VMIs are routinely generated for interpretation. However, 45- or 50-keV VMIs are likely acceptable alternatives, partly depending on the acquisition technique. It is also likely that a period of adjustment or familiarization is necessary on the part of the interpreting radiologist, because these VMIs are noisier than the typical SECT acquisition. One should note that the 40-keV VMIs may work best for the mid to upper neck, because the noise on these images may be prohibitive for the artifact-prone areas of the lower neck and thoracic inlet. For those areas, one can use either slightly higher energies or rely on the standard 65- or 70-keV acquisition for interpretation.

Evaluation of Thyroid Cartilage and Cartilage Invasion

Beyond improving tumor visualization and soft tissue boundary discrimination, a few studies also suggest that DECT could improve accuracy for the evaluation of thyroid cartilage and distinction from tumor (Figs. 5–7). In one study, the use of iodine overlay maps was investigated.[32] The authors reported that addition of iodine overlay maps (see Figs. 6 and 7) to the standard WA images generated using a dual-source scanner increased sensitivity for detection of thyroid cartilage invasion without compromising specificity. The addition of iodine maps also reduced interrater variability.

Another study compared the spectral Hounsfield attenuation curves of tumor with nonossified cartilage.[22] The pattern of ossification of the thyroid cartilage is unpredictable and varies widely from

patient to patient. Furthermore, nonossified thyroid cartilage can have attenuation similar to tumor on conventional SECT. Therefore, in the absence of prior CT imaging for comparison, it is difficult to differentiate nonossified cartilage from cartilage that was previously ossified but is now invaded by tumor. Interpretation is particularly challenging in cases where tumor abuts a focal patch of nonossification, mimicking invasion by tumor. In this study, the investigators demonstrated that nonossified thyroid cartilage has different spectral Hounsfield unit attenuation characteristics compared with HNSCC (see Figs. 5–7).[22] In particular, on high-energy VMIs, there is relative preservation of attenuation of the cartilage but relative decrease (or "suppression") of tumor attenuation as the reconstruction energy moves further away from the K-edge of iodine (see Figs. 5–7). Among the 30 patients with HNSCC evaluated in this study, there was no overlap between tumor and cartilage attenuation at VMI energies equal to or higher than 95 keV.[22] Even though the study did not directly evaluate thyroid cartilage invasion, the results suggest that high-energy reconstructions at 95 keV or higher are useful for the evaluation of thyroid cartilage invasion (see Figs. 5–7). Additional studies directly evaluating cartilage invasion and comparing high-energy VMIs with iodine maps in

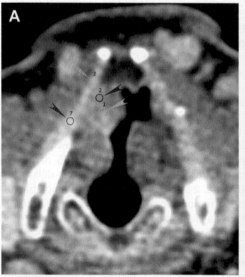
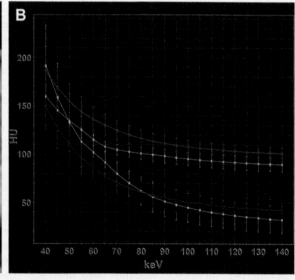

Fig. 5. Example of differential energy-dependent/spectral characteristics of nonossified thyroid cartilage (NOTC) compared with tumor. (*A*) Axial 65-keV CT image of a patient with a supraglottic tumor shows ROI analysis of NOTC (*pink/purple*) and tumor (different shades of *blue*). *Arrowheads* have been placed to help with the visualization of the ROIs. (*B*) Spectral Hounsfield unit attenuation curves from the ROI analysis in *A* are shown. Whereas the attenuation of NOTC and tumor closely overlap at 65 keV, there is increased separation of the curves in the high-energy range caused by progressive suppression of iodine within enhancing tumor but relative preservation of the intrinsic high attenuation of NOTC at higher energies. These differences suggest that high-energy virtual monochromatic images may be useful for distinguishing NOTC from tumor. The scan was acquired with a fast kVp switching scanner.

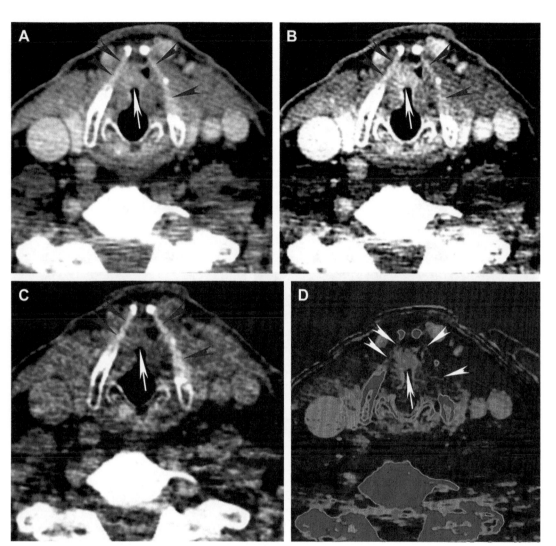

Fig. 6. Use of high-energy VMIs and iodine maps for distinction of nonossified thyroid cartilage (NOTC; *arrowheads*) from HNSCC (*arrow*). (*A*) 65-keV VMI (typically considered equivalent to a 120-kVp single-energy CT acquisition), (*B*) 40-keV VMI, (*C*) 140-keV VMI, and (*D*) iodine (iodine-water) map are shown from a patient with laryngeal HNSCC. There is partial ossification of the thyroid cartilage. Note the similarity in attenuation of normal NOTC to tumor on the 65 and 40 keV in this case (*A, B*). However, on the 140-keV VMI, there is relative preservation of high attenuation of NOTC but relative suppression of iodine within tumor, enabling much better distinction of NOTC from tumor (*C*). The iodine map provides a quantitative map of iodine distribution and relative iodine content within tissues, with higher iodine content of tumor compared with nearby normal soft tissues (*D*). There is no evidence of significant extension of tumor iodine "signal" into the NOTC (*D*). The scan was acquired with a fast kVp switching scanner.

terms of their utility and complementarity are interesting topics for future research.

Other Potential and Emerging Dual-Energy Computed Tomography Applications for the Evaluation of Head and Neck Squamous Cell Carcinoma

The use of DECT for artifact reduction and the evaluation of lymphadenopathy are discussed in detail in separate articles in this issue and therefore are only briefly discussed here in the context of HNSCC. Several studies have shown that at energies higher than the standard SECT equivalent VMIs, there is reduction of artifact associated with metal prostheses and dental materials (**Figs. 8** and **9**).[18,23,33–37] Substantial metal or dental artifact reduction has been reported in multiple studies on VMIs at 88 keV or higher energies.[18,23,33–37] However, just as with

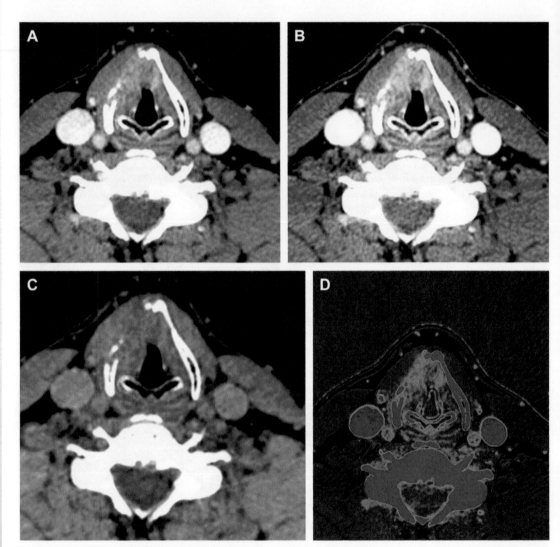

Fig. 7. Use of different DECT reconstructions for evaluation of thyroid cartilage invasion. (*A*) 65-keV VMI (typically considered equivalent to a 120-kVp single-energy CT acquisition), (*B*) 40-keV VMI, (*C*) 140-keV VMI, and (*D*) iodine (iodine-water) map are shown from a patient with laryngeal HNSCC invading the thyroid cartilage. There is an increase in tumor attenuation on the 40-keV VMI (*B*) compared with the 65-keV VMI (*A*). Conversely, there is suppression of iodine attenuation on the high-energy 140-keV VMI and the invaded portion of the thyroid cartilage appears as a relative low-attenuation defect on high-energy VMIs (*C*). This is in contradistinction to normal variants, such as nonossified thyroid cartilage, which would be expected to retain a high attenuation on high-energy VMIs (see **Fig. 6**C). The iodine map (*D*) provides a quantitative map of iodine distribution and relative iodine content within tissues, with higher iodine content of tumor compared with normal nearby soft tissues. Note the extension of iodine-containing tumor into the thyroid cartilage on the iodine map, extending through the outer cortex on the right (*D*). The scan was acquired with a fast kVp switching scanner.

low-energy VMIs, there are also trade-offs with high-energy VMIs, including suppression of iodine attenuation and a decrease in overall soft tissue contrast.

In the case of structures with high intrinsic density independent of enhancement, such as bone, the previously mentioned trade-offs may not represent a significant barrier and if the objective is to evaluate bone or bone integrity, VMIs at the

extreme of the high-energy range may be used for significant artifact reduction (see **Fig. 8**). However, if the purpose is to improve visualization of tumor obscured by artifact, such as in the oral cavity or the oropharynx, then the extremes of high-energy range may not be optimal.[38] Although these very-high-energy VMIs may result in the greatest artifact reduction, the tumor itself may no longer be clearly visible because of marked

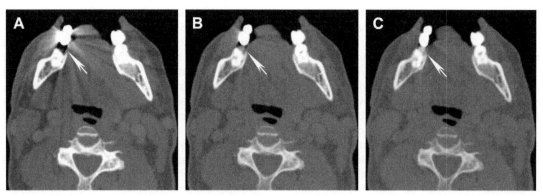

Fig. 8. Use of high-energy VMIs for dental artifact reduction. (*A*) 65-keV VMI (typically considered equivalent to a 120-kVp single-energy CT acquisition), (*B*) 95-keV VMI, and (*C*) 140-keV VMI are shown. Note the greater artifact reduction with increasing VMI energy. For example, note the much better visualization of mandible immediately adjacent to the tooth with fillings and associated artifact on high-energy VMIs (*arrow*). The trade-off is a decrease in soft tissue contrast and iodine attenuation. However, this does not pose a significant limitation for the evaluation of structures with intrinsically high attenuation independent of iodine enhancement (such as bone).

suppression of iodine attenuation within the enhancing tumor. In these cases, the trade-off between artifact suppression and iodine/enhancing tumor attenuation and soft tissue contrast needs to be considered. Based on a study of solutions with different iodine concentration obscured by artifact in a phantom, the 95-keV VMI could strike a reasonable balance between artifact

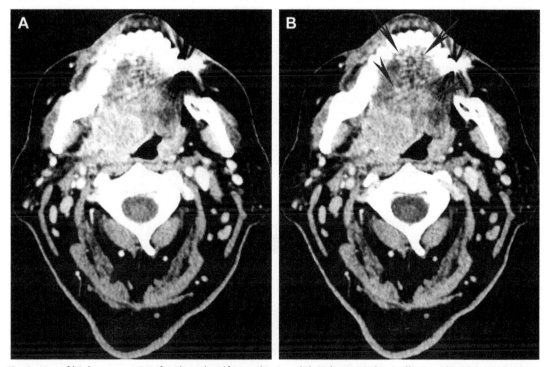

Fig. 9. Use of high-energy VMIs for dental artifact reduction. (*A*) 65-keV VMI (typically considered equivalent to a 120-kVp single-energy CT acquisition) and (*B*) 95-keV VMI are shown from a patient with a large cancer involving the oropharynx and oral tongue. Note the modest artifact reduction on the 95-keV compared with the 65-keV VMI. The anterior margin (*arrowheads*) of the tumor in the oral tongue is better delineated on the 95-keV VMI. The normal structures within the anterior part of the oral cavity (*arrows*) are also better seen on the 95-keV VMI. As expected, iodine attenuation in the tumor and other enhancing structures is diminished on the 95-keV compared with the 65-keV VMI, representing the trade-off between artifact reduction and iodine/enhancing tissue attenuation with increasing VMI energy.

suppression and preservation of soft tissue contrast and iodine attenuation when pertinent (see **Fig. 9**). Similar to other DECT reconstructions discussed previously, these are meant to complement the standard 65- or 70-keV reconstructions (see later section on multiparametric evaluation of HNSCC), and not replace them. However, it should also be noted that dental artifact is by nature highly variable, and as such, the results of interventions aimed at suppressing dental artifact are unpredictable. The final result also partly depends on the attenuation/enhancement of the lesion or structure of interest.[38] Although 95- and 140-keV reconstructions may be satisfactory in most cases for automatic generation and transfer to the picture archiving and communication system (PACS), it is likely that additional adjustments could be made on a case by case basis for best results.

Another potential application of DECT is in the evaluation of cervical lymphadenopathy. There are currently only a few studies evaluating DECT applications for metastatic HNSCC lymph nodes. However, one study showed that similar to primary tumors, low-energy VMIs can improve the conspicuity of pathologic lymph nodes (**Fig. 10**).[21] Nodal heterogeneity may also be better seen on low-energy VMIs and iodine maps (see **Fig. 10**).[9,10,39] Another study demonstrated that the iodine content of metastatic HNSCC lymph nodes (see **Fig. 10**) is significantly lower than normal or inflammatory nodes.[40] Other studies have suggested that iodine content and other DECT characteristics of lymph nodes (eg, certain features derived from

the spectral Hounsfield unit attenuation curves) may be used to distinguish different types of pathologic nodes or pathologic nodes from normal nodes.[41,42] At this time, there are few published studies, but these are interesting topics for future research and potential clinical application. Lastly, other advanced and quantitative analyses are potentially possible with DECT that may be applied either to the primary tumor or lymph nodes, and are exciting areas for future research. These include advanced DECT quantitative tissue characterization and the use of the rich quantitative spectral data for texture or radiomic analysis, some of which are discussed in greater detail elsewhere in this issue.

Multiparametric Dual-Energy Computed Tomography Approach for Head and Neck Squamous Cell Carcinoma Evaluation

At first glance, one may consider attempting to create a single DECT reconstruction that captures all of the relevant information for optimal diagnostic evaluation. However, based on careful consideration of the physical principles underlying DECT and various trade-offs at different energies, such an approach is unlikely to be successful. An alternate approach is to use the high SNR SECT equivalent 65- or 70-keV VMIs as standard reference images for routine assessment and evaluation of underlying anatomy, supplemented with other reconstructions for targeted lesion evaluation.[9,10,21,22] This multiparametric approach for

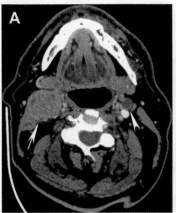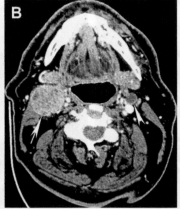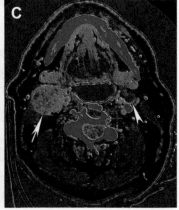

Fig. 10. Use of DECT for the evaluation of lymphadenopathy. (*A*) 65-keV VMI (typically considered equivalent to a 120-kVp single-energy CT acquisition), (*B*) 40-keV VMI, and (*C*) iodine (iodine-water) map are shown from a patient with a large internally heterogenous right level II (*arrow*) and a smaller cystic left level II (*arrowhead*) metastatic HNSCC lymph nodes. There is increase in soft tissue contrast on the 40-keV VMI (*B*) compared with the 65-keV VMI. For example, note the increased attenuation of the right level II node relative to adjacent muscle or the internal heterogeneity of the nodes on the 40-keV VMI (*B*) compared with 65-keV (*C*). The iodine map (*C*) provides a quantitative map of iodine distribution and relative iodine content within tissues, demonstrating heterogenous nodal iodine content.

Table 1
Suggested DECT reconstructions for multiparametric evaluation of HNSCC based on current evidence

Reconstructions	Comments
65- or 70-keV VMIs (or 30/70 WA images for dual-source scanners)	• Typically considered equivalent to the standard 120-kVp SECT • Used for routine clinical interpretation and as standard reference images
Supplement the standard (65 or 70 keV) VMIs with additional reconstructions for specific applications and optimal diagnostic evaluation using a multiparametric approach	
Low-energy VMIs: 40 keV (45 or 50 keV may be acceptable alternatives based on user preference)	• Enhanced tumor visibility and better visualization of tumor–normal soft tissue interface; increased visibility of pathologic lymph nodes • Higher noise levels, exacerbated in areas susceptible to artifact, such as the lower neck and thoracic inlet • Another approach for improving lesion visibility is to change the blending ratio and/or use nonlinear blending of WA images (for dual-source scanners only); same principle as use of low-energy VMIs by increasing the contribution from the lower energy spectrum
High-energy VMIs: 95 and/or 140 keV	• Reduce dental artifact • Distinction of nonossified thyroid cartilage from tumor • Simultaneous reconstruction of two sets of high-energy VMIs, one at an intermediate (95 keV) and the other at a very high (140 keV) energy, may be more practical given the variations in artifact and trade-offs with iodine suppression
Iodine maps	• Evaluate thyroid cartilage invasion

HNSCC evaluation takes advantage of the breadth of information available on different reconstructions and would be similar to the use of different MR imaging sequences for a complete diagnostic evaluation. Based on current evidence, a combination of standard images, low- and high-energy VMIs, and iodine maps could be used for the evaluation of HNSCC (summarized in **Table 1**).

MR imaging sequence to be essential for a diagnosis when using that modality. However, it is becoming increasingly clear that supplementary DECT reconstructions can help increase diagnostic accuracy or confidence in a subset of cases. In this regard, DECT has the potential to further enhance the central role of CT for the evaluation and staging of head and neck cancer and improve patient care.

SUMMARY

DECT is an exciting and evolving technology that has the potential to change the traditional approach to the use of CT in the clinical setting, providing a new layer of information previously unavailable using CT. There is increasing evidence that various supplementary DECT reconstructions can be used to improve the diagnostic evaluation of HNSCC. Different DECT reconstructions and quantitative analysis can potentially improve tissue characterization and better demonstrate tumor extent, including tumor invasion of critical anatomic structures, possibly significantly impacting patient staging and management. When implementing DECT in the clinical setting, it would not be realistic to expect the additional DECT reconstructions to make a significant impact in every case, no more than one would expect every

REFERENCES

1. Johnson TR, Krauss B, Sedlmair M, et al. Material differentiation by dual energy CT: initial experience. Eur Radiol 2007;17(6):1510–7.
2. Coursey CA, Nelson RC, Boll DT, et al. Dual-energy multidetector CT: how does it work, what can it tell us, and when can we use it in abdominopelvic imaging? Radiographics 2010;30(4):1037–55.
3. Alvarez RE, Macovski A. Energy-selective reconstructions in X-ray computerized tomography. Phys Med Biol 1976;21(5):733–44.
4. Johnson TRC, Kalender WA. Physical background. In: Johnson T, Fink C, Schönberg SO, et al, editors. Dual energy CT in clinical practice. Berlin: Springer-Verlag Berlin Heidelberg; 2011. p. 3–9.
5. Michael GJ. Tissue analysis using dual energy CT. Australas Phys Eng Sci Med 1992;15(2):75–87.

6. Johnson TR. Dual-energy CT: general principles. AJR Am J Roentgenol 2012;199(5 Suppl):S3–8.

7. Krauss B, Schmidt B, Flohr TG. Dual source CT. In: Johnson T, Fink C, Schönberg SO, et al, editors. Dual energy CT in clinical practice. Berlin: Springer-Verlag Berlin Heidelberg; 2011. p. 10–20.

8. Chandra N, Langan DA. Gemstone detector: dual energy imaging via fast kVp switching. In: Johnson T, Fink C, Schönberg SO, et al, editors. Dual energy CT in clinical practice. Berlin: Springer-Verlag Berlin Heidelberg; 2011. p. 35–41.

9. Forghani R. Advanced dual-energy CT for head and neck cancer imaging. Expert Rev Anticancer Ther 2015;15(12):1489–501.

10. Lam S, Gupta R, Kelly H, et al. Multiparametric evaluation of head and neck squamous cell carcinoma using a single-source dual-energy CT with fast kVp switching: state of the art. Cancers (Basel) 2015; 7(4):2201–16.

11. McCollough CH, Leng S, Yu L, et al. Dual- and multi-energy CT: principles, technical approaches, and clinical applications. Radiology 2015;276(3):637–53.

12. Schenzle JC, Sommer WH, Neumaier K, et al. Dual energy CT of the chest: how about the dose? Invest Radiol 2010;45(6):347–53.

13. Tawfik AM, Kerl JM, Razek AA, et al. Image quality and radiation dose of dual-energy CT of the head and neck compared with a standard 120-kVp acquisition. AJNR Am J Neuroradiol 2011;32(11):1994–9.

14. Li B, Yadava G, Hsieh J. Quantification of head and body CTDI(VOL) of dual-energy x-ray CT with fast-kVp switching. Med Phys 2011;38(5):2595–601.

15. Kamiya K, Kunimatsu A, Mori H, et al. Preliminary report on virtual monochromatic spectral imaging with fast kVp switching dual energy head CT: comparable image quality to that of 120-kVp CT without increasing the radiation dose. Jpn J Radiol 2013; 31(4):293–8.

16. Matsumoto K, Jinzaki M, Tanami Y, et al. Virtual monochromatic spectral imaging with fast kilovoltage switching: improved image quality as compared with that obtained with conventional 120-kVp CT. Radiology 2011;259(1):257–62.

17. Forghani R, Kelly H, Yu E, et al. Low-energy virtual monochromatic dual-energy computed tomography images for the evaluation of head and neck squamous cell carcinoma: a study of tumor visibility compared with single-energy computed tomography and user acceptance. J Comput Assist Tomogr 2017. in press.

18. Tanaka R, Hayashi T, Ike M, et al. Reduction of dark-band-like metal artifacts caused by dental implant bodies using hypothetical monoenergetic imaging after dual-energy computed tomography. Oral Surg Oral Med Oral Pathol Oral Radiol 2013;115(6):833–8.

19. Pinho DF, Kulkarni NM, Krishnaraj A, et al. Initial experience with single-source dual-energy CT abdominal angiography and comparison with single-energy CT angiography: image quality, enhancement, diagnosis and radiation dose. Eur Radiol 2013;23(2):351–9.

20. Patel BN, Thomas JV, Lockhart ME, et al. Single-source dual-energy spectral multidetector CT of pancreatic adenocarcinoma: optimization of energy level viewing significantly increases lesion contrast. Clin Radiol 2013;68(2):148–54.

21. Lam S, Gupta R, Levental M, et al. Optimal virtual monochromatic images for evaluation of normal tissues and head and neck cancer using dual-energy CT. AJNR Am J Neuroradiol 2015;36(8):1518–24.

22. Forghani R, Levental M, Gupta R, et al. Different spectral Hounsfield unit curve and high-energy virtual monochromatic image characteristics of squamous cell carcinoma compared with nonossified thyroid cartilage. AJNR Am J Neuroradiol 2015; 36(6):1194–200.

23. Stolzmann P, Winklhofer S, Schwendener N, et al. Monoenergetic computed tomography reconstructions reduce beam hardening artifacts from dental restorations. Forensic Sci Med Pathol 2013;9(3): 327–32.

24. Wichmann JL, Noske EM, Kraft J, et al. Virtual monoenergetic dual-energy computed tomography: optimization of kiloelectron volt settings in head and neck cancer. Invest Radiol 2014;49(11):735–41.

25. Albrecht MH, Scholtz JE, Kraft J, et al. Assessment of an advanced monoenergetic reconstruction technique in dual-energy computed tomography of head and neck cancer. Eur Radiol 2015;25(8):2493–501.

26. Graser A, Johnson TR, Hecht EM, et al. Dual-energy CT in patients suspected of having renal masses: can virtual nonenhanced images replace true nonenhanced images? Radiology 2009;252(2):433–40.

27. Tawfik AM, Kerl JM, Bauer RW, et al. Dual-energy CT of head and neck cancer: average weighting of low- and high-voltage acquisitions to improve lesion delineation and image quality-initial clinical experience. Invest Radiol 2012;47(5):306–11.

28. Scholtz JE, Husers K, Kaup M, et al. Non-linear image blending improves visualization of head and neck primary squamous cell carcinoma compared to linear blending in dual-energy CT. Clin Radiol 2015;70(2):168–75.

29. Srinivasan A, Parker RA, Manjunathan A, et al. Differentiation of benign and malignant neck pathologies: preliminary experience using spectral computed tomography. J Comput Assist Tomogr 2013;37(5): 666–72.

30. Forghani R, Roskies M, Liu X, et al. Dual-energy CT characteristics of parathyroid adenomas on 25-and 55-second 4D-CT acquisitions: preliminary experience. J Comput Assist Tomogr 2016;40(5):806–14.

31. Yamauchi H, Buehler M, Goodsitt MM, et al. Dual-energy CT-based differentiation of benign posttreatment

changes from primary or recurrent malignancy of the head and neck: comparison of spectral Hounsfield units at 40 and 70 keV and iodine concentration. AJR Am J Roentgenol 2016;206(3):580–7.

32. Kuno H, Onaya H, Iwata R, et al. Evaluation of cartilage invasion by laryngeal and hypopharyngeal squamous cell carcinoma with dual-energy CT. Radiology 2012;265(2):488–96.

33. De Crop A, Casselman J, Van Hoof T, et al. Analysis of metal artifact reduction tools for dental hardware in CT scans of the oral cavity: kVp, iterative reconstruction, dual-energy CT, metal artifact reduction software: does it make a difference? Neuroradiology 2015;57(8):841–9.

34. Komlosi P, Grady D, Smith JS, et al. Evaluation of monoenergetic imaging to reduce metallic instrumentation artifacts in computed tomography of the cervical spine. J Neurosurg Spine 2015;22(1):34–8.

35. Bamberg F, Dierks A, Nikolaou K, et al. Metal artifact reduction by dual energy computed tomography using monoenergetic extrapolation. Eur Radiol 2011; 21(7):1424–9.

36. Lee YH, Park KK, Song HT, et al. Metal artefact reduction in gemstone spectral imaging dual-energy CT with and without metal artefact reduction software. Eur Radiol 2012;22(6):1331–40.

37. Srinivasan A, Hoeffner E, Ibrahim M, et al. Utility of dual-energy CT virtual keV monochromatic series for the assessment of spinal transpedicular hardware-bone interface. AJR Am J Roentgenol 2013;201(4):878–83.

38. Nair JR, DeBlois F, Ong T, et al. Dual energy CT: balance between iodine attenuation and artifact reduction for the evaluation of head and neck cancer. J Comput Assist Tomogr 2017. [Epub ahead of print].

39. Forghani R, Srinivasan A, Levental M. Evaluation of attenuation and heterogeneity in metastatic head and neck squamous cell carcinoma lymph nodes on dual energy CT scans. Paper presented at: American Society of Head & Neck Radiology, 49th Annual Meeting. Naples Grande Beach Resort. Naples (FL), September 9-13, 2015.

40. Tawfik AM, Razek AA, Kerl JM, et al. Comparison of dual-energy CT-derived iodine content and iodine overlay of normal, inflammatory and metastatic squamous cell carcinoma cervical lymph nodes. Eur Radiol 2014;24(3):574–80.

41. Yang L, Luo D, Li L, et al. Differentiation of malignant cervical lymphadenopathy by dual-energy CT: a preliminary analysis. Sci Rep 2016;6:31020.

42. Liang H, Li A, Li Y, et al. A retrospective study of dual-energy CT for clinical detecting of metastatic cervical lymph nodes in laryngeal and hypopharyngeal squamous cell carcinoma. Acta Otolaryngol 2015;135(7):722–8.

Dual-Energy Computed Tomography Applications for the Evaluation of Cervical Lymphadenopathy

Ahmed M. Tawfik, MBBCH, MSc, MD[a],*,
Andreas Michael Bucher, MD[b], Thomas J. Vogl, MD[b]

KEYWORDS

- Dual-energy CT • Head and neck imaging • Cervical lymphadenopathy • Cervical lymph nodes

KEY POINTS

- The head and neck region is rich in lymph nodes, and cervical lymphadenopathy owing to various causes is very common.
- Imaging is frequently requested to confirm the presence of lymphadenopathy, differentiate lymph nodes from other neck masses or cysts, and characterize the nodes as benign or malignant.
- Imaging evaluation of cervical lymph nodes in patients with head and neck squamous cell carcinoma is crucial.

INTRODUCTION

The head and neck region is rich in lymph nodes, and cervical lymphadenopathy owing to various causes is very common. Imaging is frequently requested to confirm the presence of lymphadenopathy, differentiate lymph nodes from other neck masses or cysts, characterize the nodes as benign or malignant, and aid in identification of the cause. Furthermore, imaging evaluation of cervical lymph nodes in patients with head and neck squamous cell carcinoma (HNSCC) is crucial for several reasons. First, lymph node status strongly influences prognosis; the 5-year survival of patients with HNSCC and no nodal involvement is roughly twice that of patients with lymph node metastases.[1,2] Second, the patient's lymph node status is a key factor in planning of surgical selective neck dissection, and in defining the radiation field extent in patients treated with radiotherapy.[1]

Third, nonsurgical treatment options require monitoring of response and posttreatment restaging of the primary tumor and regional lymph nodes. Finally, after successful treatment resulting in disease remission, imaging surveillance is performed for early detection of tumor or nodal recurrence.

Several imaging modalities have been used for evaluation of cervical lymph nodes, especially in patients with HNSCC. Computed tomography (CT), MR imaging, ultrasound imaging, and PET-CT are currently used for this purpose.[3] The sensitivity and specificity of different imaging modalities for diagnosis of cervical lymph node metastases vary between studies, with PET-CT performing slightly better than CT or MR imaging in a number of studies.[4,5] It should be noted, however, that the diagnostic performance of all imaging modalities is nearly the same for clinically negative nodes.[6] Dual-energy (DE) CT scanning is an advanced form of CT scanning in which image acquisition

Disclosure Statement: The author has no commercial or financial conflicts of interest. The author received no funding for this article.
[a] Department of Diagnostic and Interventional Radiology, Mansoura University, 60 ElGomhoreya street, Mansoura 35516, Egypt; [b] Institute for Diagnostic and Interventional Radiology, Johann Wolfgang Goethe University Hospital, Theodor-Stern-Kai 7, 60590 Frankfurt am Main, Germany
* Corresponding author.
E-mail address: ahm_m_tawfik@hotmail.com

Neuroimag Clin N Am 27 (2017) 461–468
http://dx.doi.org/10.1016/j.nic.2017.04.002
1052-5149/17/© 2017 Elsevier Inc. All rights reserved.

is performed at 2 different energies, enabling generation of additional reconstructions and quantitative analysis not possible with single energy CT. In this article, DE CT applications for the evaluation of cervical lymphadenopathy are reviewed.

CONVENTIONAL COMPUTED TOMOGRAPHY IMAGING OF CERVICAL LYMPH NODES

CT scanning is a cornerstone of head and neck imaging and the most widely used imaging modality for evaluation of cervical lymphadenopathy. Typically, a lymph node is considered pathologic based on its size, although different size limits have been proposed.[1] A frequently used size limit defines pathologic nodes as larger than 10 mm in short axis diameter, except for retropharyngeal nodes (>5 mm), and level I and II nodes (>11 mm).[3] However, nodal size alone is neither sensitive nor specific enough; a large percentage of malignant nodes are as small as 5 mm, and many large nodes are reactive.[3] Other than size, additional criteria for the diagnosis of metastases include a rounded shape and grouping of 3 or more nodes in a drainage site for the primary tumor. Unfortunately, these criteria minimally improve the diagnostic performance of CT scanning.[1]

The presence of central necrosis is the most accurate CT sign of metastatic nodes form HNSCC,[1] and is caused by infiltration of the medulla of the node by malignant cells leading to necrosis. The center of the node is, thus, of lower attenuation than the cortex of the node, and the appearance is more conspicuous after contrast. Despite the very high specificity of this sign, the frequency of necrosis decreases in smaller nodes and so does the sensitivity of CT for its detection.[1,3]

DUAL-ENERGY COMPUTED TOMOGRAPHY SCANNING OF CERVICAL LYMPH NODES

Approaches to DE scanning include dual-source scanners with dual x-ray source-detector combinations acquiring images simultaneously at high and low energy, and single source scanners with either rapid kVp switching, split filters in the tube collimator housing, or dual layer detectors.[7] A detailed discussion of the different DE CT systems is beyond the scope of this article, but can be found in the article in this issue. Whether a dual or a single source system is used for scanning, DE postprocessing applications have been developed as a supplement to conventional CT, providing the radiologist with multiple additional sets of images, each having its own unique characteristics and potential benefits.[8,9]

Virtual Noncontrast Images

With DE CT, it is possible to identify and subtract iodine from contrast enhanced images to obtain a virtual noncontrast (VNC) image series (**Fig. 1**). An additional unenhanced scan is, thus, not needed and the radiation dose can be reduced in studies where both an unenhanced and enhanced acquisition are performed.[9] The subjective quality of VNC images in the evaluation of cervical lymphadenopathy has been reported as comparable with true unenhanced images.[10,11] Objectively, Fu and colleagues[11] analyzed the CT attenuation values of lymph nodes in 41 patients with 98 cervical lymph nodes and found no differences between VNC and true unenhanced images. In another study by Yang and colleagues,[10] lymph node attenuation values were slightly overestimated on VNC images, but

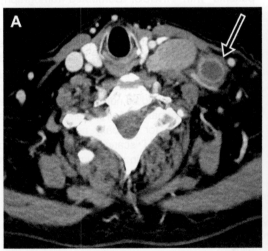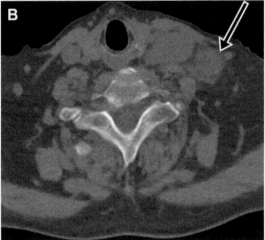

Fig. 1. Virtual noncontrast image. (*A*) Axial contrast-enhanced dual-energy computed tomography image of the neck showing a necrotic left supraclavicular metastatic lymph node (*arrow*). (*B*) Virtual noncontrast reconstruction showing subtraction of the enhancement in the cervical vessels and soft tissue. Notice the subtraction of the rim enhancement of the necrotic lymph node (*arrow*).

the mean difference in attenuation values between VNC and true unenhanced images was only 8 HU, which the authors considered as an acceptable difference, and unlikely to affect diagnosis. VNC images can be used for the detection of calcification and fatty hila in lymph nodes. As an added benefit, because the VNC images are generated from the postcontrast images, there is no misregistration in attenuation measurements made before and after contrast.[9]

Blended Images

The high and low energy components of DE acquisition have different attenuation and image noise characteristics. Image noise is less in the high energy than in the low energy component. In contrast, the contrast attenuation is higher in the low energy than in the high energy component (**Fig. 2**). Thus, by mixing or blending data from the 2 components, images can be reconstructed with greater contrast attenuation and less noise.[8]

Linear blending entails setting a blending ratio for contributions from the high and low energy components. Images reconstructed with a ratio of 0.3 (30% from the 80 kVp component and 70% from the 140 kVp component) are considered similar to the routine single energy 120 kVp CT images, and have been used for routine clinical interpretation.[12] Changing the blending ratio results in substantial changes in contrast attenuation, noise, and image quality. Tawfik and colleagues[13] investigated different blending ratios to determine an optimal linear blending ratio for head and neck imaging. Their results demonstrated that images reconstructed using a blending ratio of 0.6 (60% from the 80 kVp component and 40% from the 140 kVp component) were the best in terms of contrast attenuation and image quality. This blending ratio increased contrast attenuation compared with the 0.3 ratio, while maintaining the low image noise and optimizing the contrast-to-noise ratio.[13]

Nonlinear blending is a more sophisticated method for image blending, where contributions from the high and low energy components are not the same in all image pixels. An algorithm is used that preferentially increases the contribution of the low energy component in high attenuation pixels containing iodine; thus, contrast attenuation is maximized. Meanwhile, the contribution of the high energy component is increased in pixels with low attenuation (with no iodine) so that image noise is at its lowest level.[9] Scholtz and colleagues[14] compared nonlinear with linear blending in imaging of HNSCC and reported that nonlinear blending is superior to linear blending with different ratios in both subjective image quality and lesion delineation, as well as objective lesion enhancement and contrast-to-noise ratio.

Virtual Monochromatic Images

Virtual monochromatic or monoenergetic images are reconstructed at a specific energy level, commonly ranging between 40 and 140 keV or more (**Fig. 3**). Monochromatic images reconstructed at high energies reduce metallic artifacts compared with routine CT images, which is very useful in patients with dental fillings.[15] Furthermore, the CT attenuation of iodine and the image noise are a function of photon energy, and thus images reconstructed at optimal energy levels can improve image quality and the detection of subtle lesion enhancement. Wichmann and colleagues,[16] using dual source DE CT, compared multiple linear blending reconstructions with monochromatic reconstructions in the head and neck, and observed significant differences in image quality. In their study, monochromatic reconstruction at 60 KeV was superior to linear blended images matching routine CT acquisitions in terms of image quality and contrast-to-noise ratio.[16]

In another study using fast kVp switching scanner, Lam and colleagues[17] investigated multiple monochromatic energy levels for imaging of the head and neck. They found that tumor attenuation and conspicuity were maximized in images reconstructed at 40 keV, but image noise was high. The best image quality—in terms of image noise—was achieved when images were reconstructed at 65 KeV, which they recommended for use instead of the default 70 keV reconstructions for routine evaluation of the neck.[17] Their proposed approach is to use the 65 KeV reconstruction for routine interpretation of all cases, and to use images reconstructed at 40 keV with higher tumor conspicuity as supplement in HNSCC cases.[15]

Iodine Map and Iodine Quantification

Another common DE reconstruction is the color-coded iodine map, which can be generated by re-adding iodine to VNC images. The anatomic details are preserved, and areas of enhancement could be distinguished from nonenhancing tissue with similar attenuation[9] (**Fig. 4**). Quantification of contrast enhancement in CT is usually done by comparing attenuation values on enhanced and unenhanced images. DE postprocessing algorithms can generate a VNC image and automatically calculate the difference in attenuation owing to iodine enhancement, or the iodine overlay, in each pixel in Hounsfield units.[18]

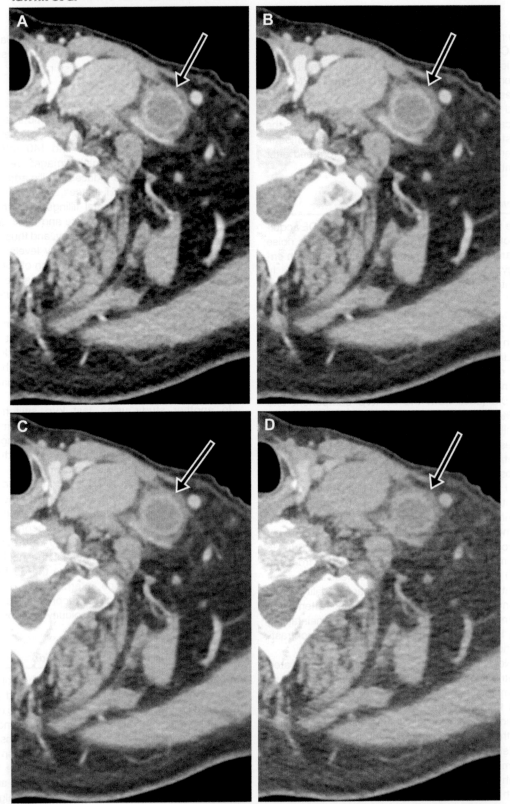

Fig. 2. Linear image blending. Left supraclavicular metastatic node (*arrows*). (*A*) Axial 80 kV computed tomography image (low tube voltage). (*B*) Linear blended image with 60% contribution from low tube voltage. (*C*) Linear blended image with 30% contribution from low tube voltage. (*D*) A 150 kV image (high tube voltage). Attenuation of iodine and tissue decreases with increasing contribution from the high tube voltage and so does image noise.

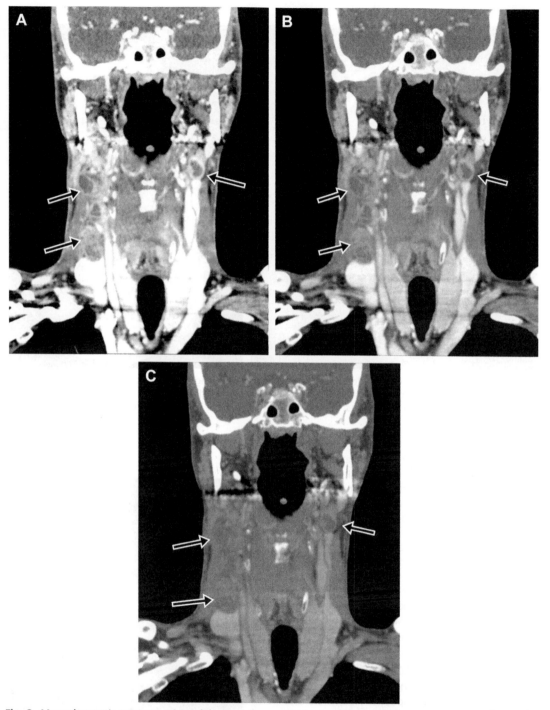

Fig. 3. Monochromatic reconstructions. (*A*) Coronal computed tomography (CT) image reconstructed at 40 keV shows increased iodine attenuation in vessels and intense rim enhancement of necrotic metastatic cervical lymph nodes (*arrows*). (*B*) CT image reconstructed at 60 keV with improved image quality and lower noise than (*A*). (*C*) CT image reconstructed at 100 KeV with lower noise and decreased iodine attenuation compared with (*A*) and (*B*).

An exciting alternative for the assessment of contrast enhancement is made possible by DE postprocessing that enables identification of iodine and a quantitative estimate of the amount of iodine in each image pixel. This process can be performed in different ways with different DE systems, but 1 method is by a "3-material decomposition." With this method, the iodine content is

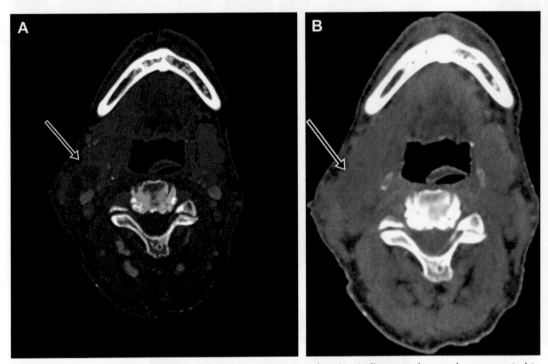

Fig. 4. Iodine map. (*A*) Axial color-coded iodine image or map showing iodine superimposed on computed to-mography image. Central necrosis and rim cortical enhancement are clearly seen in the right metastatic lymph node (*arrow*). (*B*) Axial virtual noncontrast image. Iodine enhancement is subtracted from the cortex of the lymph node (*arrow*).

measured in milligrams per milliliter rather than in Hounsfield units[18] (**Fig. 5**). Tawfik and col-leagues[18] used both iodine overlay and iodine content to measure contrast enhancement in cer-vical lymph nodes. They reported significant differ-ences in iodine overlay and iodine content between normal, inflammatory, and metastatic lymph nodes. In their study, the iodine content was more accurate in differentiation between met-astatic and nonmetastatic lymph nodes than the iodine overlay. In their study, the iodine content of metastatic lymph nodes was significantly lower than in normal and inflammatory lymph nodes.

Spectral Hounsfield Unit Attenuation Curves

DE postprocessing with region of interest analysis can be used to generate spectral Hounsfield unit attenuation curves. This process is a quantitative correlate of the different energy virtual monochro-matic images, representing the energy-dependent changes in attenuation within a region of interest across a range of virtual monochromatic energy levels, typically 40 to 140 keV. This type of analysis is readily available in the postprocessing packages of fast kVp switching scanners, but can also be performed with other scanner types. In general, and particularly for enhancing tissues, attenuation

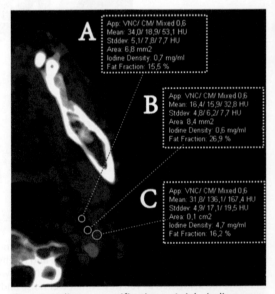

Fig. 5. Iodine quantification. Axial iodine map showing 3 regions of interest (*A*, *B*, *C*) drawn inside a left cervical metastatic lymph node for iodine quantifi-cation. The iodine content in the necrotic part is as low as 0.7 and 0.6 mg/mL (regions of interest in *A* and *B*, respectively), compared with the substantially higher iodine content in the enhancing cortex 4.7 mg/mL.

is reduced with increasing keV away from the K-edge of iodine (33.2 keV). However, the energy-dependent attenuation changes or curves of different tissues can differ.[19,20] Srinivasan and colleagues[19] investigated the use of spectral curves for differentiating between benign and malignant lesions in the neck, and reported that the spectral curves of malignant lesions had higher range and steeper decay than benign lesions curves.

Liang and colleagues[21] evaluated the spectral Hounsfield unit attenuation curves in HNSCC for differentiating metastatic and nonmetastatic lymph nodes. They calculated the slope of the spectral curve in the target lymph node and the primary lesion, and then compared the ratio between the 2 slopes. Metastatic nodes had significantly higher slope ratios than nonmetastatic nodes. In another study, Yang and colleagues[22] assessed the iodine content and the spectral curve slope of metastatic cervical lymphadenopathy from squamous cell carcinoma, thyroid and salivary carcinomas, as well as lymphoma. They reported higher iodine content and spectral curve slope in metastatic thyroid cancer than other groups, followed by metastatic lymph nodes from salivary carcinoma. There was no significant differences in iodine content and spectral curve slope between the squamous cell carcinoma and the lymphoma groups.

SUMMARY

Imaging of cervical lymphadenopathy remains a challenge and extending DE CT applications to this domain may help in overcoming some of the limitations of conventional CT imaging. With the recent increase in the number of DE-capable scanners provided by several vendors, DE CT is gaining more acceptance as a clinical and research tool in all body regions. Except for a few studies, research in DE CT of the head and neck has been largely focused on dose reduction and image quality. Therefore, future research in DE CT of cervical lymphadenopathy is encouraged and studies should concentrate more on clinical applications, with direct comparison to other imaging modalities.

REFERENCES

1. Saindane AM. Pitfalls in the staging of cervical lymph node metastasis. Neuroimaging Clin N Am 2013;23:147–66.
2. Schlumpf MF, Haerle S. The current role of imaging in head and neck cancer: a clinician's perspective. Swiss Med Wkly 2014;144:w14015.
3. Eisenmenger LB, Wiggins RH 3rd. Imaging of head and neck lymph nodes. Radiol Clin North Am 2015; 53:115–32.
4. Jeong HS, Baek CH, Son YI, et al. Use of integrated 18F-FDG PET/CT to improve the accuracy of initial cervical nodal evaluation in patients with head and neck squamous cell carcinoma. Head Neck 2007; 29:203–10.
5. Kyzas PA, Evangelou E, Denaxa-Kyza D, et al. 18F-fluorodeoxyglucose positron emission tomography to evaluate cervical node metastases in patients with head and neck squamous cell carcinoma: a meta-analysis. J Natl Cancer Inst 2008;100:712–20.
6. Liao LJ, Lo WC, Hsu WL, et al. Detection of cervical lymph node metastasis in head and neck cancer patients with clinically N0 neck-a metaanalysis comparing different imaging modalities. BMC Cancer 2012;12:236.
7. Saba L, Porcu M, Schmidt B, et al. Dual energy CT: basic principles. Chapter 1. In: De Cecco CN, Laghi A, Schoepf J, et al, editors. Dual energy CT in oncology. Heidelberg (Germany): Springer International Publishing; 2015. p. 1–20.
8. Vogl TJ, Schulz B, Bauer RW, et al. Dual-energy CT applications in head and neck imaging. AJR Am J Roentgenol 2012;199:S34–9.
9. Tawfik AM, Bodelle B, Vogl TJ. Dual energy CT in head and neck tumors. Chapter 3. In: De Cecco CN, Laghi A, Schoepf J, et al, editors. Dual energy CT in oncology. Heidelberg (Germany): Springer International Publishing; 2015. p. 31–40.
10. Yang Y, Jia X, Deng Y, et al. Can virtual non-enhanced CT be used to replace true non-enhanced CT for the detection of palpable cervical lymph nodes? A preliminary study. Jpn J Radiol 2014;32:324–30.
11. Fu F, He A, Zhang Y, et al. Dual-energy virtual non-contrast imaging in diagnosis of cervical metastasis lymph nodes. J Cancer Res Ther 2015;11:202–4.
12. Tawfik AM, Kerl JM, Razek AA, et al. Image quality and radiation dose of dual-energy CT of the head and neck compared with a standard 120-kVp acquisition. AJNR Am J Neuroradiol 2011;32:1994–9.
13. Tawfik AM, Kerl JM, Bauer RW, et al. Dual-energy CT of head and neck cancer: average weighting of low- and high-voltage acquisitions to improve lesion delineation and image quality-initial clinical experience. Invest Radiol 2012;47:306–11.
14. Scholtz JE, Hüsers K, Kaup M, et al. Non-linear image blending improves visualization of head and neck primary squamous cell carcinoma compared to linear blending in dual-energy CT. Clin Radiol 2015;70:168–75.
15. Lam S, Gupta R, Kelly H, et al. Multiparametric evaluation of head and neck squamous cell carcinoma using a single-source dual-energy CT with fast kVp switching: state of the art. Cancers (Basel) 2015;7:2201–16.
16. Wichmann JL, Nöske EM, Kraft J, et al. Virtual monoenergetic dual-energy computed tomography: optimization of kiloelectron volt settings in head and neck cancer. Invest Radiol 2014;49:735–41.

17. Lam S, Gupta R, Levental M, et al. Optimal virtual monochromatic images for evaluation of normal tissues and head and neck cancer using dual-energy CT. AJNR Am J Neuroradiol 2015;36:1518–24.

18. Tawfik AM, Razek AA, Kerl JM, et al. Comparison of dual-energy CT-derived iodine content and iodine overlay of normal, inflammatory and metastatic squamous cell carcinoma cervical lymph nodes. Eur Radiol 2014;24:574–80.

19. Srinivasan A, Parker RA, Manjunathan A, et al. Differentiation of benign and malignant neck pathologies: preliminary experience using spectral computed tomography. J Comput Assist Tomogr 2013;37:666–72.

20. Xue H, Zhu L. Dual energy CT postprocessing and images analysis strategies in oncologic imaging. Chapter 2. In: De Cecco CN, Laghi A, Schoepf J, et al, editors. Dual energy CT in oncology. Heidelberg (Germany): Springer International Publishing; 2015. p. 21–30.

21. Liang H, Li A, Li Y, et al. A retrospective study of dual-energy CT for clinical detecting of metastatic cervical lymph nodes in laryngeal and hypopharyngeal squamous cell carcinoma. Acta Otolaryngol 2015;135:722–8.

22. Yang L, Luo D, Li L, et al. Differentiation of malignant cervical lymphadenopathy by dual-energy CT: a preliminary analysis. Sci Rep 2016;6:31020.

Miscellaneous and Emerging Applications of Dual-Energy Computed Tomography for the Evaluation of Pathologies in the Head and Neck

Tommaso D'Angelo, MD[a,b], Silvio Mazziotti, MD[a],
Giorgio Ascenti, MD[a], Julian L. Wichmann, MD[b],*

KEYWORDS

- Computed tomography • Dual-energy • Head and neck • Monochromatic imaging

KEY POINTS

- Dual-energy computed tomography (DECT) scanning of the head and neck may have added value over single-source multidetector computed tomography, providing radiologists with a technology that has the potential to improve detection and characterization of benign and malignant abnormalities.
- Iodine quantification may represent an alternative imaging biomarker for differentiating head and neck tumors or monitoring their viability using DECT.
- DECT also allows for reduction of contrast material or radiation dose without compromising image quality or diagnostic accuracy.

INTRODUCTION

Multidetector computed tomography (MDCT) is a well-established method for characterizing and staging a large variety of head and neck lesions. Recent advances in MDCT have allowed for higher temporal and spatial resolution with greater anatomic coverage. Although the technical concept for dual-energy computed tomography (DECT) was originally described more than 4 decades ago, only more recently has it evolved into a multiparametric technique used increasingly in routine clinical practice[1,2] due to its quantitative imaging capabilities. The goal of this article is to briefly explain the technical principles of DECT, describe the most common postprocessing applications, provide an overview of its various clinical applications, and give an outlook on its abilities as a quantitative imaging technique.

BASIC PRINCIPLES OF DUAL-ENERGY COMPUTED TOMOGRAPHY

At x-ray energy spectra relevant to diagnostic imaging (70–150 kilovolt peak or kVp), the predominant interactions between photons and tissue

Disclosures: J. L. Wichmann received speakers' fees from GE Healthcare and Siemens Healthcare. The other authors have nothing to disclose .
[a] Section of Radiological Sciences, Department of Biomedical Sciences and Morphological and Functional Imaging, University of Messina, Via Consolare Valeria 1, 98100 Messina, Italy; [b] Department of Diagnostic and Interventional Radiology, University Hospital Frankfurt, Theodor-Stern-Kai 7, 60590 Frankfurt, Germany
* Corresponding author.
E-mail address: docwichmann@gmail.com

matter are mainly represented by the Compton effect (x-ray photons scatter with fractional loss of x-ray energy) and the photoelectric effect (complete x-ray absorption with ejection of a photoelectron). In CT, the Compton effect accounts for a large component of the attenuation but is relatively independent of beam energy. In contrast, photoelectric absorption is highly energy dependent and is therefore key for spectral tissue characterization. Normally, there is a higher probability of photoelectric interactions when the exposed material has a high atomic number. Carbon, oxygen, and nitrogen usually mainly interact with x-ray photons by Compton scattering due to their relatively low atomic number, whereas the photoelectric effect occurs more frequently with higher Z elements such calcium and iodine.[3] When biological tissues containing these materials are penetrated by photons at different energy levels, they can be characterized on the basis of the change in x-ray attenuation at the different energies used.

At higher x-ray tube voltages (eg, 140 kVp), linear attenuation values measured for iodine and calcium are similar. This phenomenon is due to the stronger weighted attenuation coefficient of mass density at higher potentials. In contrast, at lower tube potentials (eg, 80 kVp), the attenuation coefficient is stronger for iodine rather than calcium, which therefore allows for separation and identification of these materials. However, there is also increased x-ray beam tissue absorption at lower potentials, which results in higher image noise.[4]

Currently available DECT systems allow for simultaneous image acquisition using different x-ray energies, most commonly at 80 and 140 kVp. However, peak energies used for image acquisition are not pure monochromatic x-rays

beams but polychromatic spectra of photons with various energy levels. Therefore, peak tube voltage (kVp) is typically used to refer to the maximum energy reached by the photons present in each of the spectra (Table 1).

Four main different approaches for DECT imaging are currently used, and they vary depending on the manufacturer. These approaches are discussed in the detail in a separate article in this issue but will be briefly reviewed here. The first system consists of 2 x-ray tubes operating at 2 different energies with their relative opposing detectors aligned perpendicularly or nearly perpendicularly ("dual-source DECT"). The second system uses a single x-ray tube that rapidly switches between 2 different energies together with its corresponding detector ("fast-kVp switching DECT"). The third system consists of a single x-ray source, in which the beam is prefiltered and split into high- and low-energy spectra before reaching the patient ("twin-beam DECT"). Finally, the fourth type of system uses one x-ray source and one detector, the latter composed of 2 scintillation layers placed directly on top of each other ("dual-layer DECT"), with scintillation layers that are closer to the source absorbing low-energy photons, and deep layers capturing high-energy photons. Independent of the technical realization, DECT is essentially considered dose-neutral compared with standard single-energy CT.[5]

One of the goals of DECT imaging is to combine the increased iodine attenuation of the low-kVp spectrum with the lower image noise of the high-kVp spectrum in order to obtain an image with highest contrast and lowest noise possible. So far, several DECT postprocessing algorithms have been developed for this purpose.

Table 1
Different energy levels (expressed in kiloelectron volt) adopted in virtual monoenergetic image to better depict various head and neck structures and abnormality

Reference Material	Energetic Level (keV)[a]	Miscellaneous Potential Clinical Applications (eg,)
Iodine	40–60	Tumor enhancement and delineation; vascular anatomy; bleeding point of hemorrhage
Soft tissues	65–70	Best SNR and CNR for head and neck evaluation (similar image quality of single-energy MDCT)
Calcium	~80	Definition of atherosclerotic plaque calcifications; evaluation of perivascular space
Metal hardware/ implants	90–150	Minimizing beam hardening artifacts; evaluating malposition, loosening or disruption of metal implants

[a] keV values may change according to type of DECT approach or platform used. Furthermore, they represent target values based on those recently reported in the scientific literature.

DUAL-ENERGY COMPUTED TOMOGRAPHY POSTPROCESSING
Linear Blending

The principle of linear blending consists of mixing a specific fraction of each dataset at a given blending ratio. For example, using a blending ratio of 0.3 means that image characteristics of the low-energy data are blended with a weighting factor of 0.3 (30% weight from the 80-kVp dataset), whereas image characteristics of the high-energy level are blended with a factor of 0.7 (70% weight from the 140-kVp dataset). Generally, when the blending ratio moves toward lower energies, the result is an image with increased iodine attenuation but also higher image noise; in contrast, shifting the blending ratio toward higher-kV values results in low image noise but also reduced iodine signal. Linear blending is one of the most common methods for postprocessing DECT data. It is also routinely performed when performing scans in DECT mode to provide a blended image that closely resembles a standard single-energy 100-kV or 120-kV image. Typically, the recommended blending factor in head and neck imaging is 0.3.[6] Although linear blending does not require additional manual postprocessing and can be performed directly in the reconstruction settings at the scanner, it has been shown that different linear blending factors may be favorable in head and neck DECT. Tawfik and colleagues[7] compared different blending factors and found that a linear blending factor of 0.6 was superior to other factors, including the standard factor of 0.3 in dual-source DECT of the neck.

Nonlinear Blending

Nonlinear blending algorithms consist of a selective combination of information from the low- and high-kVp datasets with various weighting factors through different voxels within the same tissue. In particular, the feature of improved iodine attenuation typical of low-kVp datasets is used for imaging regions with higher x-ray attenuation, whereas the decreased noise of high-kVp dataset is used for imaging those areas with lower attenuation.[8,9] Several studies have shown that this approach may be superior to conventional linear blending algorithms with regard to image quality. Multiple algorithms are available, including slope blending, binary blending, and modified sigmoidal blending, with the latter showing the most promising results (**Fig. 1**).[10-13]

However, nonlinear blending requires the observer to manually postprocess images, because

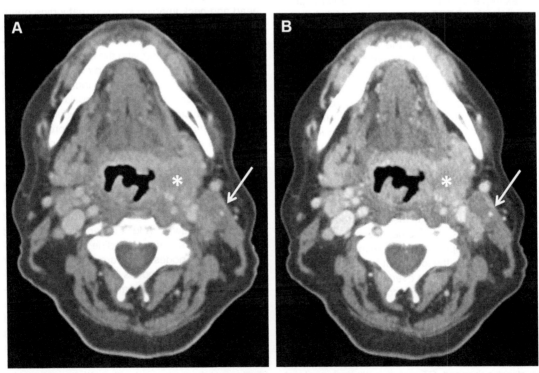

Fig. 1. Axial contrast-enhanced linearly blended (*A*) and nonlinearly blended (*B*) DECT images in a 48-year-old man with advanced oropharyngeal squamous cell carcinoma (*asterisk*) and metastatic enlarged left level IIA lymph node (*arrow*). Note the superior CNR of the nonlinearly blended (*B*) versus the linearly blended image (*A*).

the ideal blending parameters (ie, window center and width) remain an individual choice, may also be different in each case, and thus may be relatively time consuming in routine clinical practice, unless automated.

MISCELLANEOUS AND EMERGING DUAL-ENERGY COMPUTED TOMOGRAPHY CLINICAL APPLICATIONS

Among the various capabilities of DECT imaging, a key advantage is the possibility of obtaining different parameters and postprocessing data without the need for additional patient scanning or radiation exposure. DECT postprocessing applications may be divided into *material-specific* and *energy-specific applications*.

Material-Specific Applications

DECT can provide spectral information that may be used to emphasize clinically relevant characteristics of the tissue of interest, or to improve differentiation between different tissues, based on the property of certain materials to show different attenuation patterns when exposed to x-ray beams at different energy levels.

The approach to material decomposition can differ slightly among the different DECT platforms. For example, when data are acquired with "fast-kVp switching DECT," the base material decomposition is performed in the *data-domain*, whereas it is obtained by means of the *image-domain* with "dual-source DECT." With 2-material decomposition analysis, the characteristics of 2 sample materials with substantially different mass attenuation coefficients and atomic numbers (eg, iodine and water) are chosen to obtain 2 different sets of images (*material-density images*). The unique linear attenuation coefficients obtained by monochromatic imaging at 2 different energies are then used to distinguish between different materials (eg, iodine, calcium, water, fat) and can provide relatively accurate quantitative data. In 3-material decomposition analysis, the characteristics of 3 sample materials (eg, iodine, fat, and water) are used to create spectral iodine extraction images. In both methods, the iodine (or calcium) contribution to the image can be overlaid on grayscale images, creating a color-coded iodine map; alternatively, it can be subtracted, generating virtual unenhanced (VUE; or iodine-subtracted) images.[14]

Oncologic applications

Contrast-enhanced CT using iodinated contrast agents is routinely used in detection and staging of head and neck tumors, because these commonly show differences in vascularity or enhancement patterns compared with normal soft tissue. However, even on contrast-enhanced images, some neoplasms may have similar attenuation values compared with adjacent normal tissues (such as muscle), and a definitive characterization or identification may be challenging (Fig. 2).

Iodine-specific DECT images (*color-coded iodine overlay* or *iodine-density images*) allow for display of the quantitative iodine distribution within a volume in a color-coded map. This method permits not only improved direct visualization of iodine within the lesion but also a direct quantification of iodine concentration (in milligrams per milliliter) within a lesion. Application of this technique represents an alternative to conventional attenuation measurements for determining the enhancement of a lesion (Fig. 3).[15] The rationale of this method is based on the assumption that iodine is not naturally present in measurable concentrations in the normal human body (with the exception of the thyroid gland) and therefore may be thus identified using quantitative DECT. Moreover, although a standard attenuation measurement can be affected by the inclusion of necrotic or cystic areas, iodine concentration is not affected by the presence of such components as long as they do not show iodine uptake.

Preliminary studies regarding the use of DECT in head and neck imaging suggest that iodine quantification may be superior to standard attenuation measurements, especially for better estimating tumor invasion and improving the evaluation of pathologic lymph nodes.[16,17] In particular, it has been demonstrated that color-coded iodine overlay increases the specificity for diagnosis of invasion of laryngeal cartilage over single-energy MDCT with an improved interobserver reproducibility and a reduced overestimation of tumor invasion, which is crucial in preoperative workup when considering laryngectomy.[18]

Other investigators quantified the iodine content in normal and metastatic lymph nodes in patients affected by head and neck squamous cell carcinoma. Tawfik and colleagues[19] observed a significant reduction of iodine uptake in metastatic lymph nodes compared with normal or inflammatory lymph nodes (Fig. 4). Yang and colleagues[20] used iodine quantification and assessment of the slope of the spectral HU curve to distinguish different types of malignant cervical lymphadenopathy. In their study, the investigators found that metastatic lymph nodes in patients affected by thyroid cancer had a significantly higher iodine uptake compared with patients affected by lymphoma or other carcinomas, and they suggested that this may be due to richer blood supply

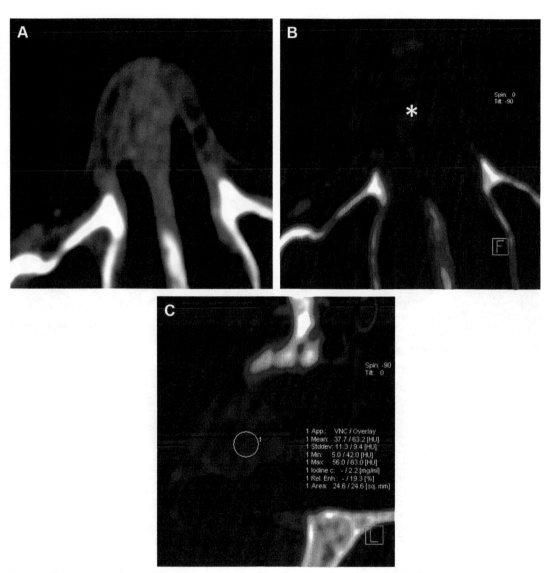

Fig. 2. Axial contrast-enhanced linearly blended (0.3 blending factor) DECT image (*A*) shows a round lesion that is not distinguishable from the septal cartilage of the nose in a 65-year-old woman. Axial (*B*) and sagittal (*C*) contrast-enhanced iodine-overlay DECT images allow for a better depiction of the enhancing lesion conspicuity (*asterisk*), aiding in the diagnosis of nasal septal squamous cell carcinoma.

of the thyroid cancer nodal metastases or to the specific iodine-absorbing features of thyroid tissue.

Finally, the adoption of iodine quantification as an imaging biomarker of tumor viability may represent a beneficial tool to depict early response to therapy beyond the mere macroscopic tumor shrinkage and instead focus on the degree of vascularization of a lesion.[21–24] This technique may be used to demonstrate the tumor-destroying activity of an agent before any morphologic change in size can be observed (**Fig. 5**). In the future, the optimal assessment of activity should combine functional and morphologic information. DECT may reveal important information about the effectiveness of

targeted molecular pharmacotherapy and may have the potential to improve noninvasive monitoring of tumor vascularity during therapy, as has been previously proposed for a variety of malignant neoplasms outside of the head and neck.[21–24]

Vascular

Computed tomographic angiography (CTA) is a routinely used method for depicting the anatomy of intracranial and extracranial vessels and has largely replaced digital subtraction angiography (DSA) for initial diagnostic imaging. Although a multitude of image reconstructions can be created using this technique, the adjacent osseous

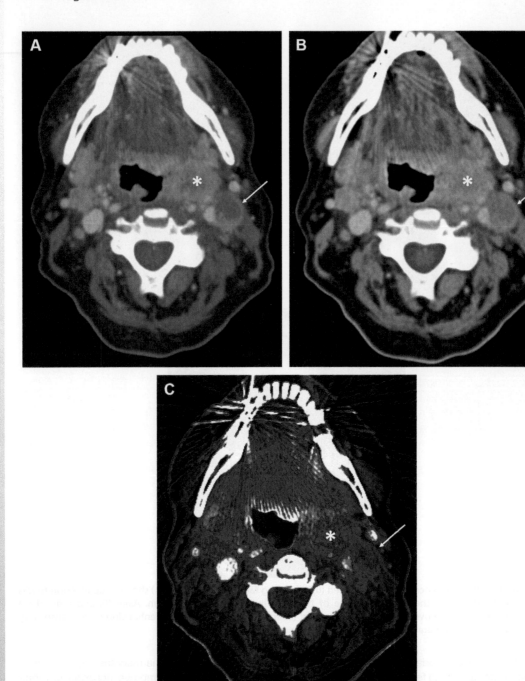

Fig. 3. Axial contrast-enhanced DECT images obtained by means of the linear blending (blending factor 0.3) algorithm (*A*) and VMI at 65 keV (*B*) in the same patient as in **Fig. 1** with advanced oropharyngeal squamous cell carcinoma (*asterisk*) and metastatic enlarged left level IIA lymph node (*arrow*). Note the better image contrast using VMI (*B*) in direct comparison. The axial contrast-enhanced iodine-overlay DECT image (*C*) well depicts the diffuse iodine uptake of the neoplasm and the necrotic core of the metastatic lymph node.

structures can often prevent accurate interpretation of the vascular anatomy. Commonly applied approaches for bone removal in single-energy MDCT include manual segmentation of bone and vessels (which may be time consuming and operator dependent) and semiautomatic segmentation (which is based on manufacturer-specific threshold-dependent software based on

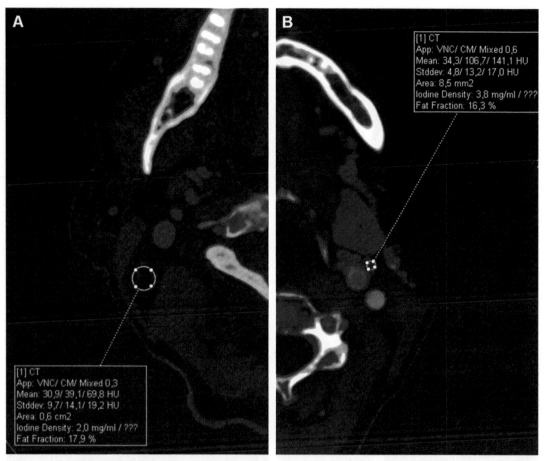

Fig. 4. Axial contrast-enhanced iodine-overlay DECT images obtained in a 57-year-old patient with metastatic melanoma to a right level IIB lymph node (*A*) and in a 67-year-old patient with a normal lymph node (*B*). Iodine quantification measuring both iodine content as well as iodine overlay values markedly differs between the 2.

differences of attenuation of the different anatomic structures). However, both of these techniques have disadvantages such as subtraction artifacts created when the HU values of vessels, calcified plaque, and bone are very similar.[25]

DECT material decomposition can provide threshold-independent bone removal, but may also highlight or remove calcified plaque, allowing for the omission of the unenhanced scan in certain cases and with a marked reduction in patient radiation exposure. However, although DECT angiography has shown improved detection and quantification of carotid artery stenosis over single-energy CTA, several studies reported that DECT-based bone-removal method leads to an overestimation of the degree of stenosis compared with DSA, likely because of the blooming effect of plaque calcifications.[26–28] Blooming artifacts caused by calcifications or nearby osseous structures (eg, the skull base) can produce artifacts due to excessive removal of bone at these locations or result in

ill-defined borders. The occurrence of such artifacts underlines the necessity to carefully check source images or to further investigate using additional DECT reconstructions (such as energy-specific applications that may be helpful in certain cases).

Skeletal
Because of its ability to detect edema and hemorrhage, MR imaging is the modality of choice in the detection of vertebral changes that may represent a "bone bruise" pattern (ie, compression fracture) without substantial disruption to the adjacent bone or overlying articular cartilage. However, advances in DECT have facilitated new approaches to the detection of subtle bone marrow lesions. In fact, trabecular microfractures, edema, and hemorrhage lead to increased amounts of interstitial fluid and blood that cause an increase in CT attenuation numbers, which is more accurately detectable by means of noncalcium DECT images compared with single-energy MDCT.[29,30]

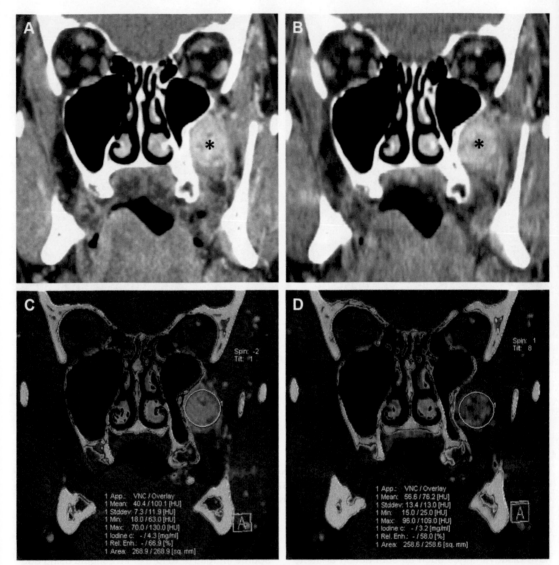

Fig. 5. Coronal contrast-enhanced linearly blended (blending factor 0.3) DECT images (*A*, *B*), obtained before (*A*) and after 6 months (*B*) of therapy with tyrosine-kinase inhibitors in a 62-year-old man with metachronous clear-cell renal cell carcinoma metastasis located in left infratemporal fossa (*asterisk*). Despite no signs of tumor shrinkage detectable after 6 months of therapy, coronal iodine-overlay follow-up imaging (*D*) shows a reduction of iodine uptake compared with the baseline examination (*C*) as a potential indicator of response to treatment.

Virtual unenhanced imaging

VUE imaging has been widely demonstrated to be quantitatively and qualitatively comparable to conventional unenhanced single-energy MDCT.[31,32] VUE HU numbers have been shown to be reproducible and similar to actual noncontrast attenuation numbers in multiple studies, not only in the various anatomic regions of head and neck but also in areas of histologic change that may lead to low attenuation (eg, liquid components, fat, or necrosis), intermediate attenuation (eg, solid components or debris), or high-attenuation areas (eg, hemorrhagic or protein-rich content, or

calcification) (**Fig. 6**). Application of this technique may allow for omitting the unenhanced scan and thus allow for substantial radiation dose savings in current clinically used head and neck MDCT protocols that include an initial noncontrast scan.

Energy-specific Applications

Virtual monoenergetic image

Using a different approach than the above-mentioned techniques, virtual monochromatic imaging (VMI; or virtual monoenergetic imaging) allows for calculating DECT spectral datasets

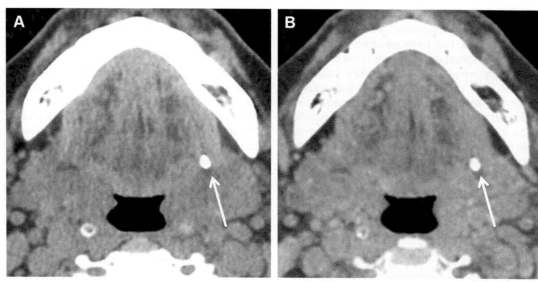

Fig. 6. An axial true unenhanced image (*A*) and VUE image (*B*) derived from contrast-enhanced DECT examination (not shown) in a 66-year-old woman with clinically suspected sialolithiasis. Both images clearly demonstrate a salivary stone in the hilum of left submandibular gland (*arrow*). As there is no discernible difference between the true unenhanced and VUE images, radiation dose could be reduced by omitting the unenhanced scan from a protocol designed for evaluation of salivary gland stones. (Courtesy of Dr Reza Forghani, Jewish General Hospital and McGill University, Montreal, Quebec, Canada.)

at a hypothetical fixed monochromatic energetic value reported in kiloelectron volt (keV). Such reconstructions can be generated directly from high- and low-kVp sinograms, before images are reconstructed (*data-domain* or *projection-space decomposition:* typically used by fast-kVp switching DECT platforms) or after high- and low-kV images are acquired (*image-domain decomposition:* typically used by dual-source platforms).[14,33,34] Information from such datasets also allows for the evaluation of the material composition in each voxel on the basis of either a 2-material or a 3-material decomposition technique.

VMI is more flexible than blending algorithms; it allows for a marked reduction of beam-hardening artifacts when using high keV levels and demonstrates the strongest iodine attenuation at the lowest virtual energy levels (eg, 40 keV), although at the cost of marked increase in image noise for most DECT platforms.[35,36] Finally, VMIs can be reconstructed automatically at a predetermined keV level without the need for time-consuming manual input.

Virtual monoenergetic image+

A noise-optimized advanced image-based reconstruction algorithm (VMI+ or Monoenergetic+; Siemens Healthcare, Forchheim, Germany) has been recently developed to overcome the limitations of traditional VMIs related to high-image noise

present on low-keV reconstructed VMIs.[37] This novel application consists of a *"frequency-split" decomposition* of the 2 spectral datasets and of a regional spatial frequency-based recombination of the high attenuation values at low energies with the noise-optimized properties of medium energy levels.[37] In phantom studies, the VMI+ algorithm demonstrated the highest contrast-to-noise ratio (CNR) at 40 keV, with a gradual decline as keV levels increased.[37,38] Consecutive phantom and clinical studies focused on the ability of this algorithm to improve image quality in examinations with low contrast and demonstrated that in a direct comparison between VMI and VMI+, the latter algorithm provided drastically higher CNR and signal-to-noise ratio (SNR).[39,40] More recent studies reported even an improvement of diagnostic accuracy when using VMI+ in DECT angiography.[41]

Oncologic

In the oncologic setting, VMI applications have been used to evaluate tumor conspicuity as well as to diagnose and distinguish metastatic lymph nodes in the head and neck.[16,19,20,42] Through the observation of the slope of spectral HU curves, calculated as the difference of the attenuation values between lower- and higher-keV images, several investigators demonstrated a better accuracy in depicting tumor conspicuity in head and neck squamous cell carcinoma.[16,17,42] Although the optimal energy level VMI for routine diagnostic evaluation of the head and neck has been reported to be 65 to 70 keV, the highest attenuation and the best tumor conspicuity were seen at lower keV values (ie, 40 keV).[17,42] These results were subsequently confirmed by the recently introduced noise-optimized VMI+ algorithm, in which the limitation of an increased noise at lower keV values has been lessened (**Fig. 7**).[16] Similar results have been reported for the evaluation of lymph nodes, in which the observation of the slope changes may help to diagnose and differentiate nodal metastases.[19,20,43]

Vascular

Multiple studies have demonstrated the beneficial value of DECT in vascular imaging, with particular regard to VMIs.[35,44–46] For traditional VMIs, the optimal energy level for the analysis of vessel anatomy has been reported to be 50 to 60 keV.[44–46] For the noise-optimized VMI+ algorithm, energy levels of 40 to 50 keV have been suggested to maximize intravascular contrast.[44–46] However, the use of higher keV levels (eg, 80–100 keV) may be useful to provide artifact-free images of the perivascular anatomic zone or allow for a better evaluation of plaque calcifications.[47]

Calcified plaques remain a problem in vascular CT because of the blooming effect of calcifications, which can obscure the vessel lumen as well as the lipid core.[27] Using VMIs at different keV ranges, Mannelli and colleagues[47] were able to demonstrate that an energy level of 80 keV best depicted the size of carotid plaque calcifications, similar to the histology reference standard. The technique and VMI reconstructions used in that study may improve the assessment of carotid calcium burden by overcoming limitations due to blooming artifacts.

Because of its ability to drastically increase the attenuation of intravascular contrast, VMI and VMI+ have also been used to reduce the amount of contrast material administered without compromising image quality.[44] Such benefits may be particularly important in patients with impaired renal function in whom contrast-enhanced CT may otherwise be contraindicated.

Artifact reduction

Reconstructing DECT datasets using VMIs at high keV level may also be a promising tool for improving lesion assessment in areas obscured by artifacts, especially the oral cavity.[48,49] Given the high prevalence of dental restorations in the

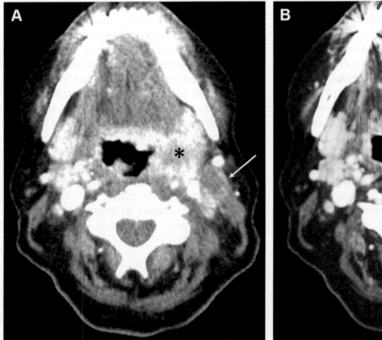

Fig. 7. Axial 40-keV standard VMI (*A*) and 40-keV noise-optimized VMI+ dataset (*B*) in a patient with advanced oropharyngeal squamous cell carcinoma (*asterisk*) and metastatic enlarged left level IIA lymph node (*arrow*) (*same patient as in* Fig. 3). Note the drastically reduced image noise of the VMI+ image compared with standard VMI, which allows for better tumor conspicuity and better delineation of the tumor margins relative to the adjacent soft tissues.

general population, there can be significant associated artifacts and image degradation, which can also vary greatly depending on the amount and type of dental material used. VMIs can improve image quality by reducing beam-hardening artifacts, with a better assessment of screws or the hardware-bone interface.[49] To date, there is no established consensus regarding the optimal VMI energy level for reduction of artifacts related to metallic hardware. Studies evaluating orthopedic hardware have found the optimal VMI energy level to be greater than 90 to 110 keV on "fast-kVp switching" DECT, and between 95 and 150 keV on "dual-source" DECT.[50–52]

However, when it comes to choosing the optimal energy level for VMI, another variable that should be considered is the location of the target region and composition of the tissue of interest. For example, if the observer needs to assess the bone texture in an area obscured by artifacts, the optimal approach may include using higher keV values, approaching or even exceeding 140 keV. On the other hand, if the aim is to better visualize the enhancement of a soft tissue tumor obscured by artifacts, then intermediate energy levels (eg, 90 keV) may be necessary in order to balance artifact reduction with the decreased contrast attenuation present on higher keV images.

Similar considerations may be appropriate in the setting of cervical spinal implants. CT imaging may be required when complications of the hardware are suspected (eg, malposition, loosening, disruption), and in such cases, a clear depiction of the spine and spinal canal can be challenging. In patients with spinal transpedicular screw fixation, Guggenberger and colleagues[50] reported an optimal image quality and artifact reduction using high keV VMI with an optimum level between 120 and 140 keV. In particular, monochromatic images at 110 keV or higher were beneficial in the reduction of streak artifacts and enabled a much better visualization of the hardware-bone interface compared with 70-keV images (considered to be the most similar to 120-kVp single-energy CT). They also stated that keV values in VMI should be individually tailored, according to the brand of the implants and type of material used. Finally, novel iterative reconstruction algorithms can further contribute to artifact reduction and may be combined with DECT (**Fig. 8**).[53]

SUMMARY

DECT and its specific algorithms and applications have been increasingly recognized in scientific studies and have been applied in clinical practice, particularly because of their beneficial impact on

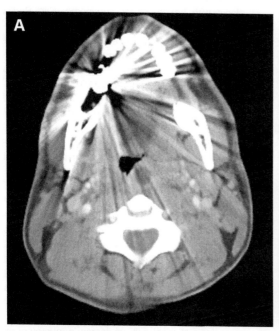
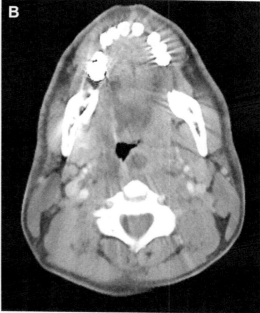

Fig. 8. Axial single-energy CT image before (*A*) and after (*B*) the application of iterative metal artifact reduction reconstruction resulting in noticeable reduction of beam-hardening artifacts from dental implants in a patient with oropharyngeal squamous cell carcinoma. (Courtesy of Dr Jakob Weiss, University Hospital Tübingen, Tübingen, Germany.)

image quality and lesion contrast in head and neck malignancy. Depending on the DECT system and generation of the scanner used, most postprocessing applications for DECT including VMI/VMI+ can be applied automatically in routine clinical practice to each imaging study without additional manual input, in order to provide images with substantially increased contrast or images highlighting other clinical features of interest. These techniques can therefore also be expected to allow for a reduction of contrast material, especially in patients with impaired renal function.

DECT may also provide additional information over standard purely attenuation-based CT imaging without any dose penalty as a material- and spectral-specific imaging method, in which iodine may be quantified as a "biological tracer" in order to accurately detect tumor conspicuity and grade of invasion, to differentiate inflammatory from neoplastic lymph nodes, or to even demonstrate early response to therapy that may go beyond macroscopic tumor reduction. Therefore, and considering all of the emerging applications of DECT in the head and neck, DECT is likely to play an increasingly important role for the diagnostic evaluation of different head and neck abnormalities.

REFERENCES

1. Marin D, Boll DT, Mileto A, et al. State of the art: dual-energy CT of the abdomen. Radiology 2014;271(2):327–42.

2. Vlahos I, Chung R, Nair A, et al. Vascular applications. AJR Am J Roentgenol 2012;199(5 Suppl):S87–97.

3. Johnson TR. Dual-energy CT: general principles. AJR Am J Roentgenol 2012;199(5 Suppl):S3–8.

4. Martin SS, Vogl TJ, Wichmann JL. Dual-energy CT post-processing applications. Curr Radiol Rep 2015;3(9):33.

5. Tawfik AM, Kerl JM, Razek AA, et al. Image quality and radiation dose of dual-energy CT of the head and neck compared with a standard 120-kVp acquisition. AJNR Am J Neuroradiol 2011;32(11):1994–9.

6. Yu L, Primak AN, Liu X, et al. Image quality optimization and evaluation of linearly mixed images in dual-source, dual-energy CT. Med Phys 2009;36(3):1019–24.

7. Tawfik AM, Kerl JM, Bauer RW, et al. Dual-energy CT of head and neck cancer: average weighting of low- and high-voltage acquisitions to improve lesion delineation and image quality-initial clinical experience. Invest Radiol 2012;47(5):306–11.

8. Ascenti G, Krauss B, Mazziotti S, et al. Dual-energy computed tomography (DECT) in renal masses: nonlinear versus linear blending. Acad Radiol 2012;19(10):1186–93.

9. Mileto A, Ramirez-Giraldo JC, Marin D, et al. Nonlinear image blending for dual-energy MDCT of the abdomen: can image quality be preserved if the contrast medium dose is reduced? AJR Am J Roentgenol 2014;203(4):838–45.

10. Kartje JK, Schmidt B, Bruners P, et al. Dual energy CT with nonlinear image blending improves visualization of delayed myocardial contrast enhancement in acute myocardial infarction. Invest Radiol 2013;48(1):41–5.

11. Wichmann JL, Hu X, Kerl JM, et al. Non-linear blending of dual-energy CT data improves depiction of late iodine enhancement in chronic myocardial infarction. Int J Cardiovasc Imaging 2014;30(6):1145–50.

12. Holmes DR 3rd, Fletcher JG, Apel A, et al. Evaluation of non-linear blending in dual-energy computed tomography. Eur J Radiol 2008;68(3):409–13.

13. Scholtz JE, Husers K, Kaup M, et al. Non-linear image blending improves visualization of head and neck primary squamous cell carcinoma compared to linear blending in dual-energy CT. Clin Radiol 2015;70(2):168–75.

14. Yu L, Leng S, McCollough CH. Dual-energy CT-based monochromatic imaging. AJR Am J Roentgenol 2012;199(5 Suppl):S9–15.

15. Ascenti G, Sofia C, Mazziotti S, et al. Dual-energy CT with iodine quantification in distinguishing between bland and neoplastic portal vein thrombosis in patients with hepatocellular carcinoma. Clin Radiol 2016;71(9):938.e1–9.

16. Lam S, Gupta R, Kelly H, et al. Multiparametric evaluation of head and neck squamous cell carcinoma using a single-source dual-energy CT with fast kVp switching: state of the art. Cancer 2015;7(4):2201–16.

17. Forghani R. Advanced dual-energy CT for head and neck cancer imaging. Expert Rev Anticancer Ther 2015;15(12):1489–501.

18. Kuno H, Onaya H, Iwata R, et al. Evaluation of cartilage invasion by laryngeal and hypopharyngeal squamous cell carcinoma with dual-energy CT. Radiology 2012;265(2):488–96.

19. Tawfik AM, Razek AA, Kerl JM, et al. Comparison of dual-energy CT-derived iodine content and iodine overlay of normal, inflammatory and metastatic squamous cell carcinoma cervical lymph nodes. Eur Radiol 2014;24(3):574–80.

20. Yang L, Luo D, Li L, et al. Differentiation of malignant cervical lymphadenopathy by dual-energy CT: a preliminary analysis. Sci Rep 2016;6:31020.

21. D'Angelo T, Blandino A, Ascenti G, et al. Solitary metastasis of renal cell carcinoma in infratemporal fossa. Clin Imaging 2015;39(1):155–7.

22. Schmid-Bindert G, Henzler T, Chu TQ, et al. Functional imaging of lung cancer using dual energy

CT: how does iodine related attenuation correlate with standardized uptake value of 18FDG-PET-CT? Eur Radiol 2012;22(1):93–103.

23. Meyer M, Hohenberger P, Apfaltrer P, et al. CT-based response assessment of advanced gastrointestinal stromal tumor: dual energy CT provides a more predictive imaging biomarker of clinical benefit than RECIST or Choi criteria. Eur J Radiol 2013; 82(6):923–8.

24. Apfaltrer P, Meyer M, Meier C, et al. Contrast-enhanced dual-energy CT of gastrointestinal stromal tumors: is iodine-related attenuation a potential indicator of tumor response? Invest Radiol 2012;47(1): 65–70.

25. Mazziotti S, Blandino A, Gaeta M, et al. Postprocessing in maxillofacial multidetector computed tomography. Can Assoc Radiol J 2015;66(3):212–22.

26. Uotani K, Watanabe Y, Higashi M, et al. Dual-energy CT head bone and hard plaque removal for quantification of calcified carotid stenosis: utility and comparison with digital subtraction angiography. Eur Radiol 2009;19(8):2060–5.

27. Morhard D, Fink C, Graser A, et al. Cervical and cranial computed tomographic angiography with automated bone removal: dual energy computed tomography versus standard computed tomography. Invest Radiol 2009;44(5):293–7.

28. Watanabe Y, Uotani K, Nakazawa T, et al. Dual-energy direct bone removal CT angiography for evaluation of intracranial aneurysm or stenosis: comparison with conventional digital subtraction angiography. Eur Radiol 2009;19(4):1019–24.

29. Na D, Hong SJ, Yoon MA, et al. Spinal bone bruise: can computed tomography (CT) enable accurate diagnosis? Acad Radiol 2016;23(11):1376–83.

30. Bierry G, Venkatasamy A, Kremer S, et al. Dual-energy CT in vertebral compression fractures: performance of visual and quantitative analysis for bone marrow edema demonstration with comparison to MRI. Skeletal Radiol 2014;43(4):485–92.

31. Ferda J, Novak M, Mirka H, et al. The assessment of intracranial bleeding with virtual unenhanced imaging by means of dual-energy CT angiography. Eur Radiol 2009;19(10):2518–22.

32. Graser A, Johnson TR, Hecht EM, et al. Dual-energy CT in patients suspected of having renal masses: can virtual nonenhanced images replace true nonenhanced images? Radiology 2009;252(2):433–40.

33. Yu L, Christner JA, Leng S, et al. Virtual monochromatic imaging in dual-source dual-energy CT: radiation dose and image quality. Med Phys 2011;38(12): 6371–9.

34. Alvarez RE, Macovski A. Energy-selective reconstructions in X-ray computerized tomography. Phys Med Biol 1976;21(5):733–44.

35. Sudarski S, Apfaltrer P, Nance JW Jr, et al. Optimization of keV-settings in abdominal and lower extremity

36. Meinel FG, Bischoff B, Zhang Q, et al. Metal artifact reduction by dual-energy computed tomography using energetic extrapolation: a systematically optimized protocol. Invest Radiol 2012;47(7):406–14.

37. Grant KL, Flohr TG, Krauss B, et al. Assessment of an advanced image-based technique to calculate virtual monoenergetic computed tomographic images from a dual-energy examination to improve contrast-to-noise ratio in examinations using iodinated contrast media. Invest Radiol 2014;49(9): 586–92.

38. Bongers MN, Schabel C, Krauss B, et al. Noise-optimized virtual monoenergetic images and iodine maps for the detection of venous thrombosis in second-generation dual-energy CT (DECT): an ex vivo phantom study. Eur Radiol 2015;25(6): 1655–64.

39. Schabel C, Bongers M, Sedlmair M, et al. Assessment of the hepatic veins in poor contrast conditions using dual energy CT: evaluation of a novel monoenergetic extrapolation software algorithm. Rofo 2014;186(6):591–7.

40. Albrecht MH, Scholtz JE, Kraft J, et al. Assessment of an advanced monoenergetic reconstruction technique in dual-energy computed tomography of head and neck cancer. Eur Radiol 2015;25(8):2493–501.

41. Wichmann JL, Gillott MR, De Cecco CN, et al. Dual-energy computed tomography angiography of the lower extremity runoff: impact of noise-optimized virtual monochromatic imaging on image quality and diagnostic accuracy. Invest Radiol 2016;51(2): 139–46.

42. Lam S, Gupta R, Levental M, et al. Optimal virtual monochromatic images for evaluation of normal tissues and head and neck cancer using dual-energy CT. AJNR Am J Neuroradiol 2015;36(8): 1518–24.

43. Liang H, Li A, Li Y, et al. A retrospective study of dual-energy CT for clinical detecting of metastatic cervical lymph nodes in laryngeal and hypopharyngeal squamous cell carcinoma. Acta Otolaryngol 2015;135(7):722–8.

44. Delesalle MA, Pontana F, Duhamel A, et al. Spectral optimization of chest CT angiography with reduced iodine load: experience in 80 patients evaluated with dual-source, dual-energy CT. Radiology 2013; 267(1):256–66.

45. Schneider D, Apfaltrer P, Sudarski S, et al. Optimization of kiloelectron volt settings in cerebral and cervical dual-energy CT angiography determined with virtual monoenergetic imaging. Acad Radiol 2014; 21(4):431–6.

46. Apfaltrer P, Sudarski S, Schneider D, et al. Value of monoenergetic low-kV dual energy CT datasets for

improved image quality of CT pulmonary angiography. Eur J Radiol 2014;83(2):322–8.

47. Mannelli L, Mitsumori LM, Ferguson M, et al. Changes in measured size of atherosclerotic plaque calcifications in dual-energy CT of ex vivo carotid endarterectomy specimens: effect of monochromatic keV image reconstructions. Eur Radiol 2013; 23(2):367–74.

48. Mazziotti S, Pandolfo I, D'Angelo T, et al. Diagnostic approach to retromolar trigone cancer by multiplanar computed tomography reconstructions. Can Assoc Radiol J 2014;65(4):335–44.

49. De Crop A, Casselman J, Van Hoof T, et al. Analysis of metal artifact reduction tools for dental hardware in CT scans of the oral cavity: kVp, iterative reconstruction, dual-energy CT, metal artifact reduction software: does it make a difference? Neuroradiology 2015;57(8):841–9.

50. Guggenberger R, Winklhofer S, Osterhoff G, et al. Metallic artefact reduction with monoenergetic dual-energy CT: systematic ex vivo evaluation of posterior spinal fusion implants from various vendors and different spine levels. Eur Radiol 2012; 22(11):2357–64.

51. Komlosi P, Grady D, Smith JS, et al. Evaluation of monoenergetic imaging to reduce metallic instrumentation artifacts in computed tomography of the cervical spine. J Neurosurg Spine 2015;22(1):34–8.

52. Mangold S, Gatidis S, Luz O, et al. Single-source dual-energy computed tomography: use of monoenergetic extrapolation for a reduction of metal artifacts. Invest Radiol 2014;49(12):788–93.

53. Weiss J, Schabel C, Bongers M, et al. Impact of iterative metal artifact reduction on diagnostic image quality in patients with dental hardware. Acta Radiol 2016;58(3):279–85.

Dual Energy Computed Tomography Applications for the Evaluation of the Spine

Peter Komlosi, MD, PhD[a],*, Max Wintermark, MD, MAS[b]

KEYWORDS

- Dual-energy computed tomography • Spine • Osteoporosis • Bone marrow • Trauma
- Bone mineral density

KEY POINTS

- Dual-energy computed tomography (CT) is a rapid and relatively inexpensive tool used to recognize marrow edema associated with acute traumatic injuries to the spine.
- Dual-energy CT can assess marrow infiltration in patients who have contraindications to MR imaging.
- Cancellous bone mineral density measurement with dual-energy CT may be a sensitive biomarker for fracture risk in patients with osteoporosis.
- Monosodium urate deposition imaging with dual-energy CT is an accurate diagnostic technique that can be used to improve our understanding of the spinal manifestations of gout.

INTRODUCTION

The spinal column encompasses in close proximity materials with vastly differing x-ray attenuation characteristics (dense cortical bone, cancellous bone, cerebrospinal fluid and, in postoperative patients, surgical metallic instruments), traditionally rendering this part of the body challenging to image with computed tomography (CT).

Dual-energy CT enables material characterization and differentiation, based on high- and low-peak voltage acquisitions. Materials with equal or near equal attenuation at a certain single energy peak voltage may be differentiated by analyzing energy-dependent changes of their attenuation. This article provides an overview of the major novel indications of dual-energy CT in the evaluation of the diseases of the spinal column.

BONE MINERAL DENSITY IMAGING

Osteoporosis, or loss of bone mass and strength, is a major risk factor for disability. Dual x-ray absorptiometry is the most ubiquitous diagnostic tool to assess bone mineral density; however, it is unable to differentiate cortical and cancellous bone, with the latter being primarily affected by the disease. Single-energy CT provides excellent spatial resolution, but quantification is difficult owing to beam-hardening artifact, x-ray scatter, and the confounding effect of varying amount of fatty bone marrow.[1] Early studies using sequential dual-energy CT yielded improved accuracy, but were limited by motion and misregistration.[2,3] The advent of simultaneous dual-energy scanners allows for significant reduction in beam-hardening artifact and more accurate separation of bone and

Disclosure Statement: M. Wintermark serves on the advisory board of the GE-NFL initiative. P. Komlosi has nothing to disclose.
[a] Department of Radiology, University of Pittsburgh, 200 Lothrop Street, 2nd Floor, Suite 200 East Wing, Pittsburgh, PA 15213, USA; [b] Department of Radiology, Stanford University School of Medicine, 300 Pasteur Drive, S047 MC 5105, Stanford, CA 94305, USA
* Corresponding author.
E-mail address: komlosip@upmc.edu

Neuroimag Clin N Am 27 (2017) 483–487
http://dx.doi.org/10.1016/j.nic.2017.04.003

marrow attenuation.[4] Owing to the volumetric nature of the technique, measurement of trabecular bone mineral density can be achieved, providing a sensitive biomarker to predict fracture risk in postmenopausal women. Dual-energy CT acquisition has also been evaluated for use in radiation therapy planning to predict proton stopping power in the vicinity of the spine.[5]

BONE MARROW IMAGING

Unenhanced single-energy CT frequently yields equivocal results in patients with suspected osteoporotic vertebral compression fractures. MR imaging is the standard for the noninvasive assessment of marrow abnormalities and can depict bone marrow edema and hemorrhages, and may clarify the diagnosis in this situation. However, issues with access and safety screening may lead to delays in the final diagnosis and ultimate treatment; in addition, MR imaging is more costly. Patients with contraindications to MR imaging (such as certain implanted devices or noncooperative patients) may benefit from CT marrow imaging as an alternative way to determine the acuity of the fracture.

Recent studies have shown that bone marrow edema after acute trauma of the spine can be detected by using the so-called virtual noncalcium technique.[6,7] Virtual noncalcium dual-energy CT can accurately depict bone marrow edema in patients with osteoporosis with acute vertebral fractures, with good correlation with MR imaging.[8] In 1 study, dual-energy–based bone marrow edema visualization significantly improved the detection rate of acute fractures and was helpful for differentiating them from older fractures compared with single-energy CT images. The investigators also found that a significant number of MR examinations could be avoided using the virtual noncalcium information. This finding is promising in light of numerous studies indicating dose-equivalence of dual-energy acquisition as compared with standard CT scans.[9-11]

Seronegative spondyloarthritis is a chronic inflammatory rheumatologic disease with sacroiliitis as the earliest clinical finding. A recent study demonstrated that dual-energy CT scanning not only depicts findings of chronic sacroiliitis (ie, bone erosion and sclerosis), but also can detect and quantify the extent of marrow edema in the subchondral bone.[12,13]

CT scanning is the primary modality in cancer staging owing to its wide availability, relatively low cost, short scanning times, and consequent high patient tolerance. A major limitation of standard CT scanning is its lower sensitivity for the detection of nonlytic bone marrow infiltration in the axial skeleton, where visualization and measurement of bone marrow attenuation are severely hampered by the dense trabecular structure of the cancellous bone. A recent study has demonstrated that bone marrow images created from dual-energy CT scanning datasets of the spine have the potential to improve the sensitivity for the detection of diffuse bone marrow infiltration in patients with multiple myeloma, especially in cases with high-grade infiltration (**Fig. 1**).[14] It remains elusive how the presence of iodine-based contrast might affect the quality of this virtual noncalcium technique. Patients with multifocal nodular bone marrow involvement may also benefit from dual-energy CT–guided bone marrow sampling.

POSTOPERATIVE SPINE

Metallic instrumentation interferes with the quality of single-energy CT imaging because of beam hardening (owing to the preferential absorption of low energy or "soft" x-rays in the polyenergetic x-ray beam spectrum as x-rays pass through the body), photon starvation, and scatter artifacts (caused by their high x-ray attenuation coefficient). Despite advances in detector technology and optimized image reconstruction, artifacts from metal implants remain a problem. Dual-energy CT scanning, allowing for analysis of energy-dependent changes in the attenuation of different materials, has been proposed as a means to reduce beam-hardening metal artifacts by generating virtual monoenergetic images.[15-17] It has been demonstrated that reconstruction of images at higher extrapolated monoenergetic x-ray energies significantly diminishes (without completely eliminating) the artifacts radially projecting from the hardware, however, at the expense of diminished soft tissue contrast.[18] A recently published reconstruction technique combines the benefits of multiple reconstructed monochromatic datasets[19] by blending the superior soft tissue and iodine contrast conspicuity at lower energies and the reduced noise and metallic artifact at medium energy images. Dual-energy CT myelography and virtual myelography are other opportunities to reduce radiation dose and minimize artifact in patients with prior osteosynthesis.[20] The assessment of the postoperative spine in patients with metallic instrumentation and various measures to reduce metallic artifact is discussed in detail (See Eric Liao and Ashok Srinivasan's article, "Applications of Dual Energy CT for Artifact Reduction in the Head, Neck, and Spine," in this issue).

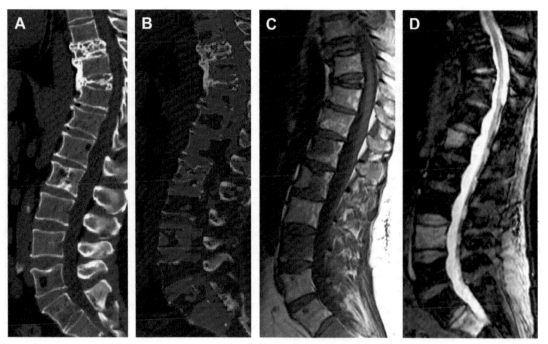

Fig. 1. Conventional computed tomography (CT) image (*A*), virtual noncalcium bone marrow overlay (*B*), T1-weighted MR imaging (*C*), and T2*-weighted MR imaging (*D*) images from a patient with multiple myeloma. The bone marrow image is displayed as color overlay with red and blue voxels indicating positive and negative signal, respectively. Red voxels in the bone marrow image represent medullary infiltration, which is not detectable on conventional CT. (*Adapted from* Thomas C, Schabel C, Krauss B, et al. Dual-energy CT: virtual calcium subtraction for assessment of bone marrow involvement of the spine in multiple myeloma. AJR Am J Roentgenol 2015;204(3):W328; with permission.)

URATE DEPOSITION IMAGING

Gout is a debilitating disease affecting primarily the musculoskeletal system, most commonly the first metatarsophalangeal joint, knees, ankles, wrist, and hand joints. The incidence of spinal gout remains elusive, but is thought to be more common than previously believed (possibly approaching 50% in patients with clinically appreciated tophi). Back pain can be the first manifestation of gouty symptoms.[21] MR imaging and single photon CT scanning are sensitive but nonspecific modalities for the identification of spinal gout. The classic imaging hallmarks of the disease on single photon CT are bone or joint erosions with well-defined sclerotic margins, facet or intervertebral new bone formation, or juxtaarticular or intraarticular masses that are denser than the surrounding muscle. Deposition of monosodium urate in cartilage and the intervertebral discs of the cervical and lumbar spine has been described, and may give rise to compressive myelopathy and spinal pain.[22,23]

The basis material decomposition feature of dual-energy CT scanning allows effective differentiation of tophi from other types of masses (**Fig. 2**).[24] The sensitivity and specificity of dual-energy CT scans in identifying gouty tophi was reported to be 92% and 85%, respectively, compared with the reference standard of crystal identification by means of polarized light microscopy.[25] However, dual-energy CT scans may be less sensitive at identifying diffuse as opposed to focal lesions.[26] Another study reported that monosodium urate signal within the intervertebral disks may be seen physiologically in older men and might not be a gout-specific finding.[27]

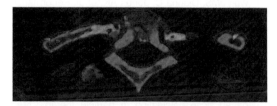

Fig. 2. Dual-energy axial computed tomography (CT) monosodium urate image showing costovertebral crystal deposition (*green*) at the level of the upper thoracic spine. (*Adapted from* Dhaese S, Stryckers M, Van Der Meersch H, et al. Gouty arthritis of the spine in a renal transplant patient: a clinical case report: an unusual presentation of a common disorder. Medicine (Baltimore) 2015;94(13):e676; with permission.)

Further studies are warranted to determine whether the sensitivity and specificity of dual-energy CT is sufficient to obviate the need for invasive procedures and tissue diagnosis in the case of a spinal mass suspicious for gout. In patients with gout who present with back pain unresponsive to conservative measures, crystal deposition in the spine should be high on the list of differentials, and dual-energy CT scanning, if available, should be considered in the workup of the patient.

SUMMARY

In this article, different dual-energy CT scanning applications for the evaluation of the spine were reviewed. In addition to the traditional strengths of CT scanning for the evaluation of the spine, dual-energy CT scanning enables the generation of additional reconstructions and quantitative analysis not possible with conventional single-energy CT scanning, with a range of potential applications such as bone and iodinated contrast removal, artifact reduction, improved bone marrow imaging, and monosodium urate imaging. Dual-energy CT scanning has the potential to become a significant complement to our tool set to diagnose the disorders of the spinal column.

REFERENCES

1. Glüer CC, Genant HK. Impact of marrow fat on accuracy of quantitative CT. J Comput Assist Tomogr 1989;13(6):1023–35.
2. Genant HK, Boyd D. Quantitative bone mineral analysis using dual energy computed tomography. Invest Radiol 1977;12(6):545–51.
3. Laval-Jeantet AM, Cann CE, Roger B, et al. A postprocessing dual energy technique for vertebral CT densitometry. J Comput Assist Tomogr 1984;8(6):1164–7.
4. Wait JMS, Dianna C, Jones AK, et al. Performance evaluation of material decomposition with rapid-kilovoltage-switching dual-energy CT and implications for assessing bone mineral density. Am J Roentgenol 2015;204(6):1234–41.
5. Hünemohr N, Paganetti H, Greilich S, et al. Tissue decomposition from dual energy CT data for MC based dose calculation in particle therapy. Med Phys 2014;41(6):061714.
6. Wang CK, Tsai JM, Chuang MT, et al. Bone marrow edema in vertebral compression fractures: detection with dual-energy CT. Radiology 2013;269(2):525–33.
7. Bierry G, Venkatasamy A, Kremer S, et al. Dual-energy CT in vertebral compression fractures: performance of visual and quantitative analysis for bone marrow edema demonstration with comparison to MRI. Skeletal Radiol 2014;43(4):485–92.
8. Kaup M, Wichmann JL, Scholtz JE, et al. Dual-energy CT-based display of bone marrow edema in osteoporotic vertebral compression fractures: impact on diagnostic accuracy of radiologists with varying levels of experience in correlation to MR imaging. Radiology 2016;280(2):510–9.
9. Pache G, Bulla S, Baumann T, et al. Dose reduction does not affect detection of bone marrow lesions with dual-energy CT virtual non-calcium technique. Acad Radiol 2012;19(12):1539–45.
10. Bauer RW, Sebastian K, Matthias R, et al. Dose and image quality at CT pulmonary angiography—comparison of first and second generation dual-energy CT and 64-slice CT. Eur Radiol 2011;21(10):2139–47.
11. Schenzle JC, Sommer WH, Neumaier K, et al. Dual energy CT of the chest: how about the dose? Invest Radiol 2010;45(6):347–53.
12. Zhang P, Ping Z, Yu KH, et al. Comparing the diagnostic utility of sacroiliac spectral CT and MRI in axial spondyloarthritis. Br J Radiol 2016;89(1059):20150196.
13. Zhang P, Yu KH, Guo RM, et al. A novel diagnostic method (spectral computed tomography of sacroiliac joints) for axial spondyloarthritis. J Formos Med Assoc 2016;115(8):658–64.
14. Thomas C, Schabel C, Krauss B, et al. Dual-energy CT: virtual calcium subtraction for assessment of bone marrow involvement of the spine in multiple myeloma. AJR Am J Roentgenol 2015;204(3):W324–31.
15. Hemmingsson A, Jung B, Ytterbergh C. Dual energy computed tomography: simulated monoenergetic and material-selective imaging. J Comput Assist Tomogr 1986;10(3):490–9.
16. Bamberg F, Dierks A, Nikolaou K, et al. Metal artifact reduction by dual energy computed tomography using monoenergetic extrapolation. Eur Radiol 2011;21(7):1424–9.
17. Srinivasan A, Hoeffner E, Ibrahim M, et al. Utility of dual-energy CT virtual keV monochromatic series for the assessment of spinal transpedicular hardware-bone interface. AJR Am J Roentgenol 2013;201(4):878–83.
18. Komlosi P, Grady D, Smith JS, et al. Evaluation of monoenergetic imaging to reduce metallic instrumentation artifacts in computed tomography of the cervical spine. J Neurosurg Spine 2015;22(1):34–8.
19. Grant KL, Flohr TG, Krauss B, et al. Assessment of an advanced image-based technique to calculate virtual monoenergetic computed tomographic

images from a dual-energy examination to improve contrast-to-noise ratio in examinations using iodinated contrast media. Invest Radiol 2014;49(9): 586–92.

20. Grams AE, Sender J, Moritz R, et al. Dual energy CT myelography after lumbar osteosynthesis. Rofo 2014;186(7):670–4.
21. Toprover M, Krasnokutsky S, Pillinger MH. Gout in the spine: imaging, diagnosis, and outcomes. Curr Rheumatol Rep 2015;17(12):70.
22. Yen HL, Cheng CH, Lin JW. Cervical myelopathy due to gouty tophi in the intervertebral disc space. Acta Neurochir 2002;144(2):205–7.
23. Nygaard HB, Shenoi S, Shukla S. Lower back pain caused by tophaceous gout of the spine. Neurology 2009;73(5):404.
24. Dhaese S, Stryckers M, Van Der Meersch H, et al. Gouty arthritis of the spine in a renal transplant patient: a clinical case report: an unusual presentation of a common disorder. Medicine 2015;94(13):e676.
25. Hu HJ, Liao MY, Xu LY. Clinical utility of dual-energy CT for gout diagnosis. Clin Imaging 2015;39(5): 880–5.
26. Dalbeth N, House ME, Aati O, et al. Urate crystal deposition in asymptomatic hyperuricaemia and symptomatic gout: a dual energy CT study. Ann Rheum Dis 2015;74(5):908–11.
27. Carr A, Doyle AJ, Dalbeth N, et al. Dual-energy CT of urate deposits in costal cartilage and intervertebral disks of patients with tophaceous gout and age-matched controls. AJR Am J Roentgenol 2016; 206(5):1063–7.

Applications of Dual-Energy Computed Tomography for Artifact Reduction in the Head, Neck, and Spine

Eric Liao, MD, Ashok Srinivasan, MD*

KEYWORDS

• Dual-energy CT • Beam-hardening artifact reduction • Virtual monochromatic imaging
• Virtual subtraction imaging

KEY POINTS

- Conventional single-energy computed tomography, using a polychromatic energy beam, is susceptible to beam-hardening artifacts as well as photon-starvation effect, which can degrade image quality in the setting of implanted metallic hardware, dense osseous structures, and dense intravenous iodinated contrast.
- Dual-energy computed tomography, by analyzing the changes in attenuation of soft tissues at disparate energies, allows for the creation of virtual monochromatic images, which can significantly improve diagnostic image quality by reducing beam-hardening artifact.
- Dual-energy computed tomography, through the process of material decomposition, can be used to virtually eliminate osseous structures as well as intravenous iodinated contrast, allowing for improved visualization of the adjacent soft tissues of interest.

INTRODUCTION

The use of computed tomography (CT) scanning in medical imaging has become ubiquitous, with an estimated 85 million CT scans performed in 2011 alone.[1] Traditional single-energy CT is able to offer exquisite anatomic detail with high contrast and spatial resolution of the structures of the neck and spine. However, despite optimization of modern single-energy CT techniques, technical challenges remain that can significantly degrade the diagnostic quality of these examinations. Especially troublesome is the evaluation of soft tissue structures adjacent to postoperative metallic hardware, dense bony structures, and in the presence of dense contrast within central venous anatomy at the level of the thoracic inlet.

Metallic artifact, in the setting of a polychromatic CT beam, results from the phenomena of beam hardening and photon starvation.[2] Beam hardening occurs as the lower-energy photons of a polyenergetic beam are preferentially absorbed by high atomic number substances, including dense metallic implants. The resultant beam is subsequently composed of only higher-energy photons, resulting in lower tissue contrast immediately adjacent to the metallic implants. The absolute number

There are no financial disclosures for either author.
Division of Neuroradiology, Department of Radiology, University of Michigan Health System, 1500 East Medical Center Drive, Ann Arbor, MI 48109, USA
* Corresponding author.
E-mail address: ashoks@med.umich.edu

neuroimaging.theclinics.com

of photons in the resultant beam is also significantly decreased as photons are attenuated by the dense metallic implants. Consequently, an insufficient number of photons are able to reach the detector to provide adequate signal, resulting in significant noise within the adjacent soft tissues, termed the photon-starvation effect.

PRINCIPLES AND STRATEGIES FOR ARTIFACT REDUCTION

The advent of dual-energy CT (DECT) has offered radiologists an additional tool with which to combat and minimize the beam-hardening and photon-starvation artifacts associated with the presence of high atomic number materials, including implanted metal, dense intravenous contrast within central venous structures at the thoracic inlet level, and inherently dense bony structures. Whether through the use of dual-source, fast-kilovoltage switching, or dual-layer detection technology, DECT analyzes the changes in attenuation of different materials at 2 disparate energy levels, and subsequently uses a process termed material decomposition to generate monochromatic DECT images.[3] The methodology of image reconstruction varies based on the acquisition method, with single-source fast-kilovoltage switching images constructed from projection space data, whereas dual-source CT (where high-energy and lower-energy acquisitions are not coincident with each other in a helical acquisition) uses image domain material decomposition.[4] A more in-depth discussion of different DECT systems and DECT postprocessing can be found in the first 2 articles in this issue (See Reza Forghani and colleagues' article, "Dual Energy CT: Physical Principles, Approaches to Scanning, Usage, and Implementation - Part 1," and Reza Forghani and colleagues' article, "Dual Energy CT: Physical Principles, Approaches to Scanning, Usage, and Implementation - Part 2," in this issue).

Virtual Monochromatic Series

In both techniques, the differential attenuation detected at lower-energy and higher-energy spectra can be used to generate mass density maps of the imaged tissues from which monochromatic images can be synthesized, and that are accurate for a wide range of atomic numbers. Monochromatic images can thus be generated for multiple different photon energy levels, to simulate how an image would look if the x-rays produced were solely of that single chosen energy level.[5] *Of considerable interest is the ability of the radiologist to choose a virtual monochromatic image (VMI) at an optimal energy level that yields the best contrast-to-noise ratio while minimizing beam-hardening artifact.* Although lower-energy imaging remains susceptible to metallic artifact (thought to be related to additional factors, such as photon starvation and nonlinear partial volume averaging), multiple studies have demonstrated virtual elimination of streak artifact adjacent to postoperative implants by using higher-energy monochromatic energies of greater than approximately 95 keV.[3,6–8]

It is not only the higher-energy VMIs that provide diagnostic benefit, however. Lower-energy monochromatic images still maintain superior tissue contrast, which can be of particular benefit in traditionally difficult to visualize regions, such as the posterior fossa, where evaluation of the parenchymal soft tissues is of primary importance. VMIs with energies in the 65-keV to 75-keV range can provide maximal signal-to-noise and contrast-to-noise ratios in the brain, while diminishing beam-hardening and streak artifacts associated with a polychromatic beam.[9] Thus, VMIs created from DECT data have the potential to markedly reduce beam-hardening artifacts and ameliorate the concomitant photon-starvation effect that degrades evaluation of the head, neck, and spine associated with a polychromatic beam. This can markedly improve the diagnostic evaluation in the setting of postoperative metallic implantation, as well as within inherently problematic areas to image, such as the posterior fossa.

Material Decomposition

The process of material decomposition also allows for the identification of tissue composition within the acquired images. This allows for the creation of material-specific images, which can show the distribution and concentration of a given material within the imaged soft tissues, and consequently also allows for the virtual elimination of the contributed attenuation of the selected material.[3] These subtraction images can allow for the formation of virtual images of the head and neck with materials such as iodinated contrast or osseous structures eliminated, improving visualization of the soft tissues immediately adjacent to these dense materials.[10] This demonstrates clinical applicability in the virtual elimination of intravenous contrast and improved visualization of the intracranial vasculature adjacent to dense osseous structures, such as the skull base.

ARTIFACT-REDUCTION STRATEGIES

In this section, different clinical applications and artifact-reduction strategies are discussed. At this time, there is no widely accepted optimal absolute energy for high-energy VMIs, and it is likely that the optimal energy can vary based on the specific application and the extent of artifact. However, some general principles should be kept in mind and can provide guidance in these applications. With increasing energy above the standard single-energy equivalent VMIs, there is greater artifact reduction but also suppression of iodine attenuation and soft tissue contrast. Therefore, for applications in which some degree of preservation of soft tissue contrast and iodine attenuation is desired, high-energy VMIs in the intermediate range, approximately close to 95 keV, may be preferred. On the other hand, in cases in which preservation of soft tissue contrast and iodine attenuation is not as important, VMIs reconstructed at higher energies than 95 keV, which can approach 140 keV or greater depending on the DECT system, may provide the best results.

BEAM HARDENING
Posterior Fossa

Utilization of virtual monochromatic series can be helpful in reduction of beam-hardening effects in the posterior intracranial compartment that commonly involve the brainstem and provide a better visualization of the anatomy (**Fig. 1**).

Aneurysm Coils and Clips

Postoperative evaluation of intracranial aneurysms following coil embolization or surgical clipping is of critical importance on follow-up examinations. Endovascular treatment of intracranial aneurysms has become an increasingly successful approach to the treatment of ruptured and nonruptured aneurysms. However, the recurrence rate of aneurysms following aneurysm coiling is markedly higher in the endovascular versus postoperative setting, with reported rates ranging from 10% to 40% in the literature,[11] and a more recent meta-analysis reporting an approximate recurrence rate of 20.8% of endovascular cases, requiring retreatment in 10.3% of cases.[12] Although treated aneurysms are often followed with conventional angiography, there is a real, albeit small, risk of neurologic complications associated with this interventional procedure.[13] Magnetic resonance (MR) angiography is an alternative examination used to evaluate patients with postoperative aneurysm. However, time of flight MR angiography can be limited by motion-related or flow-related artifacts and variable artifact from the coil material or clips, and a small subset of patients are unable to undergo MRI evaluation, such as those patients who have undergone placement of a non–MRI-compatible cardiac pacing device. For these patients, CT

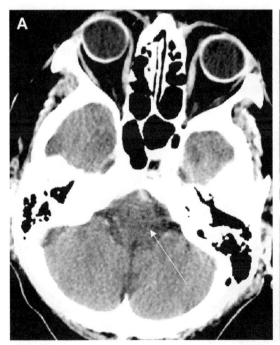
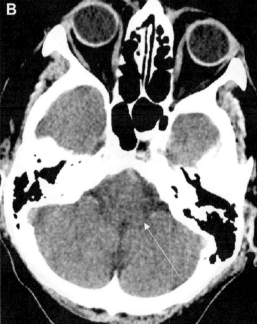

Fig. 1. Axial CT head image at 70 keV (single-energy CT equivalent) (*A*) demonstrates beam-hardening artifact overlying the lower brainstem (*arrow*). Virtual monochromatic axial CT head image at 90 keV (*B*) shows reduction of the artifact and better visualization of the brainstem anatomy (*arrow*).

angiography offers an alternate modality to evaluate intracranial vasculature in a noninvasive way. However, assessment of the soft tissues immediately adjacent to the aneurysm coil mass or clip, including any possible residual aneurysmal filling, also can be degraded due to the metallic streak artifact. Using higher monochromatic energy levels on DECT can help reduce this artifact and enable better visualization of the surrounding anatomy (**Figs. 2** and **3**). In the future, robust material density analysis algorithms could be used to selectively enhance iodine while suppressing metal, thereby providing a better visualization of recurrent or residual aneurysm opacification.

Dental Amalgam/Implants

Metallic streak artifact can also degrade evaluation of the oral cavity in the setting of dental hardware, limiting evaluation for infectious, inflammatory, and neoplastic etiologies for patient symptomatology.[14,15] Although not eliminating artifacts entirely, higher virtual monochromatic energy-level images can be very helpful in providing an improved visualization of oral cavity contents (**Figs. 4** and **5**). A more detailed discussion of the head and neck applications of DECT can be found in other articles in this issue.

Spine Hardware

One of the more common applications of CT in the neck and spine region is the postoperative evaluation of surgical hardware in the spine. Persistent back pain following spinal stabilization is a challenging diagnostic dilemma in postoperative patients, and adequate assessment of implanted hardware for complications, including hardware fracture, displacement, and loosening,[16] is often degraded on diagnostic single-energy CT due to metallic streak artifact. However, assessment of the margins of the surgical hardware remains a primary consideration on these examinations, as the incidence of screw loosening is not uncommon (with reported average rates ranging from 7.8% to 11.7%[17]), and surgical options to alleviate the symptoms associated with loosening can result in significant improvement in patient pain. **Figs. 6–8** demonstrate reduction of artifacts associated with spinal transpedicular hardware with improved visualization of the interface between bone and metal; there is also improved visualization of the spinal canal contents on the accompanying CT myelogram, all of which have been achieved using high virtual monochromatic energy levels.

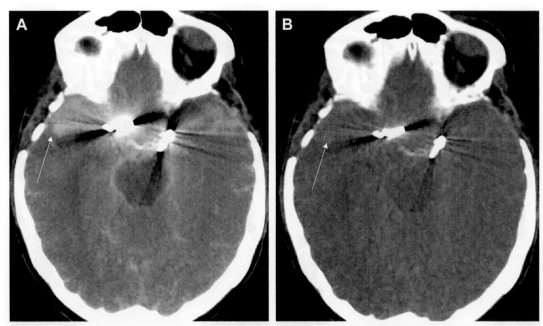

Fig. 2. Axial CT head image at 70 keV (single-energy CT equivalent) (*A*) demonstrates metallic streak artifact associated with aneurysm clips at the skull base (*arrow*), degrading evaluation of adjacent anatomy. Virtual monochromatic axial CT head image at 100 keV (*B*) demonstrates reduction of metallic streak artifact, and improved visualization of the adjacent soft tissues (*arrow*), albeit at the expense of decreased iodine attenuation and soft tissue contrast.

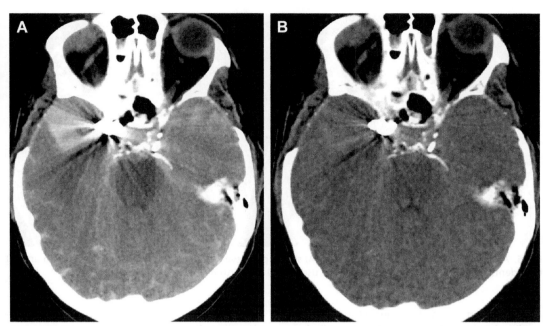

Fig. 3. Axial head CT image at 70 keV (single-energy CT equivalent) (*A*) demonstrates beam-hardening artifact that degrades evaluation of the skull base. VMI at 90 keV (*B*) with reduced artifact and superior anatomic depiction adjacent to the aneurysm clip. Creation of material density basis pairs that enhance iodine and suppress metal is the next step toward better assessment of recurrent aneurysm opacification.

Dense Iodinated Contrast and Osseous Structures

Dense contrast can be another source of artifact degradation on CT examinations of the head, neck, and spine. The relatively high atomic number of iodine allows exquisite differentiation of enhancing structures following the intravenous administration of iodinated contrast. However, concentrated contrast within the injected venous structures, as well as throughout the cervical and

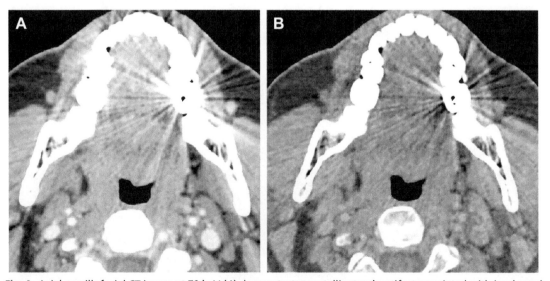

Fig. 4. Axial maxillofacial CT image at 70 keV (*A*) demonstrates metallic streak artifact associated with implanted dental hardware, which limits evaluation of the adjacent oral cavity and buccal soft tissues. VMI at 95 keV (*B*) demonstrates reduction of the streak artifact, and improved delineation of the adjacent anatomy, including the oral cavity and the adjacent buccal space fat.

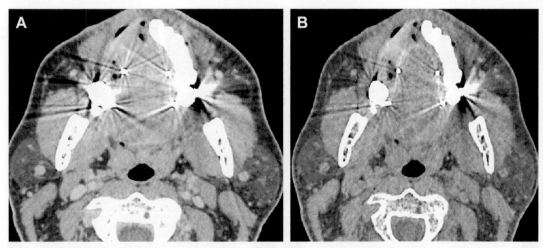

Fig. 5. Axial maxillofacial CT image at 70 keV (*A*) shows poor evaluation of oral cavity contents due to artifact from dental implants that is reduced with the use of 100 keV virtual monochromatic series (*B*).

intracranial arterial and venous structures, can result in localized streak artifact that results from both beam-hardening and photon-starvation phenomena, analogous to the streak artifact associated with implanted metallic hardware.[18,19]

An additional source of image degradation, especially prominent in imaging of the head and neck, is streak artifact associated with dense osseous structures. Evaluation of the soft tissues of the neck can be especially problematic at the level of the shoulders,[2] where the photon-starvation effect can significantly degrade assessment of the more central soft tissues of the lower neck. At the level of the head, appraisal of the intracranial vasculature can be problematic, as the osseous skull base surrounding the traversing vasculature results in both photon-starvation and beam-hardening artifact. **Fig. 9** demonstrates significant artifacts at the level of the thoracic inlet due to streak artifact from dense venous contrast

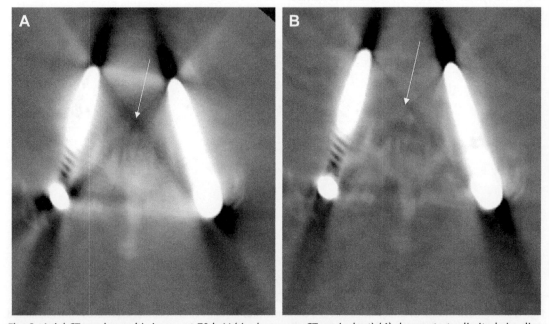

Fig. 6. Axial CT myelographic image at 70 keV (single-energy CT equivalent) (*A*) demonstrates limited visualization of the adjacent spinal soft tissues and spinal canal (*arrow*) due to metallic streak artifact from transpedicular screws. VMI at 100 keV (*B*) shows reduced artifact and improved delineation of the spinal canal anatomy (*arrow*).

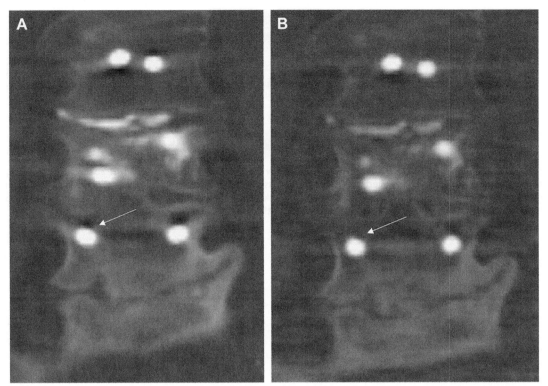

Fig. 7. Coronal spine CT image at 70 keV (*A*) demonstrates metallic streak artifact (*arrow*) associated with implanted spinal hardware. VMI at 90 keV (*B*) shows reduced streak artifact, with improved visualization of the interface between the metal and bone (*arrow*), which enables better assessment of peri-prosthetic lucencies.

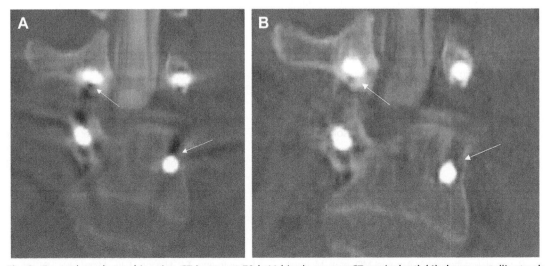

Fig. 8. Coronal myelographic spine CT image at 70 keV (single-energy CT equivalent) (*A*) shows metallic streak artifact (*arrows*) associated with implanted spinal hardware, which degrades evaluation for peri-prosthetic lucency. VMI at 100 keV (*B*) demonstrates reduction in metallic streak artifact (*arrows*), revealing subtle circumferential peri-prosthetic lucency (*right arrow*) not visible on the initial image, suggesting loosening.

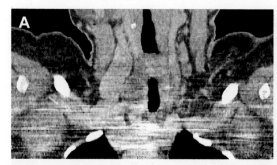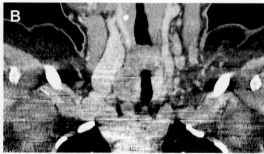

Fig. 9. Coronal CT image reconstructed at 70 keV (single-energy CT equivalent) (*A*) demonstrates beam-hardening artifact secondary to dense intravenous contrast and osseous structures at the level of the shoulders. Virtual monochromatic coronal CT image reconstructed at 95 keV (*B*) demonstrates reduced artifact and improved contrast-to-noise ratio, with improved differentiation of the soft tissue structures at the thoracic inlet.

and shoulders, which are reduced with the use of postprocessed high-energy VMIs.

SUMMARY

DECT in select clinical settings adds a powerful tool to the arsenal of the diagnostic radiologist in the evaluation of the head, neck, and spine. Analysis of the differential attenuation of the scanned soft tissues at varied energy levels allows for the creation of a range of VMIs, from which the radiologist has the ability to select the energy level at which the contrast-to-noise ratio is optimized, while minimizing beam-hardening artifact. This technique is especially valuable in the setting of implanted surgical hardware, where beam-hardening artifact can markedly degrade evaluation of the immediately adjacent regions of interest, as well as in areas of the body susceptible to both beam-hardening and photon-starvation effect, such as the posterior fossa and the thoracic inlet. The material decomposition process by which this occurs also allows for the creation of material-specific images, from which virtual subtraction images can be obtained, eliminating substances such as dense osseous structures and concentrated intravenous contrast, to allow for improved visualization of adjacent soft tissues.

REFERENCES

1. IMV Medical Information Division. IMV 2012 CT market outlook report. Des Plaines (IL): IMV Medical Information Division; 2012.
2. Barrett JF, Keat N. Artifacts in CT: recognition and avoidance. Radiographics 2004;24(6):1679–91.
3. Patino N, Prochowski A, Agrawal MD, et al. Material separation using dual-energy CT: current and emerging applications. Radiographics 2016;36: 1087–105.
4. Yu L, Leng S, McCollough CH. Dual-energy CT-based monochromatic imaging. AJR Am J Roentgenol 2012;199:S9–15.
5. Goodsitt MM, Christodoulou EG, Larson SC. Accuracies of the synthesized monochromatic CT numbers and effective atomic numbers obtained with a rapid kVp switching dual energy CT scanner. Med Phys 2011;38:2222–32.
6. Srinivasan A, Hoeffner E, Ibrahim M, et al. Utility of dual-energy CT virtual keV monochromatic series for the assessment of spinal transpedicular hardware-bone interface. AJR Am J Roentgenol 2013;201: 878–83.
7. Shinohara Y, Sakamoto M, Iwata N, et al. Usefulness of monochromatic imaging with metal artifact reduction software for computed tomography angiography after intracranial aneurysm coil embolization. Acta Radiol 2014;55(8):1015–23.
8. McLellan AM, Daniel S, Corcuera-Solano I, et al. Optimized imaging of the postoperative spine. Neuroimaging Clin N Am 2014;24:349–64.
9. Postma AA, Das M, Stadler AAR, et al. Dual-energy CT: what the neuroradiologist should know. Curr Radiol Rep 2015;3:16.
10. Postma AA, Hofman PA, Stadler AA, et al. Dual-energy CT of the brain and intracranial vessels. AJR Am J Roentgenol 2012;199:S26–33.
11. Wallace RC, Karis JP, Partovi S, et al. Noninvasive imaging of treated cerebral aneurysms, part I: MR angiographic follow-up of coiled aneurysms. AJNR Am J Neuroradiol 2007;28:1001–8.
12. Crobeddu E, Lanzino G, Kallmes DF, et al. Review of 2 decades of aneurysm-recurrence literature, part 2: managing recurrence after endovascular coiling. AJNR Am J Neuroradiol 2013;34:266–70.
13. Kaufmann TJ, Huston J III, Mandrekar JN, et al. Complications of diagnostic cerebral angiography: evaluation of 19 826 consecutive patients. Radiology 2007;243(3):812–9.

14. Lam S, Gupta R, Kelly H, et al. Multiparametric evaluation of head and neck squamous cell carcinoma using a single-source dual-energy CT with fast kVp switching: state of the art. Cancer 2015;7: 2201–16.

15. Ginat DT, Mayich M, Daftari-Besheli L, et al. Clinical applications of dual-energy CT in head and neck imaging. Eur Arch Otorhinolaryngol 2016;273:547–53.

16. Hayashi D, Roemer FW, Mian A, et al. Imaging features of postoperative complications after spinal surgery and instrumentation. AJR Am J Roentgenol 2012;199(1):W123–9.

17. Pham MH, Mehta VA, Patel NN, et al. Complications associated with the Dynesys dynamic stabilization system: a comprehensive review of the literature. Neurosurg Focus 2016;40(1):E2.

18. Takeyama N, Ohgiya Y, Itokawa H, et al. Comparison of 40 and 60 milliliters of contrast in assessment of the carotid artery by computed tomography angiography. Acta Radiol 2008;49(9):1068–78.

19. Xu Y, Wei L, Xin-ye N. Spectral imaging technology-based evaluation of radiation treatment planning to remove contrast agent artifacts. Technol Cancer Res Treat 2016;15(5):NP17–26.

Dual-Energy Computed Tomography of the Neck

A Pictorial Review of Normal Anatomy, Variants, and Pathologic Entities Using Different Energy Reconstructions and Material Decomposition Maps

Almudena Pérez-Lara, MD, PhD[a], Reza Forghani, MD, PhD[a,b],*

KEYWORDS

- Pictorial review • Dual-energy CT • Head and neck imaging • Virtual monochromatic images
- Material decomposition maps • Iodine overlay maps • Virtual unenhanced or noncontrast images
- Head and neck cancer

KEY POINTS

- Head and neck anatomy is complex and may be difficult to differentiate from the diverse range of pathologic entities that may be encountered and can make scan interpretation challenging.
- Dual-Energy Computed Tomography (DECT) enables the creation of additional reconstructions not available with conventional single-energy computed tomography that may help diagnostic evaluation in the neck.
- Radiologists using DECT must be familiar with the appearance of normal anatomy and different pathologic entities on specialized DECT reconstructions for optimal use and diagnosis.
- This article provides a practical, pictorial review of the appearance of normal anatomy and diverse pathologic entities of the neck on different DECT reconstructions.

INTRODUCTION

There is increasing use of dual-energy computed tomography (DECT) for the evaluation of head and neck pathologic entities.[1-13] To take full advantage of DECT, radiologists must be familiar with the appearance of normal tissues and pathologic entities on the various reconstructions that can be generated for use in clinical practice. This article provides a practical, pictorial review of the appearance of normal anatomic structures and a broad range of different head and neck pathologic

Disclosures: R. Forghani has acted as a consultant for GE Healthcare and has served as a speaker at lunch and learn sessions titled "Dual-Energy CT Applications in Neuroradiology and Head and Neck Imaging" sponsored by GE Healthcare at the 27th and 28th Annual Meetings of the Eastern Neuroradiological Society in 2015 and 2016 (no personal compensation or travel support for these sessions). A.P. Lara declares no relevant conflict of interest.
[a] Department of Radiology, Jewish General Hospital, McGill University, 3755 Cote Sainte-Catherine Road, Montreal, Quebec H3T 1E2, Canada; [b] Department of Radiology, Segal Cancer Centre and Lady Davis Institute for Medical Research, Jewish General Hospital, McGill University, Room C-212.1, 3755 Cote Sainte-Catherine Road, Montreal, Quebec H3T 1E2, Canada
* Corresponding author.
E-mail address: rforghani@jgh.mcgill.ca

Neuroimag Clin N Am 27 (2017) 499–522
http://dx.doi.org/10.1016/j.nic.2017.04.005

entities, both neoplastic and nonneoplastic, on commonly used DECT reconstructions using a fast kilovolt peak switching DECT scanner (GE Healthcare, Waukesha, WI).

OVERVIEW OF DIFFERENT DUAL-ENERGY COMPUTED TOMOGRAPHY RECONSTRUCTIONS

Different DECT approaches and systems, the fundamental principles behind DECT and DECT material characterization, and a detailed review of the evidence behind specific head and neck applications can be found in separate articles in this issue and will not be discussed here. However, the different types of reconstructions commonly generated when using fast kilovolt peak switching DECT systems are briefly reviewed. These include virtual monochromatic images (VMIs) and basis material decomposition maps.

VMIs are images reconstructed at predetermined or prescribed energies that are possible using DECT. Essentially, these are reconstructed based on the data acquired at the 2 different energies and simulate what an image would look like if the scan was acquired with a monoenergetic beam at a given energy. VMIs at 65 or 70 keV are typically considered equivalent to a standard 120 kilovolt peak [kVp] single-energy computed tomography (SECT) acquisition and can be used as a replacement for the latter for routine clinical interpretation when obtaining DECT scans.[6,9] At the authors' institution, where a fast kilovolt peak switching DECT scanner is used, 65 keV VMIs are generated for every neck scan for routine clinical interpretation, based on 2 prior studies evaluating the signal-to-noise ratio and other parameters specifically for neck scans using this type of scanner.[5,7]

In addition to the standard SECT equivalent VMIs, VMIs can be reconstructed at a wide range of energies, between 40 and 140 keV, with this type of scanner. Different energy reconstructions can be used to supplement 65 or 70 keV VMIs for specific clinical applications to improve diagnostic evaluation. For example, VMIs reconstructed at energies lower than 65 or 70 keV can increase iodine attenuation and soft tissue contrast. These have been shown to improve visibility of enhancing structures and lesions, such as head and neck squamous cell carcinoma (HNSCC), although with most DECT systems, this comes at the expense of increased image noise.[5,10,11] At the authors' center, 40 keV VMIs are reconstructed automatically for all neck DECT scans (in addition to the 65 keV VMIs).

VMIs reconstructed at high energies can help with the distinction of nonossified thyroid cartilage

(NOTC) from tumor and for reduction of artifact from metallic hardware or dental material.[4,14–20] The tradeoff with increasing VMI energies is a decrease in the attenuation of iodine and, therefore, tissue enhancement, along with decreased soft tissue contrast.

A third type of reconstruction generated with DECT is the basis material decomposition map.[21,22] These maps use differences in the energy-dependent attenuation of materials for identification and classification of their various composite elements based on their relation to the expected energy-dependent characteristics of known materials. In simple terms, these maps can be used to demonstrate the distribution of a material of interest and provide an estimate of its concentration within tissues. They can also be used to remove or subtract a given material from the images. Some common examples of material decomposition maps are iodine (or iodine overlay) maps representing the distribution and estimated content of iodine within different tissues or the virtual unenhanced or noncontrast images that remove iodine from images (eg, for creation of an image set equivalent to a noncontrast acquisition from a single contrast-enhanced study, eliminating the need for a multiphase protocol in some situations).

Although basis material decomposition maps can be very useful for characterization of materials, the radiologist must be aware of their limitations. In contradistinction to well-controlled experimental conditions, materials or fluids in vivo are mixtures and not pure solutions. Material decomposition maps are very useful for distinguishing elements with significant differences in their spectral or energy-dependent attenuation properties. However, the presence of other materials in solution can potentially affect the results, depending on their respective energy-dependent characteristics. Furthermore, the radiologist must keep in mind that material characterization is performed by cross-correlating the attenuation properties to that of known materials and these images should not be interpreted as the physical distribution of a pure solution. As an example, calcified tissues or bones have high signal both on the iodine and water axes of an iodine-water basis decomposition map and, therefore, will retain high signal on an iodine-water map that should not be misinterpreted as high iodine content (eg, high signal of bone on the iodine map in **Fig. 1** and other figures that follow). However, this pitfall can be easily avoided by cross-correlating with the standard 65 keV images. When necessary, additional maps (eg, calcium maps) may be generated for more accurate tissue

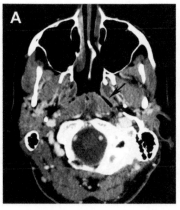
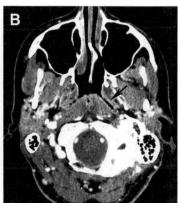
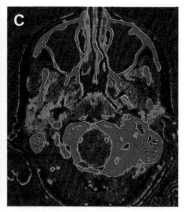

Fig. 1. Normal neck anatomy on different energy VMIs and iodine maps at the level of the nasopharynx. (A) 65 keV VMI (typically considered equivalent to a standard 120 kVp SECT acquisition), (B) 40 keV VMI, and (C) iodine (iodine-water) map reconstructed from the same contrast-enhanced DECT scan are shown. Note the differences in the appearance of different tissues on the various reconstructions. Iodine attenuation and soft tissue contrast increase on the 40 keV VMI compared with that at 65 keV, but this comes at the expense of increased image noise. The black arrows point to the mucosal lining of the nasopharynx at the left fossa of Rosenmüller.

characterization.[23] A more detailed discussion of the intricacies of these maps and how they are derived can be found in elsewhere in the literature.[21,22,24] (See Reza Forghani and colleagues' article, "Dual Energy CT: Physical Principles, Approaches to Scanning, Usage, and Implementation - Part 2," in this issue.)

The previous point emphasizes the importance of interpreting basis material decomposition maps (or different energy VMIs, for that matter) in conjunction with the standard 65 or 70 keV reconstructions to avoid pitfalls and misinterpretations. The radiologist must also keep in mind that the presence of artifact can introduce significant errors in material decomposition maps, and these

maps should be interpreted with caution in areas where there is significant artifact on the standard 65 or 70 keV images.

NORMAL HEAD AND NECK ANATOMY ON DUAL-ENERGY COMPUTED TOMOGRAPHY

There are differences in the attenuation and enhancement of different tissues at different energy levels. Therefore, certain characteristics may be accentuated on low-energy VMIs or the differences in enhancement of different tissues may become more apparent on iodine maps. Fig. 1; Figs. 2–6 demonstrate examples of the normal appearance of different tissues at different

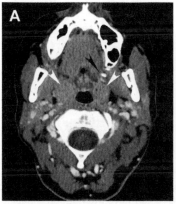
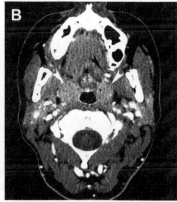
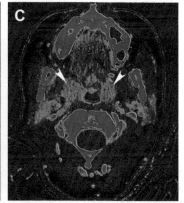

Fig. 2. Normal neck anatomy on various VMIs and iodine maps at the level of the oropharynx. (A) 65 keV VMI, (B) 40 keV VMI, and (C) iodine (iodine-water) map reconstructed from the same contrast-enhanced DECT scan are shown. Note the accentuation of differences in the appearance of tissues, for example, palatine tonsils (white arrowheads), on the 40 keV VMI or iodine map. The black arrowheads point to a small focus of calcification or ossification that could be mistaken for iodine signal if the iodine map is interpreted in isolation but is clearly evident as calcification on the 65 keV image.

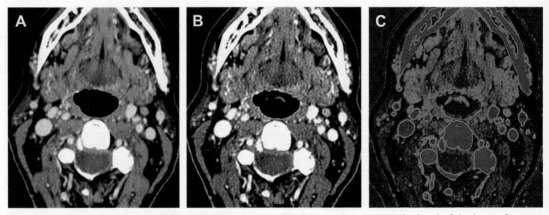

Fig. 3. Normal neck anatomy on different energy VMIs and iodine overlay maps at the level of the base of tongue and floor of the mouth. (*A*) 65 keV VMI, (*B*) 40 keV VMI, and (*C*) iodine (iodine-water) map reconstructed from the same contrast-enhanced DECT scan are shown.

levels in the neck from the nasopharynx superiorly to the level of the thyroid gland inferiorly. The purpose of these figures is to familiarize the reader with general appearances and concepts. However, the radiologist should keep in mind that, just like with conventional computed tomography (CT) images, there can be variations in the appearances of normal tissues and, therefore, the relationships discussed should not be overtly generalized or considered absolute.

Starting with vascular structures, note the much higher attenuation of enhancing large or medium-size vessels on the 40 keV compared with 65 keV VMI (see **Figs. 1–3**). Now compare the

VMIs to the iodine maps, on which various colors and hues are used to demonstrate the relative distribution and concentration of iodine in those vessels (see **Figs. 1–3**). As previously discussed, calcified tissue will retain high signal on iodine-water maps, explaining the high signal mapped to the osseous structures of the neck (see **Figs. 1–3**). When there is doubt, such as for the small focus of ossification shown in **Fig. 2** (black arrowhead), correlation with the 65 keV image will typically enable ready distinction and avoid misinterpretation. When the distinction is not readily evident, for example, when attempting to distinguish intracranial calcium from hemorrhage,

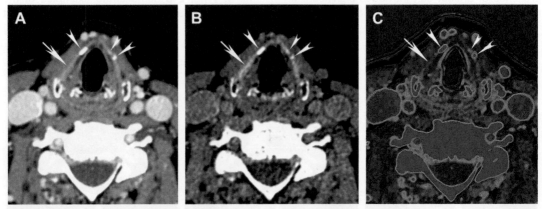

Fig. 4. Variations in the appearance of thyroid cartilage and use of high-energy VMIs and iodine maps for evaluation. (*A*) 65 keV VMI, (*B*) 140 keV VMI, and (*C*) iodine (iodine-water) map demonstrate heterogeneous thyroid cartilage ossification with a large nonossified component (eg, *arrows*). NOTC can have attenuation similar to muscle (and tumor) on 65 keV or standard SECT images. On the other hand, on the 140 keV VMIs, it has higher attenuation compared with muscle (*arrow in B*). On the iodine map, NOTC should not have significant iodine signal (*arrow in C*). However, ossified components will have high signal (*arrowheads*) and the signal can vary depending on the degree of calcification or ossification (eg, note lower signal on the iodine map for the faint focus of calcification on the left (*small arrowhead*) compared with the more heavily ossified components (*large arrowheads*). Correlation with the 65 keV is helpful for avoiding mischaracterization.

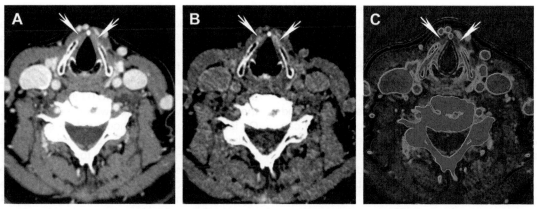

Fig. 5. Variations in the appearance of thyroid cartilage and use of high-energy VMIs and iodine maps for evaluation. (*A*) 65 keV VMI, (*B*) 140 keV VMI, and (*C*) iodine (iodine-water) map demonstrate predominantly ossified thyroid cartilage with small focal nonossified components anteriorly (*arrows*). Normal nonossified cartilage may be similar in attenuation to muscle (and enhancing tumor, if present) on the 65 keV VMIs but, unlike enhancing tumor, will also have high attenuation on the 140 keV VMIs (*arrows, B*), but virtually no iodine content on the iodine map (*arrows, C*).

other maps such as calcium maps may be generated for more accurate characterization.

The pharyngeal mucosa and lymphatic tissues of Waldeyer ring typically enhance to a greater degree than normal muscle,[25,26] but these differences can be subtle and very similar in attenuation on SECT. The use of DECT reconstructions may better demonstrate the increased enhancement of the pharyngeal mucosa and lymphatic tissues of the Waldeyer ring. For example, the thin enhancing pharyngeal mucosa may be better appreciated on the 40 keV VMI or iodine map compared with 65 keV VMI, in some cases (see **Fig. 1**, black arrow). In **Fig. 2**, note how the difference in attenuation or iodine content of the palatine tonsils (white arrowheads) relative to that of muscle is better seen on the 40 keV VMI and iodine map, compared with the 65 keV VMI.

Different normal muscle groups in the neck have relatively similar attenuation and relatively similar iodine signal on the iodine map, typically lower than that of tonsillar tissues, pharyngeal mucosa, and the major salivary glands (see **Figs. 1** and **2**). However, there can still be variations in the appearance of different muscles, including differences in iodine content (eg, note the relatively higher iodine signal in the genioglossus and mylohyoid muscles relative to the paraspinal muscles in **Fig. 3**C).

The appearance and attenuation of the parotid and submandibular glands can vary on CT, partly depending on the degree of fatty infiltration. In elderly patients, the overall density of the gland

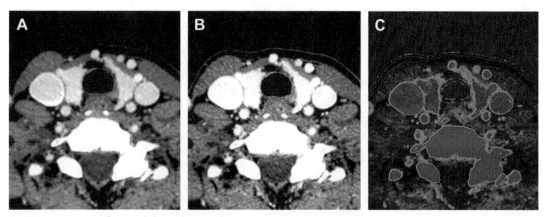

Fig. 6. Appearance of normal thyroid parenchyma on various VMIs and iodine overlay maps. (*A*) 65 keV VMI, (*B*) 40 keV VMI, and (*C*) iodine (iodine-water) map reconstructed from the same contrast-enhanced DECT scan are shown.

may be lower than in younger patients. However, in the absence of significant fat infiltration, the salivary glands may have higher attenuation than muscle[27] and these differences may be better seen on DECT reconstructions compared with SECT or the SECT-equivalent 65 keV VMIs. For example, note the higher iodine content of the parotid glands compared with muscle in **Figs. 1** and **2**. Iodine distribution and signal (or content) can also be quite heterogeneous, as seen in **Figs. 1** and **2**.

Accurate determination of thyroid cartilage invasion is essential for appropriate staging of laryngeal or hypopharyngeal cancers. A few studies have suggested that DECT is useful for distinguishing tumor from NOTC and for the determination of thyroid cartilage invasion.[1,4] Therefore, familiarity with the normal appearance of the thyroid cartilage on various DECT reconstructions is important. One challenge when evaluating the thyroid cartilage is that normal patterns of ossification can be variable and unpredictable from patient to patient (see **Figs. 4** and **5**). Because NOTC can have attenuation similar to tumor, tumor abutting the nonossified component of a partially ossified thyroid cartilage can mimic tumor invading (and replacing) ossified cartilage, presenting a diagnostic challenge.

NOTC does not enhance but has intrinsic high attenuation that persists at high energies. As a result, on very-high-energy VMIs, there is relative preservation of its attenuation but relative suppression of the attenuation of iodine within enhancing normal structures (or tumor), helping to distinguish these 2 entities.[4] For example, in **Figs. 4** and **5**, note the greater contrast or attenuation difference between NOTC and muscle on the 140 keV VMI compared with the 65 keV VMI. On iodine maps, there should not be significant iodine signal in NOTC because it does not enhance. However, similar to what was previously discussed for bone, a pitfall is that the calcified or ossified components will have high signal on the iodine maps (see **Figs. 4** and **5**). These are typically readily identifiable by their very high signal but, occasionally, especially if faint (see **Fig. 4**, small arrowhead) they could be mistaken for enhancement. This pitfall can be avoided by correlating with the 65 keV VMI.

The thyroid gland is intrinsically hyperdense due to its inherent iodine content but also enhances after administration of contrast. Therefore, as expected, its attenuation will be higher on the 40 keV VMIs compared with 65 keV VMIs (see **Fig. 6**). Iodine maps demonstrate the high iodine content of the thyroid gland (see **Fig. 6**), whereas virtual unenhanced images remove the iodine attenuation from thyroid and other enhancing tissues (**Fig. 7**).

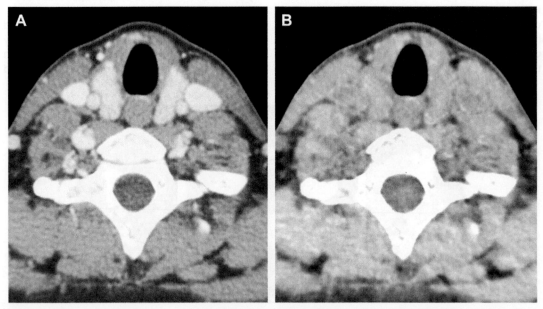

Fig. 7. (*A*) 65 keV VMI and (*B*) virtual unenhanced or noncontrast image (water-iodine map) reconstructed from the same contrast-enhanced DECT scan are shown. Note the suppression and removal of the attenuation of iodine from different tissues and vessels on the virtual unenhanced image (*B*).

HEAD AND NECK LESIONS AND VARIANTS ON DUAL-ENERGY COMPUTED TOMOGRAPHY
Inflammatory and Infectious Diseases

There are studies demonstrating that additional DECT reconstructions, such as low-energy VMIs, can improve visualization of HNSCC and its borders along adjacent normal soft tissues.[5,10,11] Although there are no published data on DECT for evaluation of inflammatory disease in the neck other than its use for characterization of pathologic and inflammatory lymph nodes,[13] the same principles may apply. **Figs. 8–13** demonstrate examples of inflammatory disease in the soft tissues of the neck on standard SECT equivalent 65 keV VMIs, 40 keV VMIs, and iodine maps or virtual unenhanced images. As illustrated by the cases presented, inflammatory tissue enhancement may be better seen on the 40 keV VMIs compared with 65 keV VMIs. Also, the iodine maps may in some instances more clearly demonstrate inflammatory changes. Iodine maps can also be used to confirm absence of iodine or enhancement within abscesses or retropharyngeal edema (see **Figs. 8–11** and **13**). Sometimes, the abscess capsule may be better seen on the 40 keV VMIs and iodine maps. Virtual unenhanced images can be generated to confirm calcifications or salivary stones (see **Fig. 12**) and help distinguish them from enhancing tissues.

Benign Neck Lesions and Variants

Parathyroid adenoma
Multiphasic multidetector-row (MDCT), or 4-dimensional (4D)-CT, is an emerging technique that is increasingly used for preoperative localization of parathyroid adenomas (PAs) (**Fig. 14**). Preliminary studies using DECT demonstrate that there can be differences in the energy-dependent attenuation of PAs compared with the normal thyroid gland or lymph nodes, which can potentially help in challenging cases.[8,28] However, unlike cases in which virtual unenhanced images are used to distinguish calcifications from enhancement and may be used to replace the true unenhanced acquisition, these reconstructions are unlikely to represent a satisfactory replacement for the true unenhanced acquisition for PA identification.[8,28] The iodine in intravenously administered CT contrast is not distinguishable from the intrinsic iodine within the thyroid gland and both will be suppressed or removed on virtual unenhanced images, making differentiation of a PA from an exophytic thyroid nodule or normal thyroid parenchyma very difficult on the virtual unenhanced images (**Fig. 15**).

Vallecular cyst
Also known as epiglottic mucous retention cysts or base of tongue cysts, vallecular cysts are covered by normal mucosa (ductal cells) and filled with fluid.[29] They can have mild enhancement of their mucosal layer but should not have any solid or nodular enhancing components. DECT reconstructions may provide greater confidence that a vallecular lesion has no solid enhancement, confirming this benign diagnosis. Note the lack of iodine signal within such a cyst on the iodine map in **Fig. 16**.

Ranula
Ranulas, also referred to as mucoceles or mucous retention cysts, of the floor of mouth are believed to occur as a result of obstruction or trauma to

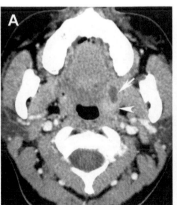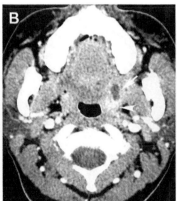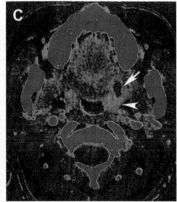

Fig. 8. Left peritonsillar abscess. Axial (A) 65 keV VMI, (B) 40 keV VMI, and (C) iodine (iodine-water) map demonstrate a small collection with peripheral enhancement in the region of the left palatine tonsil (*white arrows*). The enhancing capsule and adjacent inflammatory changes or phlegmon (*arrowheads*) are more conspicuous on the 40 keV VMI and on the iodine map compared with the 65 keV VMI.

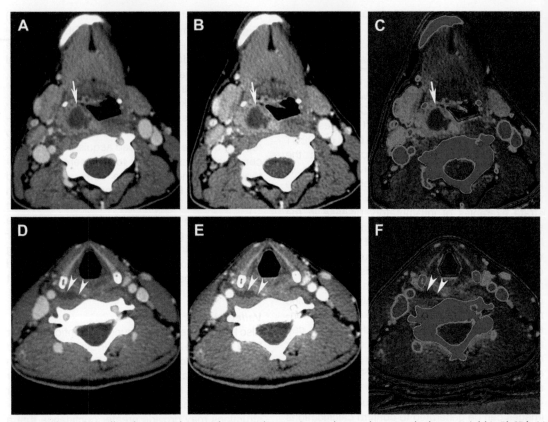

Fig. 9. Right peritonsillar abscess with retropharyngeal extension and retropharyngeal edema. Axial (*A, D*) 65 keV VMIs, (*B, E*) 40 keV VMIs, and (*C, F*) iodine (iodine-water) maps from a contrast-enhanced neck CT. There is a rim-enhancing collection extending from the region of the lower right palatine tonsil to the right retropharyngeal space (*white arrow*). Note how the enhancing capsule and surrounding inflammatory changes are better defined on the 40 keV VMI (*B*) and iodine-overlay map (*C*). More caudally, there is retropharyngeal edema (*D–F; white arrowheads*). Note absence of any rim-enhancing capsule or surrounding iodine signal.

the sublingual glands or minor salivary glands.[30] They can be classified as a simple ranula, confined to the floor of the mouth above the mylohyoid muscle or sublingual space, or a plunging ranula,

extending below the mylohyoid muscle into the submandibular space (**Fig. 17**). Note the increased contrast between the cystic lesion or ranula and adjacent enhancing normal tissues on the 40 keV

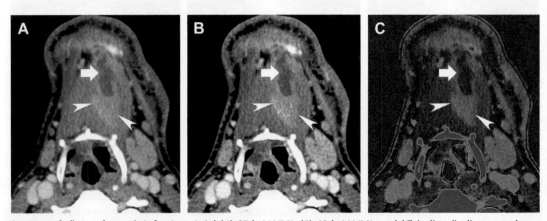

Fig. 10. Left floor of mouth infection. Axial (*A*) 65 keV VMI, (*B*) 40 keV VMI, and (*C*) iodine (iodine-water) map demonstrate a left floor of mouth abscess (*thick arrows*) with surrounding inflammatory and phlegmonous changes, most prominent posteriorly (*arrowheads*).

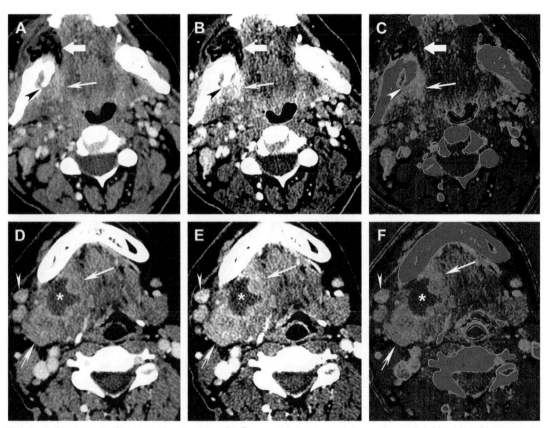

Fig. 11. Odontogenic abscess and extension of inflammation to surrounding spaces. Axial (*A, D*) 65 keV VMIs, (*B, E*) 40 keV VMIs, and (*C, F*) iodine (iodine-water) maps from a contrast-enhanced neck CT. This patient had a recent tooth extraction with postprocedure changes (*thick arrows*). Note the presence of a small defect (*A–C; arrowheads*) in the lingual cortex of the right mandible providing a communication between inflammatory changes in the tooth socket and bone with the adjacent soft tissues. This is associated with a right submandibular space abscess (*D–F; asterisks*). There are enhancing phlegmonous changes in the adjacent soft tissues (*long thin arrows*). There is also asymmetric enlargement and enhancement of the right submandibular gland (*D–F; short thin arrows*), compare to the left submandibular gland). Note the relative hyperenhancement of a nearby reactive (inflamed) right level IB lymph node (*D–F; arrowheads*), not readily evident on the 65 keV VMI (*D*) but seen on the 40 keV VMI (*E*) and iodine map (*F*). Overall, the inflammatory changes are better delineated on the 40 keV VMIs and iodine overlay maps compared with the 65 keV VMIs.

image as well as absence of iodine signal within the ranula on the iodine map. Low-energy VMIs and iodine maps may help demonstrate associated inflammation, if present (as previously discussed) or may highlight any solid enhancing component that would suggest an alternative diagnosis.

Thyroglossal duct cyst
Thyroglossal duct cysts are the most common congenital neck masses, representing a remnant of the thyroglossal duct (**Fig. 18**). They typically have a thin wall that may demonstrate mild peripheral rim enhancement.[31] On the other hand, they should not have any internal nodular enhancing components that would suggest the rare coexistent papillary thyroid carcinoma.

Thornwaldt cyst
Thornwaldt cysts are relatively common benign developmental lesions that occur at the midline in the nasopharynx (**Fig. 19**).[27] They can have simple fluid density or may have increased internal attenuation due to proteinaceous content. Similar to the thyroglossal duct cyst previously discussed, they should not have solid internal enhancement. There should be no iodine signal within these cysts on the iodine map, which may help differentiate this benign entity from an enhancing nasopharyngeal lesion.

Laryngocele
Laryngocele is a dilatation of the laryngeal saccule that can present as a thin-walled lesion that is, either air-filled or fluid-filled and communicates with the laryngeal ventricle (**Fig. 20**).[27] Unless superinfected,

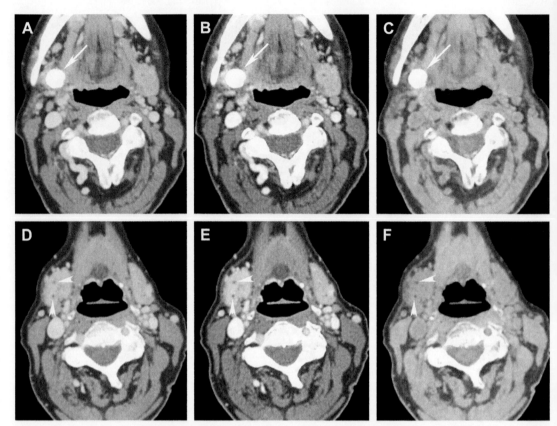

Fig. 12. Right submandibular stone with intraglandular ductal dilatation. Axial (*A, D*) 65 keV VMIs, (*B, E*) 40 keV VMIs, and (*C, F*) virtual unenhanced (water-iodine) maps from the same contrast-enhanced neck CT are shown. There is a large right submandibular stone (*A–C; arrows*) with intraglandular ductal dilatation (*D–F; arrowheads*). The contrast between the dilated ducts and adjacent parenchyma is greater on the 40 keV images. Note suppression of iodine attenuation in enhancing structures on the virtual unenhanced images (*C, F*).

they should not have significant peripheral enhancement.[27] Laryngoceles can be internal (or simple; extending in the paraglottic space), external (saccule herniates through the thyrohyoid membrane with a dilated superficial portion), or they can be mixed (extralaryngeal extension from the paraglottic space through the thyrohyoid membrane with dilation of the internal and external components). When evaluating fluid-filled laryngoceles, it is imperative to exclude a secondary laryngocele resulting from an obstructive laryngeal cancer. Low kiloelectron volt VMIs and iodine maps can potentially improve diagnostic evaluation by excluding or identifying subtle enhancing tumor in the larynx.

Branchial cleft cyst

Branchial cleft cysts are developmental cysts related to incomplete obliteration of the branchial apparatus (**Fig. 21**).[27] Uncomplicated cysts should have simple fluid density without a perceptible enhancing wall. However, if superinfected, the cysts can have variable rim enhancement and/or internal debris. The radiologist must exercise extreme caution in diagnosing a branchial cleft cyst in an adult presenting with a neck mass for the first time because cystic metastatic lymphadenopathy can mimic a branchial cleft cyst. It is important to evaluate for any features that warrant further evaluation, especially in the era of human papillomavirus (HPV)-associated oropharyngeal squamous cell carcinoma, which are commonly presenting in younger patients without the traditional risk factors of alcohol and tobacco use.

Lipoma

Head and neck lipomas most frequently arise from the subcutaneous soft tissues of the posterior neck, although less frequently they may be present elsewhere in different spaces of the neck (**Fig. 22**).[32] CT is helpful for the diagnosis of lipomas, determination of their extent, and identification of any complex soft tissue components that may suggest a more aggressive lesion, such as liposarcoma.

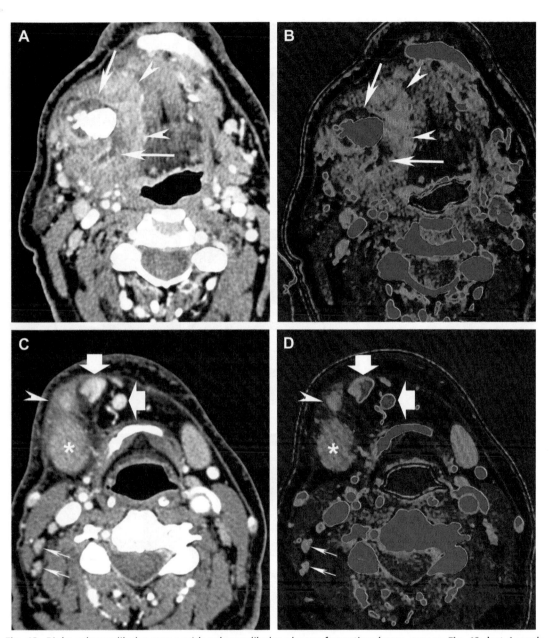

Fig. 13. Right submandibular stone with submandibular abscess formation (same case as **Fig. 12**, but 1 week later). Axial (*A, C*) 40 keV VMIs and (*B, D*) iodine (iodine-water) maps from a contrast-enhanced neck CT. There has been formation of a rim-enhancing fluid collection (*A, B; thin long arrows*) around the stone representing an abscess. There are surrounding inflammatory and phlegmonous changes (*white arrowheads*) in the adjacent soft tissues, including inflammatory changes of the right submandibular gland (*C, D; asterisks*). Note the hetero-geneous attenuation and iodine content of the surrounding inflammation, especially well-appreciated on the iodine map. Also note the increased iodine content within a few adjacent reactive (inflamed) lymph nodes (*C, D; some examples marked by wide short arrows*): for example, compare the iodine signal in 2 level IB lymph nodes (*C, D; wide short arrows*) to that of some right level IIB nodes on the same image (*C, D; thin short arrows*).

Herniation of the sublingual gland through a mylohyoid boutonnière

There are frequently small defects in the mylo-hyoid, especially along its thinner anterior part, and these have sometimes been referred to as boutonnières.[30,33] Sometimes, these contain fat or vessels but, at other times, the sublingual gland may herniate through these defects (**Fig. 23**). These may come to clinical attention as a palpable mass in the submandibular space,

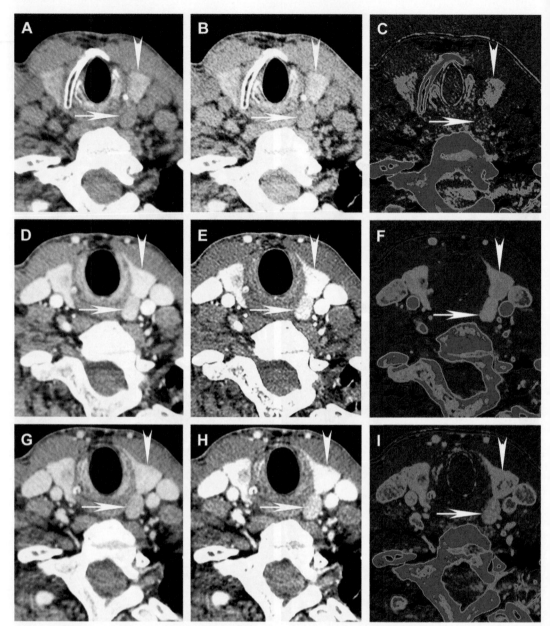

Fig. 14. Left PA on multiphasic DECT performed before IV contrast (*top row*; *A–C*), in an arterial phase after contrast administration (*middle row*; *D–F*), and after a 65-second delay (*bottom row*; *G–I*). Images shown are 65 keV VMIs (*left column*; *A, D, G*), 40 keV VMIs (*middle column*; *B, E, H*), and iodine overlay maps (*right column*; *C, F, I*). Note the differences in attenuation or iodine signal between the normal left thyroid lobe (*arrowhead*) and the left PA (*arrow*). Incidentally, there is a small thyroid nodule on the right that is better seen on the postcontrast 40 keV images and iodine maps compared with the 65 keV VMIs.

and the radiologist should take care to recognize these normal variants and not mistake a normal sublingual gland for tumor or other pathologic entities. On the various dual-energy reconstructions, these should follow the attenuation, tissue architecture, and iodine signal (iodine maps) of normal salivary glands.

Salivary Gland Tumors

Most salivary gland tumors are benign. In general, benign lesions are well-circumscribed, whereas malignant lesions tend to have infiltrative, invasive, and/or other aggressive features.[34] The role of CT is to identify and characterize the lesion, localize

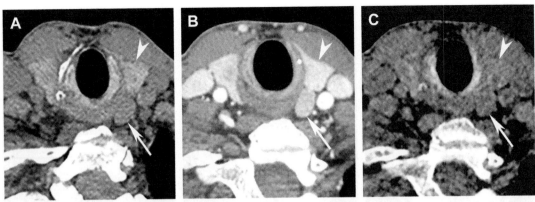

Fig. 15. PA (same patient as in **Fig. 14**). (*A*) True unenhanced CT, (*B*) 65 keV VMI from an arterial phase DECT acquisition, and (*C*) virtual unenhanced (water-iodine) image derived from the contrast-enhanced DECT are shown. On the true unenhanced image, the PA (*arrows*) has lower attenuation than the thyroid gland (*arrowheads*), which is useful for distinguishing the 2 structures and accurate PA identification. However, because the intravenously administered contrast is not distinguishable from the intrinsic iodine of the thyroid gland, all iodine attenuation is suppressed on the virtual unenhanced image and the 2 structures are no longer distinguishable from each other based on their attenuation. Therefore, virtual unenhanced images are unlikely to be useful as a replacement for the true unenhanced acquisition in 4D-CT for PA localization.

the tumor, and define its relation to important anatomic landmarks, such as the plane of the facial nerve. CT may also suggest the presence of perineural spread, although typically MR imaging is superior for this indication.[34,35] Because there can be significant variation in the attenuation of the normal parotid gland, tumor-gland soft tissue contrast can be unpredictable and defining the anatomic boundaries of a salivary gland tumor may be difficult. Low-energy VMIs and iodine maps have the potential to improve the visualization of salivary gland tumors or associated perineural spread of tumor in some cases (**Figs. 24–26**).

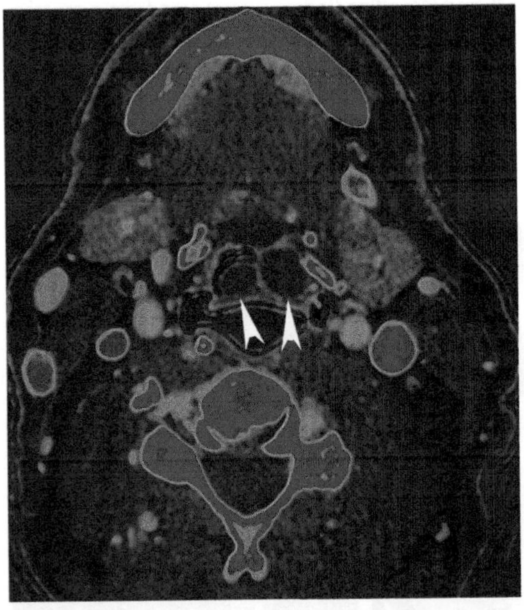

Thyroid Carcinoma

The most common malignancy in the thyroid gland is papillary carcinoma with other histologic types, such as follicular, medullary, and anaplastic types, being much less common.[36] In addition to enlarged lymph nodes, papillary thyroid cancer nodal metastases can present with cystic changes, may contain calcifications, and may enhance avidly.[36] At least 1 investigation using DECT for analysis of pathologic lymph nodes has shown that thyroid cancer nodal metastases have higher iodine concentration compared with normal nodes or other pathologic lymph nodes, such as those from HNSCC.[37] The intrinsic iodine content of most thyroid carcinomas as well as the intense enhancement of some of these tumors,[36] can potentially be exploited using DECT to improve visualization of the primary tumor or metastatic lymph nodes on low-energy VMIs and iodine maps (**Fig. 27**). Virtual unenhanced images can be used to confirm the presence of calcifications (see **Fig. 27**).

Lymphoma

CT is commonly used for the initial evaluation and follow-up of lymphoma. It is used for characterization and determination of the extent of

Fig. 16. Vallecular cysts. Iodine (iodine-water) map from a contrast-enhanced neck CT does not show any significant iodine signal in the vallecular cysts (*white arrowheads*).

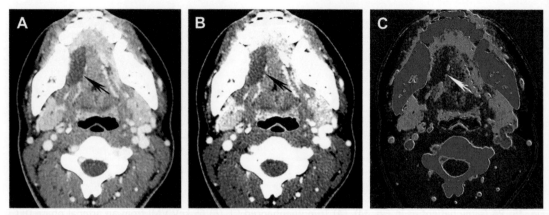

Fig. 17. Ranula. (*A*) 65 keV VMI, (*B*) 40 keV VMI, and (*C*) iodine (iodine-water) map demonstrate a well-defined nonenhancing cystic lesion in the right floor of mouth (*arrows*).

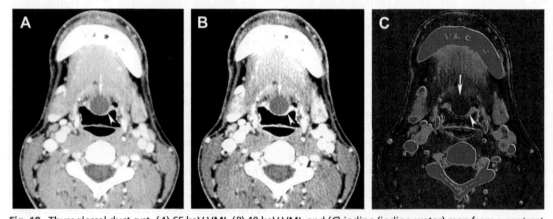

Fig. 18. Thyroglossal duct cyst. (*A*) 65 keV VMI, (*B*) 40 keV VMI, and (*C*) iodine (iodine-water) map from a contrast-enhanced neck CT demonstrate a cystic midline lesion partially protruding into the pre-epiglottic space and vallecula (*white arrows*). Note displaced adjacent enhancing lymphoid tissue (*arrowheads*). On the conventional SECT equivalent 65 keV image, the internal contents are mildly complex or hyperattenuating but without any evidence of iodine signal on the iodine map, consistent with mildly proteinaceous content. The 40 keV VMI and iodine map provide reassurance that there is no enhancing solid component and that this is a simple, benign cyst.

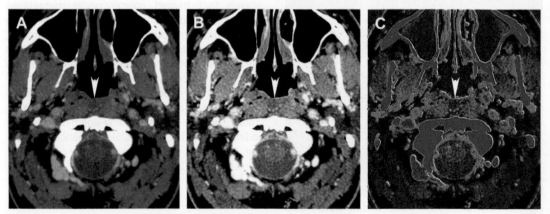

Fig. 19. Thornwaldt cyst. (*A*) 65 keV VMI, (*B*) 40 keV VMI, and (*C*) iodine (iodine-water) map from a contrast-enhanced neck CT demonstrate a well-circumscribed nonenhancing cyst in the midline posterior nasopharyngeal wall (*white arrowheads*).

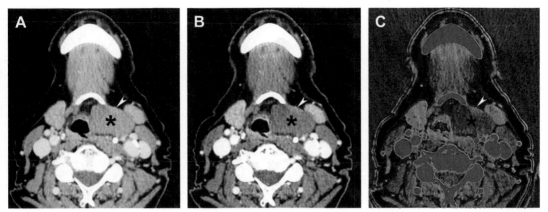

Fig. 20. Fluid-filled mixed laryngocele. (*A*) 65 keV VMI, (*B*) 40 keV VMI, and (*C*) iodine (iodine-water) map from a contrast-enhanced neck CT demonstrate a cystic left paraglottic lesion (*asterisks*) with extralaryngeal extension into the low left submandibular space, consistent with a mixed laryngocele. Note the flattened strap muscle (*arrowheads*) anterior to the lesion, only distinctly visible on the high-contrast 40 keV VMI and iodine map and not well seen on the 65 keV VMI. The cyst is otherwise simple without solid nodular components.

lymphadenopathy as well as evaluation of extranodal involvement, such as involvement of Waldeyer ring and the orbits.[38] Similar to other pathologic entities in the neck, some of the features may be more evident or further characterized on low-energy VMIs and iodine overlay maps (**Fig. 28**).

Head and Neck Squamous Cell Carcinoma

Low-energy VMIs have been shown to improve visibility and contour delineation of HNSCC[5–7,9–11] and iodine maps have been shown to increase accuracy for determination of thyroid cartilage

invasion.[1] Low-energy VMIs may also improve visualization of abnormal lymph nodes[5] and potentially internal nodal heterogeneity or cystic change.[6,9] Preliminary studies suggest that some nodal characteristics on DECT scans, such as their iodine content, may also be helpful for distinguishing different types of pathologic nodes.[13,37] Applications of DECT for the evaluation of HNSCC are shown in **Figs. 29–33**. For a more detailed review (See Reza Forghani and colleagues' article, "Applications of dual energy CT for the evaluation of head and neck squamous cell carcinoma," in this issue.).

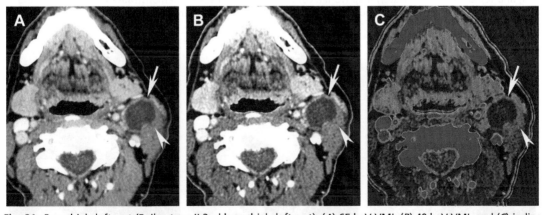

Fig. 21. Branchial cleft cyst (Bailey type II 2nd branchial cleft cyst). (*A*) 65 keV VMI, (*B*) 40 keV VMI, and (*C*) iodine (iodine-water) map from a contrast-enhanced neck CT demonstrate a well-defined cystic lesion (*arrows*) anterior to the left sternocleidomastoid muscle, posterior to the submandibular gland, and lateral to the carotid sheath representing a superinfected Bailey type II 2nd branchial cleft cyst that required surgical drainage (*white arrows*). On the 65 keV image (*A*), mild wall-thickening, irregularity, and enhancement is barely visible. The inflammatory changes in the cyst wall and surrounding tissues (*arrowheads*) are slightly better appreciated on the 40 keV image (*B*) but best seen on the iodine map (*C*). Note the presence of a thickened enhancing wall, better shown on the iodine overlay maps. It is noteworthy that in cases such as this, tissue sampling is likely necessary to exclude nodal metastatic disease.

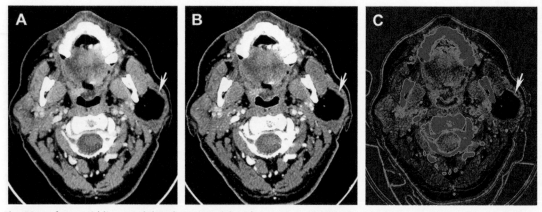

Fig. 22. Left parotid lipoma. (*A*) 65 keV VMI, (*B*) 40 keV VMI, and (*C*) iodine (iodine-water) map from a contrast-enhanced neck CT demonstrate a lipoma (*white arrows*) centered in the superficial lobe of the left parotid gland and crossing the expected plane of the facial nerve. There are a few tiny vessels and/or soft tissue septations within the lesion but otherwise it does not enhance.

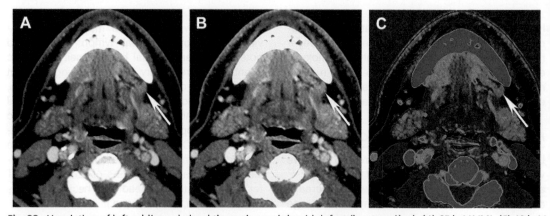

Fig. 23. Herniation of left sublingual gland through a mylohyoid defect (boutonnière). (*A*) 65 keV VMI, (*B*) 40 keV VMI, and (*C*) iodine (iodine-water) map from a contrast-enhanced neck CT demonstrate extension of sublingual gland tissue into the left submandibular space (*white arrows*) through a mylohyoid defect.

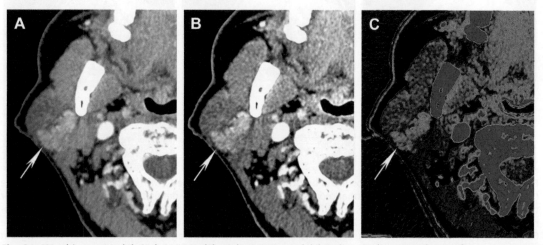

Fig. 24. Warthin tumor. (*A*) 65 keV VMI, (*B*) 40 keV VMI, and (*C*) iodine (iodine-water) map from a contrast-enhanced neck CT demonstrate a relatively well-defined lesion (*white arrows*) centered in the superficial lobe of the right parotid gland but approaching the plane of the facial nerve.

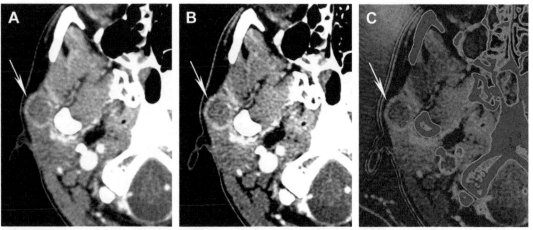

Fig. 25. Pleomorphic adenoma. (*A*) 65 keV VMI, (*B*) 40 keV VMI, and (*C*) iodine (iodine-water) map from a contrast-enhanced neck CT demonstrate a rim enhancing lesion (*white arrows*) in the superficial lobe of the right parotid gland.

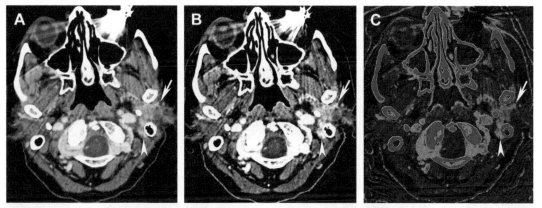

Fig. 26. Left parotid adenocarcinoma with perineural spread of tumor. (*A*) 65 keV VMI, (*B*) 40 keV VMI, and (*C*) iodine (iodine-water) map from a contrast-enhanced neck CT demonstrate an invasive enhancing lesion (*white arrows*) centered in the superficial lobe of the left parotid gland and crossing the plane of the facial nerve. Abnormal enhancement is also demonstrated along the course of the facial nerve adjacent to the mastoid tip (*white arrowheads*); this finding is more conspicuous on 40 keV and on iodine overlay maps. Perineural tumor spread along the facial nerve was subsequently confirmed on MR imaging and pathologic specimens. (*Courtesy of* Dr Reza Forghani, MD, PhD, Montreal, Quebec, Canada.)

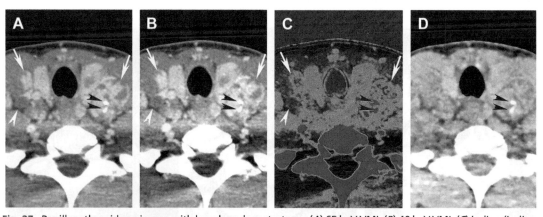

Fig. 27. Papillary thyroid carcinoma with lymph node metastases. (*A*) 65 keV VMI, (*B*) 40 keV VMI, (*C*) iodine (iodine-water) map, and (*D*) virtual unenhanced image (water-iodine map) from a contrast-enhanced neck CT demonstrate multiple nodal metastases with marked but heterogeneous enhancement (*white arrows*), calcifications (*black arrowheads*), and variable cystic components (*white arrowheads*). Note suppression or removal of iodine signal with preservation and confirmation of calcifications on the virtual unenhanced image (*black arrowheads, D*). As previously discussed, calcifications retain high signal on iodine-water maps (*C; black arrowheads*) but can be correctly identified in conjunction with the standard images, such as 65 keV VMIs or other maps, such as virtual unenhanced images (*D*).

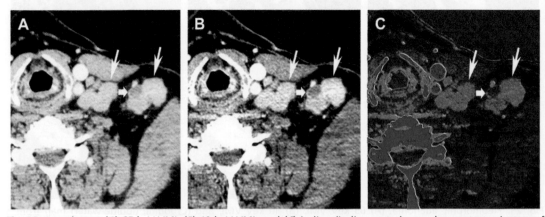

Fig. 28. Lymphoma. (*A*) 65 keV VMI, (*B*) 40 keV VMI, and (*C*) iodine (iodine-water) map demonstrate clusters of abnormal left level III and VA lymph nodes (*arrows*). Note the increased attenuation and contrast on the 40 keV compared with 65 keV VMI (relative to the cystic component [*wide short arrows*] or nearby muscle). On the iodine map, most nodes have relatively homogenous iodine content but 1 node demonstrates heterogeneity, with a clear focus of cystic internal change (*wide short arrow*).

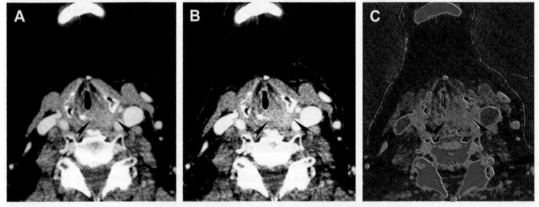

Fig. 29. Squamous cell carcinoma of the hypopharynx. (*A*) 65 keV VMI, (*B*) 40 keV VMI, and (*C*) iodine (iodine-water) map demonstrate a left hypopharyngeal mass (*arrowheads*) with erosion of the cricoid cartilage. The lesion has higher attenuation on the 40 keV VMI and its extent and margins are better appreciated on 40 keV VMI and iodine overlay map compared with the 65 keV VMI.

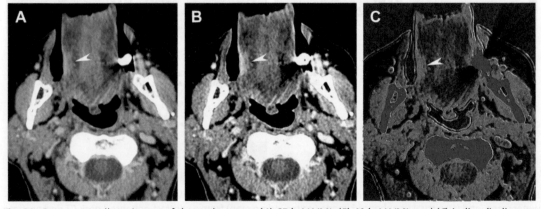

Fig. 30. Squamous cell carcinoma of the oral tongue. (*A*) 65 keV VMI, (*B*) 40 keV VMI, and (*C*) iodine (iodine-water) map demonstrate an enhancing lesion along the right lateral margin of the oral tongue (*arrowhead*). Note improved visibility of the lesion and its margins on the 40 keV VMI compared with the more subtle findings on the 65 keV VMI. (*Courtesy of* Dr Reza Forghani, MD, PhD, Montreal, Quebec, Canada.)

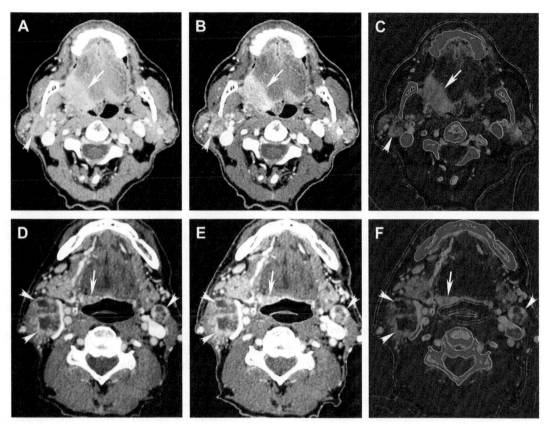

Fig. 31. Squamous cell carcinoma of the tongue base with metastatic lymphadenopathy. Axial (*A, D*) 65 keV VMIs, (*B, E*) 40 keV VMIs, and (*C, F*) iodine (iodine-water) maps from a contrast-enhanced neck CT demonstrate a large lesion at the right base of tongue (*white arrows*). There are bilateral pathologic lymph nodes with internal cystic change or necrosis (*D–F; arrowheads*). The primary tumor has higher attenuation and its margin is better delineated on the 40 keV VMI and iodine map compared with the 65 keV VMI.

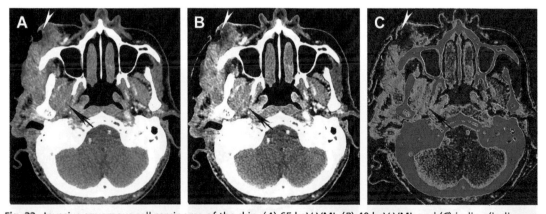

Fig. 32. Invasive squamous cell carcinoma of the skin. (*A*) 65 keV VMI, (*B*) 40 keV VMI, and (*C*) iodine (iodine-water) map demonstrate an invasive mass involving a large part of the face with deep extension, including infiltration and abnormal enhancement in the right masticator space (*black arrows*). Note the increased attenuation in the medial right masticator space compared with the contralateral side, much better appreciated on the 40 keV compared with 65 keV VMI. The asymmetry in this case is perhaps best seen on the iodine map. Note the clearly higher iodine signal on the right (*black arrows*) compared with the normal contralateral left side. The white arrowheads point to an area of skin ulceration within the area involved by tumor. (*Courtesy of* Dr Reza Forghani, MD, PhD, Montreal, Quebec, Canada.)

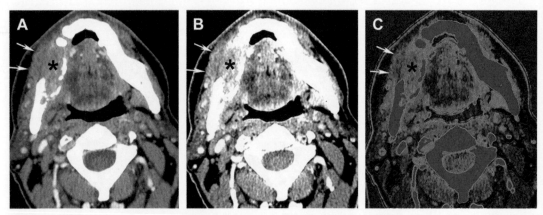

Fig. 33. Squamous cell carcinoma of the buccal mucosa with bone invasion. (*A*) 65 keV VMI, (*B*) 40 keV VMI, and (*C*) iodine (iodine-water) map demonstrate a large infiltrative mass (*arrows*) invading and destroying a portion of the adjacent right hemimandible (*asterisks*).

Recurrent Head and Neck Squamous Cell Carcinoma and Post-treatment Changes

Local recurrence of HNSCC may not be evident on clinical examination, particularly if it occurs along the deep aspect of the surgical flap.[39] On imaging, evaluation for recurrence can sometimes be challenging against the background of postsurgical and postradiation changes and distortion of normal anatomy. Recurrent lesions frequently present as expansile tumors in the surgical site or as thickening of the soft tissues of the flap.[39] On CT, the lesions can have ill-defined margins and diffuse enhancement and can invade nearby structures such as bone.[39] Similar to primary untreated HNSCC, low kiloelectron volt VMIs can improve visibility and contour delineation of recurrent tumors (**Fig. 34**).[5,7] One study also demonstrated a statistically significant difference with higher attenuation and iodine content of tumor compared with benign post-treatment changes on 40 kiloelectron volt VMIs and iodine maps, respectively (see **Fig. 34**).[12]

Perineural Spread of Tumor

Perineural tumor spread (PNS) is an important prognostic factor in malignant tumors of the head and neck.[40] MR imaging is considered the optimal modality for the evaluation of PNS but PNS may also be evident on CT, especially if advanced. Supplemental DECT reconstructions can be used in the evaluation and identification of PNS (see **Fig. 26**; **Fig. 35**), and may be helpful in identifying

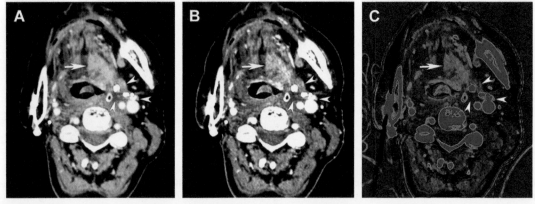

Fig. 34. Recurrent squamous cell carcinoma. (*A*) 65 keV VMI, (*B*) 40 keV VMI, and (*C*) iodine (iodine-water) map demonstrate a mass adjacent to the site of previous surgery and flap reconstruction on the left (*white arrows*). Note the presence of surgical clips with postsurgical and radiation changes posterior and lateral to the mass (*white arrowheads*). In particular, note how the posterolateral margin of the recurrence is better distinguished from nearby post-treatment changes on the 40 keV VMI or iodine map compared with the 65 keV VMI. (*Courtesy of* Dr Reza Forghani, MD, PhD, Montreal, Quebec, Canada.)

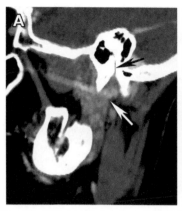
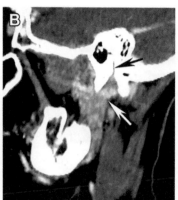
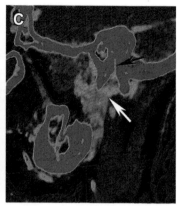

Fig. 35. PNS. Sagittal reformatted (*A*) 65 keV VMI, (*B*) 40 keV VMI, and (*C*) iodine (iodine-water) map from a contrast-enhanced neck CT demonstrate abnormal enhancement and iodine signal along the vertical (mastoid) segment of the facial nerve (*black arrows*), representing PNS from a left parotid adenocarcinoma (*white arrows; same case as shown in* **Fig. 26**), subsequently confirmed on MR imaging and pathologic specimens. (*Courtesy of Dr Reza Forghani, MD, PhD, Montreal, Quebec, Canada.*)

abnormal skull base foramina, as well as the presence of enhancement along the course of the involved nerve.

ARTIFACT REDUCTION

This pictorial essay concludes with a few examples of artifact reduction using DECT (See discussion of artifact reduction using DECT, other articles in this issue.) As previously discussed in the section on different DECT reconstructions, in addition to helping distinguish NOTC from tumor, high-energy VMIs can be used to reduce artifacts, including those from metallic hardware or dental material.[4,14–20]

The effectiveness of artifact reduction depends on the type and degree of artifact, but modest reduction is achievable (**Figs. 36–38**). It is also noteworthy that although artifact is reduced with increasing VMI energy, so is iodine attenuation and soft tissue contrast. Therefore, if the target of interest is visualization of a structure with high

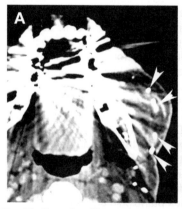
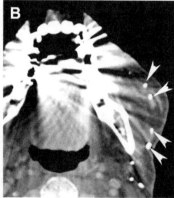
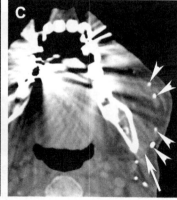

Fig. 36. Dental artifact reduction using high-energy VMIs. (*A*) 40 keV VMI, (*B*) 65 keV VMI, and (*C*) 95 keV VMI from a contrast-enhanced neck CT with extensive and severe dental artifact. In addition to marked obscuration of the oral cavity, artifact partially obscures the left parotid bed in this patient with prior resection of a left parotid squamous cell carcinoma. Although low-energy VMIs, such as 40 keV, increase iodine attenuation and soft tissue contrast, they also increase image noise and certain artifacts; compare the 40 keV VMI (*A*) to the 65 keV VMI (*B*). On the other hand, increasing VMI energy above that used for routine interpretation can result in modest artifact reduction; compare the 95 keV VMI (*C*) with the 65 keV VMI (*B*). Note improved visualization and, therefore, assessment of the surgical bed for recurrence on the 95 keV VMI (*long arrow* in *C* points to an example of an area of artifact reduction and improved visualization of the underlying tissues and post-treatment changes. *Arrowheads* point to surgical clips within the surgical bed).

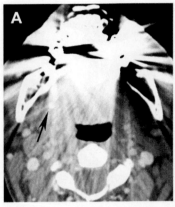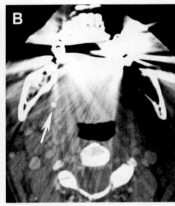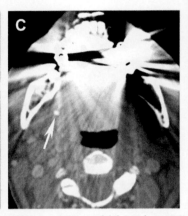

Fig. 37. Dental artifact reduction using high-energy VMIs. (*A*) 65 keV VMI, (*B*) 95 keV VMI, and (*C*) 140 keV VMI from a contrast-enhanced neck CT with extensive and severe dental artifact. Note artifact reduction on the 95 and 140 keV VMIs, enabling confident identification of a small right submandibular stone (*arrows*) that is much less well-seen on the 65 keV VMI. There is slightly better artifact reduction on the 140 compared with the 95 keV VMI.

attenuation independent of iodine enhancement, then very-high-energy VMIs, 130 to 140 keV (or even greater with some DECT systems) may be useful. However, if the objective is better visualization of an enhancing lesion where preserving some degree of enhancement or soft tissue contrast is important, then high-energy VMIs in a more intermediate range (for example 95 keV) may be more suitable.[17] The application of high-energy VMIs need not be limited to metallic implant and dental artifacts, and these reconstructions may also be useful for reduction of other artifacts, such as those from dense venous contrast or bones at the thoracic inlet (see **Fig. 38**).

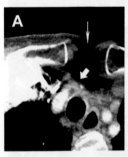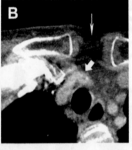

Fig. 38. Artifact reduction using high-energy VMIs. (*A*) 65 keV VMI and (*B*) 95 keV VMI from a contrast-enhanced neck CT demonstrate significant artifact secondary to dense venous contrast, as well as the clavicles obscuring the thoracic inlet. Note significant artifact reduction on 95 keV VMI compared with the 65 keV VMI, enabling visualization of the brachiocephalic trunk (*thick white arrows*). The fat between the clavicular heads (*long thin arrows*) also becomes at least partially visible on the 95 keV VMI. The trade-off is lower iodine attenuation with increasing VMI energy, as can be seen by comparison of enhancing structures such as vessels.

SUMMARY

There are increasing DECT applications for the evaluation of head and neck pathologic entities. Various DECT reconstructions can be used to improve visualization of enhancing lesions and soft tissue contrast; provide a topographic distribution of materials, such as iodine within tissues; reduce artifact; and create virtual unenhanced or noncontrast images from a contrast-enhanced acquisition. These reconstructions can aid diagnostic interpretation, but optimal implementation and use of DECT requires familiarity with the appearance of normal tissues and pathologic entities on various DECT reconstructions. This article provides a pictorial review that includes examples of the appearance of normal anatomic structures and a multitude of neoplastic and nonneoplastic pathologic entities on commonly used DECT reconstructions, as well as other DECT applications, such as artifact reduction. These should help familiarize the reader with the expected appearance of normal structures and lesions in the head and neck on DECT, and serve as a reference. Also, the authors hope that this article will stimulate interest in the use of this technology and provide an impetus for further research into known and novel applications of DECT for the evaluation of head and neck pathologic entities.

REFERENCES

1. Kuno H, Onaya H, Iwata R, et al. Evaluation of cartilage invasion by laryngeal and hypopharyngeal squamous cell carcinoma with dual-energy CT. Radiology 2012;265(2):488–96.
2. Srinivasan A, Parker RA, Manjunathan A, et al. Differentiation of benign and malignant neck

pathologies: preliminary experience using spectral computed tomography. J Comput Assist Tomogr 2013;37(5):666–72.

3. Tawfik AM, Kerl JM, Bauer RW, et al. Dual-energy CT of head and neck cancer: average weighting of low- and high-voltage acquisitions to improve lesion delineation and image quality-initial clinical experience. Invest Radiol 2012;47(5):306–11.

4. Forghani R, Levental M, Gupta R, et al. Different spectral hounsfield unit curve and high-energy virtual monochromatic image characteristics of squamous cell carcinoma compared with nonossified thyroid cartilage. AJNR Am J Neuroradiol 2015; 36(6):1194–200.

5. Lam S, Gupta R, Levental M, et al. Optimal virtual monochromatic images for evaluation of normal tissues and head and neck cancer using dual-energy CT. AJNR Am J Neuroradiol 2015;36(8): 1518–24.

6. Forghani R. Advanced dual-energy CT for head and neck cancer imaging. Expert Rev Anticancer Ther 2015;15(12):1489–501.

7. Forghani R, Kelly H, Yu E, et al. Low-energy virtual monochromatic dual-energy Computed Tomography Images for the evaluation of head and neck squamous cell carcinoma: a Study of tumor visibility compared with single-energy computed tomography and user acceptance. J Comput Assist Tomogr 2017. in press.

8. Forghani R, Roskies M, Liu X, et al. Dual-energy CT characteristics of parathyroid adenomas on 25-and 55-second 4D-CT acquisitions: preliminary experience. J Comput Assist Tomogr 2016;40(5):806–14.

9. Lam S, Gupta R, Kelly H, et al. Multiparametric evaluation of head and neck squamous cell carcinoma using a single-source dual-energy CT with Fast kVp switching: State of the Art. Cancers 2015;7(4): 2201–16.

10. Albrecht MH, Scholtz JE, Kraft J, et al. Assessment of an advanced monoenergetic reconstruction technique in dual-energy computed tomography of head and neck cancer. Eur Radiol 2015;25(8):2493–501.

11. Wichmann JL, Noske EM, Kraft J, et al. Virtual monoenergetic dual-energy computed tomography: optimization of kiloelectron volt settings in head and neck cancer. Invest Radiol 2014;49(11):735–41.

12. Yamauchi H, Buehler M, Goodsitt MM, et al. Dual-Energy CT-based differentiation of benign posttreatment changes from primary or recurrent malignancy of the head and neck: comparison of spectral hounsfield units at 40 and 70 keV and iodine concentration. AJR Am J Roentgenol 2016;206(3):580–7.

13. Tawfik AM, Razek AA, Kerl JM, et al. Comparison of dual-energy CT-derived iodine content and iodine overlay of normal, inflammatory and metastatic squamous cell carcinoma cervical lymph nodes. Eur Radiol 2014;24(3):574–80.

14. Bamberg F, Dierks A, Nikolaou K, et al. Metal artifact reduction by dual energy computed tomography using monoenergetic extrapolation. Eur Radiol 2011; 21(7):1424–9.

15. De Crop A, Casselman J, Van Hoof T, et al. Analysis of metal artifact reduction tools for dental hardware in CT scans of the oral cavity: kVp, iterative reconstruction, dual-energy CT, metal artifact reduction software: does it make a difference? Neuroradiology 2015;57(8):841–9.

16. Lee YH, Park KK, Song HT, et al. Metal artefact reduction in gemstone spectral imaging dual-energy CT with and without metal artefact reduction software. Eur Radiol 2012;22(6):1331–40.

17. Nair JR, DeBlois F, Ong T, et al. Dual energy CT: Balance between iodine attenuation and artifact reduction for the evaluation of head and neck cancer. J Comput Assist Tomogr 2017. [Epub ahead of print].

18. Srinivasan A, Hoeffner E, Ibrahim M, et al. Utility of dual-energy CT virtual keV monochromatic series for the assessment of spinal transpedicular hardware-bone interface. AJR Am J Roentgenol 2013;201(4):878–83.

19. Tanaka R, Hayashi T, Ike M, et al. Reduction of dark-band-like metal artifacts caused by dental implant bodies using hypothetical monoenergetic imaging after dual-energy computed tomography. Oral Surg Oral Med Oral Pathol Oral Radiol 2013;115(6): 833–8.

20. Stolzmann P, Winklhofer S, Schwendener N, et al. Monoenergetic computed tomography reconstructions reduce beam hardening artifacts from dental restorations. Forensic Sci Med Pathol 2013;9(3): 327–32.

21. McCollough CH, Leng S, Yu L, et al. Dual- and multi-energy CT: principles, technical approaches, and clinical applications. Radiology 2015;276(3):637–53.

22. Forghani R, De Man B, Gupta R. Dual energy CT: physical principles, approaches to scanning, usage, and implementation - Part 2. Neuroimaging Clin N Am 2017. in press.

23. Hu R, Daftari Besheli L, Young J, et al. Dual-energy head CT enables accurate distinction of intraparenchymal hemorrhage from calcification in emergency department patients. Radiology 2016;280(1): 177–83.

24. Hu R, Padole A, Gupta R. Dual energy CT applications for differentiation of intracranial hemorrhage, calcium, and iodine. Neuroimaging Clin N Am 2017. in press.

25. Hoang JK, Glastonbury CM, Chen LF, et al. CT mucosal window settings: a novel approach to evaluating early T-stage head and neck carcinoma. Am J Roentgenol 2010;195(4):1002–6.

26. Wippold FJ. Head and neck imaging: the role of CT and MRI. J Magn Reson Imaging 2007;25(3): 453–65.

27. Branstetter Iv BF, Weissman JL. Normal anatomy of the neck with CT and MR imaging correlation. Radiol Clin North Am 2000;38(5):925–40.

28. Roskies M, Liu X, Hier MP, et al. 3-phase dual-energy CT scan as a feasible salvage imaging modality for the identification of non-localizing parathyroid adenomas: a prospective study. J Otolaryngol Head Neck Surg 2015;44:44.

29. Berger G, Averbuch E, Zilka K, et al. Adult vallecular cyst: thirteen-year experience. Otolaryngol Head Neck Surg 2008;138(3):321–7.

30. Forghani R, Smoker WRK, Curtin HD. Pathology of the oral region. Head and neck imaging. 5th edition. St Louis (MO): Mosby; 2011. p. 1643–748.

31. Woo E, Connor S. Computed tomography and magnetic resonance imaging appearances of cystic lesions in the suprahyoid neck: a pictorial review. Dentomaxillofac Radiol 2014;36:451–8.

32. El-Monem MHA, Gaafar AH, Magdy EA. Lipomas of the head and neck: presentation variability and diagnostic work-up. J Laryngol Otol 2006;120(1): 47–55.

33. White DK, Davidson HC, Harnsberger HR, et al. Accessory salivary tissue in the mylohyoid boutonniere: a clinical and radiologic pseudolesion of the oral cavity. AJNR Am J Neuroradiol 2001;22(2): 406–12.

34. Choi DS, Na DG, Byun HS, et al. Salivary gland tumors: evaluation with two-phase helical CT. Radiology 2000;214(1):231–6.

35. Yousem DM, Kraut MA, Chalian AA. Major salivary gland imaging. Radiology 2000;216(1):19–29.

36. Hoang JK, Branstetter BF, Gafton AR, et al. Imaging of thyroid carcinoma with CT and MRI: approaches to common scenarios. Cancer Imaging 2013;13(1): 128–39.

37. Yang L, Luo D, Li L, et al. Differentiation of malignant cervical lymphadenopathy by dual-energy CT: a preliminary analysis. Sci Rep 2016;6:31020.

38. Weber AL, Rahemtullah A, Ferry JA. Hodgkin and non-Hodgkin lymphoma of the head and neck: clinical, pathologic, and imaging evaluation. Neuroimaging Clin N Am 2003;13(3):371–92.

39. Saito N, Nadgir RN, Nakahira M, et al. Posttreatment CT and MR imaging in head and neck cancer: what the radiologist needs to know. Radiographics 2012; 32(5):1261–82 [discussion: 1282–4].

40. Brea Alvarez B, Tunon Gomez M. Perineural spread in head and neck tumors. Radiologia 2014;56(5): 400–12.

Routine Dual-Energy Computed Tomography Scanning of the Neck in Clinical Practice: A Single-Institution Experience

Almudena Pérez-Lara, MD, PhD[a], Mark Levental, MD[a],
Lorne Rosenbloom, MD[a], Gary Wing, RT[a],
Reza Forghani, MD, PhD[a,b],*

KEYWORDS

- Dual-energy CT • Spectral CT • Head and neck • Workflow • Radiology department productivity
- Optimized DECT protocols • Virtual monochromatic images • Material decomposition maps

KEY POINTS

- Implementation of routine dual-energy computed tomography (DECT) scanning in a radiology department poses unique challenges for the technologists (production) and radiologists (interpretation).
- A properly trained and engaged team of technologists having access to clear preset protocols is helpful for maintaining a smooth and efficient operation.
- Predetermined DECT protocols resulting in automatic reconstruction of image sets at the computed tomography scanner console that are sent to the picture archiving and communication system can reduce or eliminate the need for additional manipulations, promoting routine use and enhancing the efficiency of radiologist workflow.
- Ultimately, vendor solutions for integrated and seamless workflow will likely be key for widespread use and to take advantage of the full range of DECT diagnostic capabilities.

INTRODUCTION

There are multiple emerging clinical applications for dual-energy computed tomography (DECT), including many applications in neuroimaging and head and neck imaging, which are discussed in detail in many of the accompanying articles in this issue. The various clinical applications and the potential added value of DECT for diagnostic evaluation of our patients will ultimately be the main drivers for routine and widespread use of this technology in the clinical setting. However, implementation of DECT in routine clinical practice has specific requirements and poses certain challenges that

Disclosures: R.F. has acted as a consultant for GE Healthcare and has served as a speaker at lunch and learn sessions titled "Dual-Energy CT Applications in Neuroradiology and Head and Neck Imaging" sponsored by GE Healthcare at the 27th and 28th Annual Meetings of the Eastern Neuroradiological Society in 2015 and 2016 (no personal compensation or travel support for these sessions).
The other authors declare no relevant conflict of interest.
[a] Department of Radiology, Jewish General Hospital, McGill University, 3755 Cote Sainte-Catherine Road, Montreal, Quebec H3T 1E2, Canada; [b] Department of Radiology, Segal Cancer Centre and Lady Davis Institute for Medical Research, Jewish General Hospital, McGill University, Room C-212.1, 3755 Cote Sainte-Catherine Road, Montreal, Quebec H3T 1E2, Canada
* Corresponding author.
E-mail address: rforghani@jgh.mcgill.ca

Neuroimag Clin N Am 27 (2017) 523–531
http://dx.doi.org/10.1016/j.nic.2017.04.006
1052-5149/17/© 2017 Elsevier Inc. All rights reserved.

should not be ignored.[1] This is especially true in the current health care environment, with progressively increasing volumes in diagnostic radiology departments resulting in demands for increased productivity, from both the technologists and the radiologists interpreting these examinations. Widespread adoption of DECT in routine clinical practice will likely at least in part depend on seamless, workflow-friendly integration.

Routine use of DECT scanning can be challenging because it can affect the normal departmental workflow at multiple levels, both on the production (technologist) and interpretation (radiologist) side. Consequently, successful implementation in the clinical setting requires the development of algorithms for patient selection, optimization of scanning protocols, and establishment of an integrated working team composed of highly trained technologists and radiologists working closely together to ensure smooth workflow and optimal results.[1,2] The purpose of this article is to review the practical workflow implications of routine DECT scanning based on the experience at a single institution where a large percentage of elective neck computed tomography scans (CTs) are acquired in DECT mode using a fast kVp switching scanner (GE Healthcare, Waukesha, WI). This article provides an overview of the challenges encountered based on this experience and discusses strategies for addressing these challenges and enabling seamless workflow integration.

PROSPECTIVE SCAN ACQUISITION IN DUAL-ENERGY COMPUTED TOMOGRAPHY MODE

The various commercially available DECT scanning systems are discussed in detail in the first 2 articles in this issue and are not reviewed here (See Reza Forghani and colleagues' article, "Dual Energy CT: Physical Principles, Approaches to Scanning, Usage, and Implementation - Part 1," and Reza Forghani and colleagues' article, "Dual Energy CT: Physical Principles, Approaches to Scanning, Usage, and Implementation - Part 2," in this issue). However, the topic of acquisition modes is central to DECT workflow and is briefly discussed. As discussed in other articles in this series, most of the current clinical DECT systems enable scan acquisition in either DECT or single-energy computed tomography (SECT) mode. This means that the decision to acquire scans in DECT mode must be made prospectively. For these systems, a preset algorithm or protocol can simplify the process of determining which cases will be scanned in DECT mode. Scanners with a layered or "sandwich" detector (Philips Healthcare, Andover, MA) are the exception to

this rule. Because spectral separation for these scanners is achieved at the level of the detector arrays, these scanners practically always acquire in "DECT mode."

DUAL-ENERGY COMPUTED TOMOGRAPHY SCAN SELECTION ALGORITHMS

Because most clinical DECT systems, including fast kVp switching scanners, enable acquisition in DECT or SECT modes, it is not unusual to have a subset of studies performed in SECT mode on these scanners. However, using a DECT scanner *exclusively* in SECT mode defeats the purpose of having such a scanner, and does not take advantage of its full potential. The only possible exception would be the use of a *dual-source* type of DECT scanner primarily devoted to cardiac imaging with the 2 sources being used simultaneously to improve temporal resolution.

The decision on whether or not to perform scans in DECT mode can be based on several factors, as with any other protocoling algorithm (**Box 1**). This could be based on specific referral patterns (eg, all brain oncology or head and neck oncology studies) or based on highly selective clinical indications (eg, all brain CT scans after intra-arterial interventions for ischemic stroke to distinguish hemorrhage from iodinated contrast). Alternatively, it may be done more broadly, based on the body area and/or certain general indications (eg, all adult neck studies, all brain CTs, all oncology studies). For scan protocols consisting of multiple acquisitions, a decision also has to be made regarding which phases should be acquired in DECT mode.

The indications for clinical use of DECT are currently based on studies demonstrating the

---

Box 1
Decision making for scan acquisition in dual-energy computed tomography (DECT) mode

- Most DECT scanners provide the option for scanning in DECT or single-energy computed tomography (SECT) mode and therefore the decision to acquire DECT images must be made prospectively (the exception being the layered or sandwich detector systems that essentially always acquire in DECT mode)

- Therefore, algorithms need to be in place for protocoling studies as DECT acquisitions prospectively

- Selection could be based on specific referral patterns, selective clinical indications, or more broadly based on the body area and/or certain general indications

usefulness of various DECT reconstructions as supplements for diagnostic interpretation. These indications are likely to evolve and will most likely expand with additional studies verifying the usefulness of existing applications or demonstrating new clinical applications. Routine use of DECT, regardless of indication, is another approach that could be more straightforward to implement, assuming there is not a prohibitive impact on production and technologist workflow (discussed in the following sections). This approach can be justified and is feasible because it is possible to routinely acquire scans in DECT mode with acceptable radiation doses that are similar to those of SECT scans. Nonetheless, for departments implementing DECT for the first time, it is advisable that benchmarks be observed based on current radiation doses at that institution or those published in the literature, and that the acquisition protocols are evaluated to ensure that the radiation exposure is as low as reasonably achievable.

In our department, a large percentage of elective neck CT scans are performed in DECT mode (57% based on a recent audit). Currently, the CT scanner located in our emergency department is not a DECT scanner and therefore those scans cannot be acquired in DECT mode. Priority is given to primary head and neck cancer studies and scans performed for the evaluation of salivary gland disease; however, neck CTs for other indications also may be performed in DECT mode. The reason for this flexibility is that DECT can negatively impact CT productivity and technologist workflow (as discussed in the following sections), which must be taken into account to ensure sustainable practices in a high-volume environment. **Table 1** provides a breakdown of DECT scans performed in our department, stratified by clinical indication based on a recent audit.

COMPUTED TOMOGRAPHY DEPARTMENT PRODUCTIVITY AND TECHNOLOGIST WORKFLOW
Initial Scan Organization and Scheduling

Implementation of DECT in the clinical setting requires careful attention to every step involved in organizing and performing these scans (**Box 2**). Depending on the organization of a department, and the physical location of different CT scanners, the need for adjustments may start at the time of scheduling, unless every CT scanner in the health care facility is a DECT scanner (currently not the case in most departments). In our hospital, the outpatient SECT and DECT scanners are in the same physical location. Therefore, we usually

Table 1
Percentage of neck computed tomography (CT) studies acquired in dual-energy CT mode by clinical indication

Reason for Consultation	Frequency, %
Head and neck cancer staging (other than thyroid)	10
Head and neck cancer surveillance and follow-up	17
Suspected salivary gland tumor	6
Parathyroid adenoma	4
Thyroid cancer	4
Lymphoproliferative disorder	16
Other malignancies	7
Infectious/inflammatory process	12
Other	24

have the flexibility to change protocols at the last minute, if necessary. However, attempts are made to limit the number of DECT scans performed in a given shift, and ideally stagger them between SECT acquisitions, to minimize the impact of the increased scan processing time required with DECTs on throughput, as is discussed later in this article. For departments

Box 2
DECT acquisition assessment

- The need for DECT acquisition may have to be taken into account at the time of scan scheduling
- This is most important for centers with multiple physical sites in which patients need to be directed to a specific location to obtain the appropriate study
- Appropriate scheduling also should take into account the longer scan processing times, especially for busy departments operating at or near full capacity
- Practices that can help mitigate impact on productivity and workflow and help to maintain a smooth operation are as follows:
  - Limit the number of DECT scans performed within a given shift
  - Stagger or mix DECT and SECT acquisitions
- Ideally, future development of systems with more powerful processing capabilities will result in reduced processing times and will minimize the impact of DECT scans on scheduling and productivity

offering CT services at different physical locations, especially those with multiple outpatient facilities that may be distant from one another, predetermination of the mode of acquisition is required at the time of scheduling to ensure that the patient is scheduled at the appropriate facility.

Computed Tomography Technologist Training and Engagement

DECT technique has multiple potential applications and offers various reconstruction algorithms, requiring specific and specialized training for the CT technologist. At our center, 16 CT technologists have been trained to perform DECT scans autonomously, some as "super users" who can be approached by other technologists for questions or for support in complex cases. Appropriate technologist training and engagement is essential and has been central to the success of our DECT program and the ability to incorporate this into the clinical workflow on a routine basis. Moreover, it has been our experience that active CT technologist engagement, including feedback on the value of the work they perform, is also an important part of this process.

Preset Dual-Energy Computed Tomography Protocols, Generation of Different Dual-Energy Computed Tomography Reconstructions, and Scan Processing Times

In addition to the protocols and technical details of how to perform scans (eg, scan coverage, administration of intravenous contrast, number of phases, additional acquisitions such as angled neck acquisitions for patients with dental fillings), many of which are not unique to DECT, it is advisable to predetermine which additional or specialized DECT reconstructions should be generated at the CT console and sent to the picture archiving and communication system (PACS) as part of a given protocol (**Box 3**). Routine reconstructions equivalent to those typically generated for an SECT acquisition differ based on the scanner type. For fast kVp switching DECT scanners, 70 or 65 keV virtual monochromatic images (VMIs) are generally considered similar to a 120-kVp SECT acquisition and are typically generated for routine clinical interpretation.[3–6] However, the main advantage of DECT is the ability to perform additional analysis and generate supplemental reconstructions not possible with SECT. Although one could rely solely on postprocessing by the radiologist for additional reconstructions, this would not be workflow friendly on the radiologist (interpretation) side and is likely to reduce the

---

> **Box 3**
> **Preset DECT image reconstruction sets**
>
> - In addition to routine reconstructions replacing those obtained with SECT, specialized DECT reconstructions that have been shown to be clinically useful for specific indications can be generated automatically and sent to the picture archiving and communication system (PACS) so that they are readily available at the time of interpretation
> - Such preset DECT protocols with predetermined image reconstruction sets can help minimize additional image postprocessing by the radiologist at the time of interpretation and improve interpretation workflow

use of specialized DECT reconstructions and its additional postprocessing capabilities.

Therefore, one possible approach would be to routinely generate those reconstructions that are most likely to be clinically useful at the CT console and send them to PACS so they are readily available for interpretation.[7,8] This is our preferred approach, although in the ideal setting a combination of preset reconstructions and seamless PACS integration with advanced image analysis software, allowing the radiologist to quickly perform additional analysis and/or generate nonroutine reconstructions when needed, would be optimal. Examples of reconstructions that can be created based on specific clinical indications include generation of low-energy VMI image sets to supplement the standard 65-keV or 70-keV VMIs for improving visibility and contour delineation of head and neck squamous cell carcinoma[6–10] or the generation of high-energy VMIs and iodine maps for improving evaluation of thyroid cartilage invasion by head and neck cancer[7,8,11,12] (as discussed in detail in a separate article on head and neck squamous cell carcinoma evaluation in this issue). At our center, low-energy VMIs (40 keV) are generated for every neck scan and sent to PACS so that they are readily available for interpretation.

The ease of generating supplemental DECT reconstructions such as VMIs at different energies or basis material decomposition maps (eg, iodine maps) varies based on the scanner type and can even vary depending on the model of the scanner console. For our scanner, many reconstructions, including 40-keV VMIs, can be programmed and generated automatically without additional technologist manipulation. For some other console models or scanner types, variable degrees of technologist manipulation will be required to create such reconstructions. These factors can clearly impact technologist workflow and CT productivity. In general, greater automation is likely to increase widespread adoption and help with the implementation and use of DECT in the clinical setting.

In addition to specific image manipulations required by CT technologists, in our experience, another important factor that can impact CT productivity and DECT scanning is the scan processing time. Once again, this can vary significantly between scanner types and generations/models. It can also vary depending on the type of scan performed. For example, large angiographic studies would require more processing time than basic body or neck DECT scans. The time required per scan may be as little as 5 to 10 minutes or more than 15 to 20 minutes for large studies or studies with multiple acquisitions. For some scanner types, one must allow the postprocessing to proceed without interruption; this means that further scanning cannot be performed until the queue has been cleared and the current study completed and closed. Although technologist engagement is not required for the entire processing duration and the technologist may be free to perform other tasks, it can nonetheless impact and strain workflow by delaying the initiation of the following scan. This can negatively impact busy departments operating at or near capacity. If the delays become extensive, this could also pose a challenge for studies performed in the emergency setting by delaying final interpretation.

One way to deal with the effects of increased scan processing times is to limit the number of DECT scans scheduled within a given shift. Another workaround to improve workflow is to avoid scheduling of multiple, especially "processing-heavy" examinations back to back. Interleaving DECT and SECT acquisitions also can be helpful. However, the ideal solution, especially for more widespread use of DECT, will ultimately have to come from the vendors. Optimally, systems should have more robust computing and processing power that shorten scan processing times, ideally to the point that scan processing time does not have to be a significant consideration in deciding whether or not to perform a DECT scan. Various vendor solutions are under way to address the issue of workflow as well as processing time. For example, with newer-generation consoles of fast kVp switching DECT scanners, many DECT reconstructions can be generated automatically. Furthermore, some of the newer systems being introduced into the market may enable simultaneous image processing to enable automatic reconstruction of large DECT image sets without significant additional time penalty for image processing beyond a certain number of initial image sets. These are welcome refinements that will aid routine clinical implementation.

Overview of Scan Acquisition and Processing Times for Neck Computed Tomography Scans

We recently conducted an evaluation of technologist time spent on neck DECT scans. Based on the evaluation of a total of 137 patient scans, the average time to perform a standard DECT of the neck is 5 to 10 minutes. This includes the time required to carefully position the patient and the time to check the acquired images once the examination is finished. Subsequently, the technologist is free to perform other tasks while the automatic image reconstruction process is performed and images are transferred to PACS. This process required an average of 18.6 minutes to be completed (range of 14–23 minutes, median of 18.3 minutes), as measured from the moment that the CT scan was acquired until all the reformatted images were successfully transferred to PACS and were available for visualization from any workstation.

As expected, the processing time depends on the number of CT acquisitions performed, and if ancillary techniques or dynamic maneuvers are obtained, the required time to reformat the images increases. For example, as dental fillings are so common, most of our neck scans include a second, angled acquisition. Other scans may have additional acquisitions based on our standard protocols as well (eg, tongue-out views for patients with tongue cancers, phonation views for the evaluation of the larynx). Network speed can also impact the time to availability on PACS and likewise should be optimized to ensure rapid transfer of the additional image sets created with DECT.

With our system, while these reconstructions are being generated at the CT console, it is not advisable to scan other patients, as this would significantly slow down the reconstruction process. This has an unavoidable impact on CT scan workflow and patient scheduling, which must be taken into consideration to adapt the expected examination times and estimate the working capacity of the CT scan equipment.

Spectral Image Datasets

One final important consideration on the production side is the storage of the spectral datasets. It is important for users new to DECT to keep in mind that the specific reconstructions created for clinical interpretation (eg, 65 keV or 70 keV VMIs) do not contain the full complement of "spectral" data. To take full advantage of spectral datasets and different DECT analytical tools for clinical or research use at the time of interpretation or at a later time, the specific spectral dataset containing this information must be preserved. The most common options are to send the dataset to an advanced processing workstation (eg, Advantage Workstation; GE Healthcare, Waukesha, WI) where these can also be analyzed or used to generate other reconstructions or to send this dataset to PACS for permanent storage. If the advanced workstation is used for storage, there must be a mechanism in place for long-term storage (if that is desired), to avoid eventual overwriting of older scans due to storage limits on the workstation.

DUAL-ENERGY COMPUTED TOMOGRAPHY SCAN INTERPRETATION: RADIOLOGIST WORKFLOW
Automatically Generated Advanced Dual-Energy Computed Tomography Reconstructions and Tailored Evaluation Using Advanced Dual-Energy Computed Tomography Processing Software

As discussed earlier, one approach for facilitating integration of DECT into routine clinical workflow is to stipulate that specific sets of reconstructions be generated as part of the CT protocol and have the technologists routinely send them to PACS so that they are readily available for review at the time of interpretation. These reconstructions would be incorporated into such protocols based on existing literature demonstrating their utility. An example is the use of different energy reconstructions for evaluating head and neck cancer, as discussed in a separate article in this issue or elsewhere.[7,8] The advantage of this approach is that the reconstructions that are mostly likely to be of clinical utility are readily available for use. The disadvantage of this approach (without easy access to advanced postprocessing software) is that the radiologist is limited to preselected reconstructions and cannot perform more advanced quantitative analysis, such as region of interest analysis and/or derivation of spectral Hounsfield unit attenuation curves, in a workflow-friendly manner. Depending on the vendor, certain reconstructions, such as material decomposition maps, are also best viewed at the advanced image workstation rather than on PACS, due to limitations with windowing or other manipulations, representing another limitation.

When implementing DECT for the first time or introducing a new DECT application in the clinical setting, it is important to ensure proper communication to radiologist colleagues, including the rationale and potential utility of the various specialized reconstructions. This is important, as not all members may be up to date with the literature on the applications of this emerging technology. This will help ensure optimal use and enhance user acceptance. Another factor to consider when implementing DECT is that some reconstructions may require a period of adjustment for a radiologist to be comfortable using them in routine interpretation. For example, 40 keV VMIs are more noisy than standard reconstructions and it may take some time before one is used to "reading through" the noise to extract maximal information and benefit from these reconstructions. Of course, one must ensure that they are appropriately displayed using optimal window-level settings. Like any other image set, one must also get used to the appearance of normal structures, artifacts, and so forth on these various specialized DECT reconstructions.

The approach of sending preselected reconstructions to PACS can ease workflow and is likely to be sufficient in most cases (**Box 4**). It is also likely to promote the use of advanced DECT reconstructions in routine clinical practice. For cases in which additional image reconstructions or advanced spectral analysis is required, the radiologist has the option to use an advanced workstation or advanced integrated software (if available) (see **Box 4**). In the ideal setting, the radiologist should have access to advanced DECT processing software that is integrated into PACS, enabling the radiologist to take advantage of the full complement of DECT analytical tools without the need to physically displace and use a separate workstation. The aim is to minimize the impact of this technology on radiologist productivity, which

---

Box 4
Factors enabling seamless DECT radiologist workflow

- Automatic generation of specialized DECT reconstructions that are most likely to be of utility based on current literature is possible with newer DECT systems

- Availability of those reconstructions that are most likely to be needed at the time of interpretation in PACS can ease integration into radiologist workflow

- In the ideal setting, predetermined reconstructions would be sent to PACS but the radiologist would also have access to advanced DECT processing software integrated into PACS for rapid use, if required, without the need for physical displacement and interruption of normal workflow

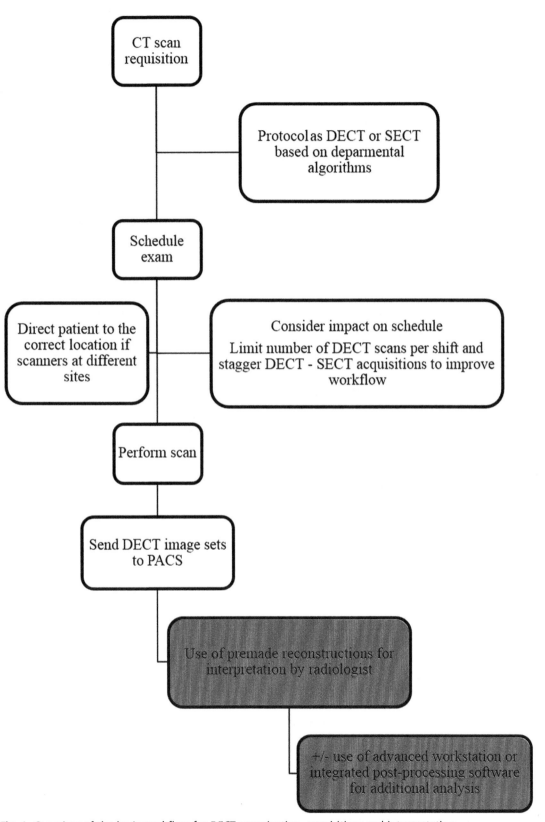

Fig. 1. Overview of the basic workflow for DECT organization, acquisition, and interpretation.

in turn will increase user acceptance. The impact of smooth and seamless workflow-friendly integration on widespread adoption and use of this technology should not be underestimated. **Fig. 1** summarizes the different steps for DECT organization, acquisition, and interpretation.

Advanced Dual-Energy Computed Tomography Postprocessing Software

Currently, the postprocessing software for advanced DECT data analysis is proprietary and vendor-specific. We are not aware of a vendor-neutral independent platform that offers the full spectral analytical and reconstruction capabilities for scans generated by different DECT systems at this time. This is important to consider when planning acquisition of a DECT system, especially for vendors that may not include the full software capabilities as part of their basic or standard package. It also implies that, at least in the short term, innovations and development of integrated analytical platforms for improving workflow will depend primarily on the scanner vendors. Depending on the scanner vendor and type, these may include physical workstations and/or "thin client" models providing access to advanced DECT analysis and processing software running on a specialized server that can be remotely accessed from the PACS workstation. Technological developments and refinements that enable complete interpretation of studies on the PACS workstation are likely to have a positive impact on the use and widespread adoption of DECT in busy clinical practice.

Overview of the Use of Specialized Low-Energy Neck Reconstructions Available Through the Picture Archiving and Communication System: A Single-Institution Experience

It has been our experience that the ready availability of multiple DECT reconstructions in PACS promotes their use. For example, we implemented automatic generation and transfer of low-energy (40 keV) VMIs to PACS more than 1 year ago (initially this required manual reconstruction by technologists at the CT console but later became automated after a console upgrade). These are sent in addition to and are meant to supplement the standard 65 keV VMIs used for routine interpretation.[6–8,13] In our department, all elective neck CTs are interpreted by 1 of 3 dedicated head and neck radiologists, who were recently surveyed on the use of low-energy (40 keV) VMIs. All 3 radiologists responded that 40 keV VMIs can provide additional useful information/value for the evaluation of head and neck

pathology. One of the radiologists reported reviewing the 40-keV VMIs in nearly all (90% or greater) cases when available. A second head and neck radiologist used these reconstructions in more than 50% of cases, whereas the third radiologist reported reviewing these VMIs in 10% to 50% of cases.

The 3 radiologists agreed that the low-energy VMI is useful in evaluating squamous cell carcinoma of the head and neck, in assessing the presence of pathologic lymph nodes, and in detecting other malignancies. However, 1 of the 3 radiologists also reported using the 40-keV VMI to assess other pathology, including benign disorders; for example, for the evaluation and determination of the extent of inflammatory changes. Two of the radiologists indicated that they also use the 40-keV VMIs for general screening of the neck, to help avoid overlooking important pathology. The same 2 radiologists indicated that reviewing the 40 keV VMIs could increase interpretation time, but felt it was worth the additional information. However, 1 of 3 felt that that these VMIs increased interpretation time excessively. The latter point is important and needs to be taken into consideration, especially in busy high-volume settings. Of course, the additional reconstructions are meant to supplement the standard 65 keV or 70 keV VMIs for specific applications, and are generated from the same acquisition. Therefore, one has the option to tailor the time spent on these reconstructions according to the complexity of the case and their additional potential value. The approach of using multiple DECT reconstructions for diagnostic interpretation can be viewed as analogous to using multiple MRI sequences for optimal interpretation.[7,8]

Overall, there was agreement among the 3 head and neck readers that the automatic transfer of the low-energy VMIs is useful and facilitates the evaluation of these images, as they are available to rapidly review on PACS. There was also general agreement that, if there was an advanced analysis software accessible from PACS, the utility of DECT would be even greater for the evaluation of the neck.

SUMMARY

DECT scanners have become increasingly available, with the number of clinical applications steadily rising. As a result, the use of this technology is expanding both for clinical research and for routine use in the clinical setting. DECT implementation for routine clinical use can pose certain challenges that can impact production and radiologist workflow. These challenges should be anticipated and planned for to ensure orderly and smooth integration into the clinical departmental workflow. In this review, we discussed our experience with the use of this technology, with the intention to provide practical tips that help minimize any potentially negative impact as well as short-term and long-term suggestions for seamless integration into clinical practice.

Despite these challenges, routine DECT scanning using current technology is feasible in the clinical setting. Several steps can be taken to help integration into the clinical workflow and reduce impact on departmental productivity, and the remaining challenges will hopefully be resolved with future technical innovations. Ultimately, widespread adoption and maximal use of this exciting technology in routine clinical practice is likely to at least in part depend on seamless workflow integration.

REFERENCES

1. Tamm EP, Le O, Liu X, et al. "How to" incorporate dual-energy imaging into a high volume abdominal imaging practice. Abdom Radiol (New York) 2017; 42(3):688–701.
2. Megibow AJ, Sahani D. Best practice: implementation and use of abdominal dual-energy CT in routine patient care. AJR Am J Roentgenol 2012; 199(5 Suppl):S71–7.
3. Matsumoto K, Jinzaki M, Tanami Y, et al. Virtual monochromatic spectral imaging with fast kilovoltage switching: improved image quality as compared with that obtained with conventional 120-kVp CT. Radiology 2011;259(1):257–62.
4. Patel BN, Thomas JV, Lockhart ME, et al. Single-source dual-energy spectral multidetector CT of pancreatic adenocarcinoma: optimization of energy level viewing significantly increases lesion contrast. Clin Radiol 2013;68(2):148–54.
5. Pinho DF, Kulkarni NM, Krishnaraj A, et al. Initial experience with single-source dual-energy CT abdominal angiography and comparison with single-energy CT angiography: image quality, enhancement, diagnosis and radiation dose. Eur Radiol 2013;23(2):351–9.
6. Lam S, Gupta R, Levental M, et al. Optimal virtual monochromatic images for evaluation of normal tissues and head and neck cancer using dual-energy CT. AJNR Am J Neuroradiol 2015;36(8): 1518–24.
7. Forghani R. Advanced dual-energy CT for head and neck cancer imaging. Expert Rev Anticancer Ther 2015;15(12):1489–501.
8. Lam S, Gupta R, Kelly H, et al. Multiparametric evaluation of head and neck squamous cell carcinoma using a single-source dual-energy CT with fast kVp switching: state of the art. Cancers 2015;7(4): 2201–16.
9. Albrecht MH, Scholtz JE, Kraft J, et al. Assessment of an advanced monoenergetic reconstruction technique in dual-energy computed tomography of head and neck cancer. Eur Radiol 2015;25(8):2493–501.
10. Wichmann JL, Noske EM, Kraft J, et al. Virtual monoenergetic dual-energy computed tomography: optimization of kiloelectron volt settings in head and neck cancer. Invest Radiol 2014;49(11):735–41.
11. Kuno H, Onaya H, Iwata R, et al. Evaluation of cartilage invasion by laryngeal and hypopharyngeal squamous cell carcinoma with dual-energy CT. Radiology 2012;265(2):488–96.
12. Forghani R, Levental M, Gupta R, et al. Different spectral Hounsfield unit curve and high-energy virtual monochromatic image characteristics of squamous cell carcinoma compared with nonossified thyroid cartilage. Am J Neuroradiol 2015;36(6): 1194–200.
13. Forghani R, Kelly H, Yu E, et al. Low-energy virtual monochromatic dual-energy computed tomography images for the evaluation of head and neck squamous cell carcinoma: a study of tumor visibility compared with single-energy computed tomography and user acceptance. J Comput Assist Tomogr 2017. http://dx.doi.org/10.1097/RCT.0000000000000571.

Advanced Tissue Characterization and Texture Analysis Using Dual-Energy Computed Tomography
Horizons and Emerging Applications

Reza Forghani, MD, PhD[a],*, Ashok Srinivasan, MD[b],
Behzad Forghani, M.Eng[c]

KEYWORDS

- Dual-energy CT • Head and neck squamous cell carcinoma • Virtual monochromatic images
- Material decomposition iodine maps • Spectral Hounsfield unit attenuation curves
- Machine learning • Texture analysis • Radiomic analysis

KEY POINTS

- The rich quantitative data acquired using dual-energy computed tomography (DECT) lends itself to a variety of advanced analyses not possible with conventional single-energy CT (SECT).
- Spectral Hounsfield unit attenuation curves represent plots of predicted attenuations within a region of interest at different energies and are a quantitative corollary of virtual monochromatic images.
- Basis material decomposition and a number of other DECT analytical methods are available and enable tissue characterization not possible with SECT.
- The rich quantitative data available with DECT scans, such as the spectral Hounsfield unit attenuation curves, may further be analyzed using various statistical and mathematical methods for tissue characterization.
- An exciting emerging application is the use of quantitative spectral DECT datasets for texture or radiomic analysis.

INTRODUCTION

Dual-energy computed tomography (DECT) is an advanced form of CT in which image acquisition is performed at 2 different energies, instead of a single peak energy acquisition as is used in conventional single-energy CT (SECT).[1–5] As a result, the attenuation data from the different energy acquisitions can be combined to generate various

Disclosures: R. Forghani has acted as a consultant for GE Healthcare and has served as a speaker at lunch and learn sessions titled "Dual-Energy CT Applications in Neuroradiology and Head and Neck Imaging" sponsored by GE Healthcare at the 27th and 28th Annual Meetings of the Eastern Neuroradiological Society in 2015 and 2016 (no personal compensation or travel support for these sessions).

[a] Department of Radiology, Segal Cancer Centre and Lady Davis Institute for Medical Research, Jewish General Hospital, McGill University, Room C-212.1, 3755 Cote Sainte-Catherine Road, Montreal, Quebec H3T 1E2, Canada; [b] Division of Neuroradiology, Department of Radiology, University of Michigan Health System, 1500 East Medical Center Drive, Ann Arbor, MI 48109, USA; [c] Reza Forghani Medical Services Inc, Cote St-Luc, Quebec H3X 4A6, Canada
* Corresponding author.
E-mail address: rforghani@jgh.mcgill.ca

Neuroimag Clin N Am 27 (2017) 533–546
http://dx.doi.org/10.1016/j.nic.2017.04.007
1052-5149/17/© 2017 Elsevier Inc. All rights reserved.

neuroimaging.theclinics.com

reconstructions (including virtual monochromatic images and material decomposition maps, among others) that cannot be created using conventional SECT. DECT also can be used to quantitatively evaluate the energy-dependent attenuation characteristics of various component materials beyond what is possible with conventional SECT. Since its introduction into clinical practice, there have been ongoing technical improvements in the available DECT systems and an increase in their availability. As a result, multiple clinical applications have emerged in neuroradiology and head and neck imaging using this exciting technology that are covered in the other articles in this issue. In the final article of this series, we discuss in greater detail some of the advanced analytical tools for DECT quantitative analysis that are available using a fast kVp switching DECT scanner (GE Healthcare, Waukesha, WI) and explore exciting developments and applications combining DECT with advanced image processing (texture or radiomic analysis) and machine learning methods.

BASIC PRINCIPLES OF MATERIAL CHARACTERIZATION IN DUAL-ENERGY COMPUTED TOMOGRAPHY SCANNING

The different commercially available and experimental spectral CT scanning approaches and systems are reviewed in detail in separate articles in this issue and are not discussed here. However, understanding the fundamental principles behind DECT scan acquisitions and material characterization is essential for its successful application and is briefly reviewed.[1–4] In clinical CT scanning, attenuation is achieved by 2 main physical mechanisms. These are Compton scatter, which is based on the electron density of the tissue elements, and the photoelectric effect (PE), which is strongly dependent on the atomic number or Z of the tissue elements. A third physical mechanism, Rayleigh or coherent scatter, accounts for only a small percentage of the attenuation and is generally considered negligible.

Although the Compton effect accounts for significant attenuation in clinical CT scanning, it is nearly independent of photon energy. Therefore, it is not the main physical mechanism exploited by DECT approaches. On the other hand, the PE is strongly energy dependent and a key underlying physical process for DECT material characterizations that rely on energy-dependent attenuation changes of elements or tissues. Photoelectric interactions refer to the ejection of an electron from the innermost shell, or K-shell, of an atom by an incident photon. For this to occur, the incident photon must have a minimum energy that is equal to the binding energy of the electron to its shell. The K-shell has the most strongly bound electrons and the probability of photoelectric interactions, and consequently the degree of attenuation, is highest when the incident photon energy just exceeds the binding energy of K-shell electrons. This energy represents the K-edge of an element, at which there is a sudden increase or spike in attenuation, followed by a rapid drop with further increases in energy above the K-edge. Understanding the energy-dependent attenuation characteristics and behavior of elements, including the relation to the K-edge, is essential for understanding the behavior of materials or tissues with DECT.

One way to predict which materials or elements will have significant energy-dependent changes in their attenuation and therefore likely to be amenable to additional characterization using DECT approaches is to look at their atomic number or Z.[1,6] The probability of the PE is proportional to approximately the third power of an element's atomic number (Z).[1] Because photoelectric interactions are the main underlying physical process accounting for the *energy-dependent* attenuation changes seen in DECT scanning, elements with a higher atomic number would be expected to have greater energy-dependent changes in their attenuation or strong "spectral properties" (**Fig. 1**). These elements are good candidates for evaluation and characterization based on their energy-dependent attenuation characteristics using DECT. Iodine (Z = 53), present in the body within the thyroid gland and the main constituent of most CT contrast agents, is an example of one such element (see **Fig. 1**). Another element with a relatively high atomic number is calcium (Z = 20). As would be expected and discussed in multiple accompanying articles in this issue, iodine's strong "spectral" properties can be exploited in several applications in neuroradiology and head and neck imaging.

Elements with a small atomic number, on the other hand, typically exhibit little change in attenuation at different energies and therefore are not good candidates for characterization based on their energy-dependent (or "spectral") properties.[1] Relevant examples are common elements found in the human body, such as hydrogen (Z = 1), carbon (Z = 6), nitrogen (Z = 7), and oxygen (Z = 8).[1] For example, note how, unlike iodine within the thyroid gland, there is little change in energy-dependent attenuation of muscle on the noncontrast CT shown in **Fig. 2**. Because these would not be expected to exhibit sufficient changes in their attenuation at different energies, one would not expect to characterize such materials based on their

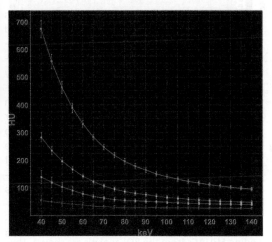

Fig. 1. Example of energy-dependent attenuation changes of iodine. SHUACs derived from ROI analysis of 4 solutions containing different concentrations of iodine, imaged within a phantom, are shown. Iodine has a high atomic number (Z = 53) and therefore exhibits significant changes in attenuation at different energies or has "strong spectral" properties. Note the increase in attenuation with decreasing energies approaching the K-edge of iodine (33.2 keV). For example, note the much higher attenuation at 40 keV compared with 65 or 70 keV (generally considered similar to a conventional 120 kVp SECT acquisition). With most DECT systems, this comes at the expense of greater image noise at low energies, as represented by the error bars depicting standard deviation of attenuation within the ROI evaluated. The scan was acquired with a fast kVp switching scanner.

spectral or energy-dependent characteristics.[1,7] Of course, when evaluating attenuation curves, one also needs to consider particularities of the specific material or tissue being analyzed, including relative contribution from each process (ie, photoelectric and Compton effects) to the attenuation coefficient, and the way CT numbers are calculated (ie, normalized relative to water). The latter accounts for the fact that the CT number of fat in **Fig. 2** decreases with decreasing energy; that is, even though fat attenuation increases at lower energies, its CT number *decreases* relative to water.

Last, it is worth noting that although the energy dependency of the attenuation of elements or materials is a key component of material characterization by DECT, the attenuation information from other physical processes, namely Compton scatter, is not ignored and also can be used as part of the material characterization algorithms with DECT. This will become more evident during the discussion of material decomposition maps in the sections that follow, but is important to keep in mind. For example, an element with little energy

dependency of its attenuation may nonetheless be readily distinguishable from another element that has strong spectral properties with significant energy-dependent changes in its attenuation. This is readily evident by examination of the attenuation curves in **Fig. 2**; even if muscle shows little energy-dependent changes in its attenuation, it is readily distinguishable from the other tissues.

Therefore, if the objective is to distinguish 2 materials or use 2 materials as basis pairs (see next section), what is important is that there are sufficient *differences* in the attenuation or energy-dependent attenuation characteristics of 2 materials of interest for reliable distinction by DECT. If there is sufficient difference in the Z and K-edge of 2 materials, DECT can be used to separately identify and differentiate them based on the differences in their attenuation at various energies. On the other hand, if one is specifically trying to exploit the spectral characteristics of an element, such as using low-energy reconstructions to increase iodine attenuation, then the element or material should have sufficient energy dependency of its attenuation. Such manipulations work best with elements with high atomic numbers and generally would not be expected to be successful with low atomic number elements.

DUAL-ENERGY COMPUTED TOMOGRAPHY POSTPROCESSING: QUANTITATIVE ANALYSIS AND DIFFERENT DUAL-ENERGY COMPUTED TOMOGRAPHY RECONSTRUCTIONS FOR MATERIAL CHARACTERIZATION

In this section, different DECT quantitative analytical tools are discussed. Different types of DECT reconstructions are discussed in detail in the first 2 articles in this issue (See Reza Forghani and colleagues' article, "Dual Energy CT: Physical Principles, Approaches to Scanning, Usage, and Implementation - Part 1," and Reza Forghani and colleagues' article, "Dual Energy CT: Physical Principles, Approaches to Scanning, Usage, and Implementation - Part 2," in this issue) but are briefly reviewed here, focusing on their derivation and relation to the quantitative attenuation curves or other quantitative graphic tools. For the purposes of this article, the DECT postprocessing tools discussed are those available using a fast kVp switching DECT scanner (GE Healthcare). However, the fundamental principles are the same for other DECT systems and many of the reconstructions or postprocessing tools are also available with other systems. Therefore, it is likely that many of the DECT applications discussed can be applied across different DECT platforms, although fine tuning or optimization may be necessary.

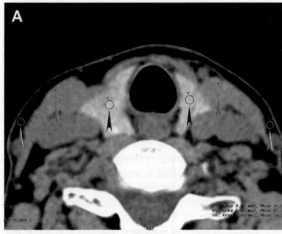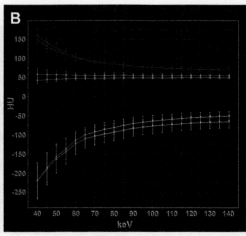

Fig. 2. Example of energy-dependent attenuation of different tissues. (*A*) Axial noncontrast neck CT image showing ROI analysis of different tissues and (*B*) the corresponding SHUACs from the ROI analysis are shown. Thyroid tissue (*blue* ROIs and curves) contains iodine, which has a high atomic number (Z = 53), with strong "spectral properties" or energy-dependent attenuation changes due to the PE. Note the pronounced increase in thyroid attenuation at low energies approaching the K-edge of iodine (33.2 keV). On the other hand, most of the soft tissues in the human body, such as muscle, are composed of low atomic number materials (eg, oxygen [Z = 8], carbon [Z = 6], and hydrogen [Z = 1]). As a result, there is much less propensity for PE contribution to their attenuation and consequently little energy dependency of their attenuation. For example, note how muscle (*green* ROIs and curves) has little change in attenuation at different energies on noncontrast CT. Other tissues, like fat, have completely different attenuation characteristics with a decrease in their attenuation at lower energies (*yellow* ROIs and curves), as discussed in greater detail in the text. Arrowheads are used in (*A*) to improve visibility of ROIs. The scan was acquired with a fast kVp switching scanner.

Spectral Hounsfield Unit Attenuation Curves and Virtual Monochromatic Images

In earlier examples discussing the energy-dependent changes of different materials or tissues, graphs were shown that display attenuation as a function of energy (see **Figs. 1** and **2**). These can be referred to as spectral Hounsfield unit attenuation curves (SHUACs) and are very useful for demonstrating and comparing the energy-dependent changes in attenuation of different materials or tissues of interest (see **Figs. 1** and **2**; **Fig. 3**).[8–10] These graphs are also the quantitative correlate of virtual monochromatic images (VMIs). Briefly, VMIs simulate what the actual image would look like if the study was acquired with a monoenergetic X-ray beam at a prescribed or predicted X-ray energy level (**Fig. 4**). The SHUAC represents what the measured attenuation would be within a region of interest (ROI) on VMIs at those energies (see **Figs. 3** and **4**).

Inspection of the SHUACs demonstrates well the rich quantitative information available on DECT scans. For example, if ROI analysis is performed on a conventional SECT scan, the main quantitative information obtained is a single mean density or attenuation (as well as a single standard deviation, minimum, maximum attenuation). Typically, this is considered similar or close to what would be observed at 65 or 70 keV on VMIs derived from a DECT scan. In contradistinction, an ROI placed on image sets obtained with DECT provides a wide range of predicted attenuations from 40 to 140 keV for fast kVp switching systems (see **Figs. 1–3**). In the graphs shown, attenuation measurements were obtained at intervals of 5 keV but the interval can be reduced to 1 keV if needed.

It should be readily apparent how in some cases this additional information can be advantageous. Different tissues may have similar attenuation at a single energy, such as 65 or 70 keV, but have different SHUACs, enabling differentiation by DECT not possible with SECT (see **Fig. 3; Fig. 5**). For example, in **Fig. 5**, note how nonossified thyroid cartilage (NOTC) has attenuation very similar to enhancing head and neck squamous cell carcinoma (HNSCC) at 65 or 70 keV, but significantly different attenuation at higher energies. This observed difference is due to "suppression" of attenuation of iodine within the enhancing tumor at high energies (much greater than the K-edge of iodine) but relative preservation of the intrinsically high attenuation of NOTC.[9]

Basis Material Decomposition Maps and Material Labeling

Basis material decomposition (BMD) maps and different ways of deriving these maps are also discussed in detail in a separate article in this issue

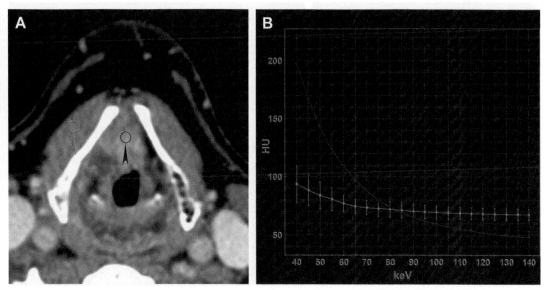

Fig. 3. SHUACs demonstrating an example of differences in the energy-dependent attenuation characteristics of a laryngeal cancer compared with normal prelaryngeal strap muscles. (*A*) Axial contrast-enhanced neck CT showing ROI analysis and (*B*) the corresponding SHUACs derived from the ROI analysis are shown. Enhancing tumor (*blue* ROI and curve) has very different energy-dependent attenuation characteristics compared with muscle (*green* ROI and curve) in this case. Although both tumor and muscle attenuation increase at lower energies approaching the K-edge of iodine (33.2 keV), the attenuation increase is much greater for tumor. For example, note how at 65 or 70 keV (virtual monochromatic image energies typically considered similar to a standard 120-kVp SECT acquisition), there is only a small difference in the attenuation of tumor compared with muscle. On the other hand, there is a progressive increase in the attenuation difference between tumor and muscle with decreasing energy, most pronounced at 40 keV. These quantitative changes are reflected in the changes in the appearance of tissues seen on the corresponding VMIs and form the basis for the use of low-energy reconstructions for improving tumor visibility and soft tissue contrast, as shown in **Fig. 4**. The increased attenuation at lower energies comes at the expense of image noise, represented by the error bars (standard deviation of attenuation within the ROI). Arrowheads are used in (*A*) to improve visibility of ROIs. The scan was acquired with a fast kVp switching scanner.

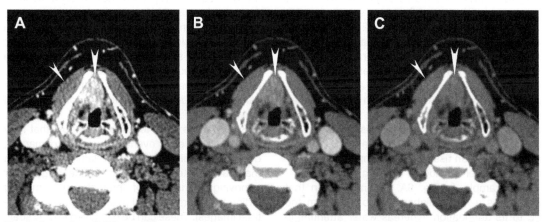

Fig. 4. Examples of VMIs at different energies reconstructed from a contrast-enhanced neck CT of a patient with laryngeal cancer (*arrow*; same patient as in **Fig. 3**). Shown are VMIs at (*A*) 40 keV, (*B*) 65 keV (typically considered equivalent to a standard 120-kVp SECT acquisition), and (*C*) 95 keV. To emphasize the differences between different VMI energies, all images are displayed using the same window-level setting. Note the much higher attenuation of enhancing tumor (large *arrowhead*) as well the much greater attenuation difference or soft tissue contrast compared with normal muscle (small *arrowhead*) with decreasing VMI energy, most pronounced on the 40-keV VMI (*A*). This reflects and provides a qualitative correlate of what is seen on the SHUACs in **Fig. 3**. The increased attenuation at lower energies comes at the expense of greater image noise. The scan was acquired with a fast kVp switching scanner.

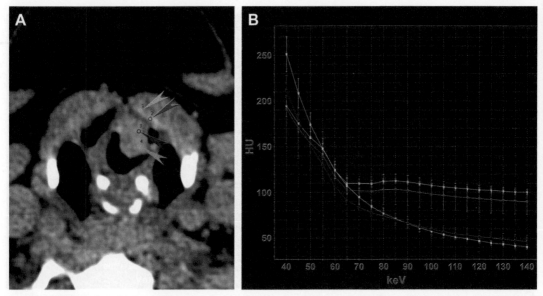

Fig. 5. SHUACs demonstrating differences in the energy-dependent attenuation characteristics of a laryngeal cancer compared with normal NOTC. (*A*) Axial contrast-enhanced neck CT showing ROI analysis and (*B*) the corresponding SHUACs derived from the ROI analysis are shown. Enhancing tumor (*pale* and *dark blue* ROIs and curves) has different energy-dependent attenuation characteristics compared with NOTC (*pink* and *red* ROIs and curves). Note how at 65 or 70 keV (virtual monochromatic image energies typically considered similar to a standard 120-kVp SECT acquisition), the attenuation of tumor is very similar to that of NOTC with overlap in their standard deviations. On the other hand, there is attenuation separation at higher energies. This occurs because the spectral curve of NOTC flattens out with relative preservation of high attenuation even at high energies. However, at energies further away from the K-edge of iodine, the attenuation of the enhancing tumor continues to drop, resulting in increased separation of the attenuation curves in the high-energy range. Arrowheads are used in (*A*) to improve visibility of ROIs. The scan was acquired with a fast kVp switching scanner.

but is briefly reviewed here. As discussed earlier, in the range of energies used for diagnostic CT scanning, the X-ray attenuation of any material is mainly due to a combination of Compton scatter and PE. The energy dependence of these 2 effects can be assumed to be fixed across all materials, but the relative contribution to the overall attenuation changes depending on the material. Therefore, Compton scatter and PE can form a *material basis pair* in which other materials can be expressed (**Fig. 6**). However, it should be noted that in DECT, it is more common to express materials using material basis pairs that are more closely related to human tissues, for example, the combination of water and iodine (see **Fig. 6A**).

For example, in **Fig. 6A**, it can be seen that iodine has a much higher contribution from the PE to its attenuation, whereas water attenuation is dominated by Compton scatter with a much smaller component of the PE. The water-iodine material basis pair can be used to represent different materials as a linear combination of water and iodine (see **Fig. 6A**). For instance, the attenuation of blood within vessels is close to that of water (blue dot). By definition, blood would be considered 100% water and 0 mg/mL iodine.

Other materials can be expressed as different weighted combinations of water and iodine and the dashed lines represent how each material is mapped in this BMD coordinate system. It is important to understand that this does not mean that they physically consist of water and iodine; that is, these should not be interpreted as the physical distribution of pure water and pure iodine. It simply means that their X-ray attenuation is the same as a specific combination of water and iodine.

BMD can be used to generate maps (that may be superimposed or overlaid on standard images), depicting the distribution and relative content of a material of interest such as iodine (**Fig. 7**) or removing a material of interest (eg, removing iodine to generate virtual unenhanced or noncontrast images). These can be displayed in gray scale or in color, with different colors and hues representing the estimated relative concentration of the material of interest in different tissues. In addition, ROI analysis of these maps can be performed and will provide an estimate of the concentration of the material of interest within a tissue.

BMD coordinate systems can be very useful for material characterization, by cross-correlating

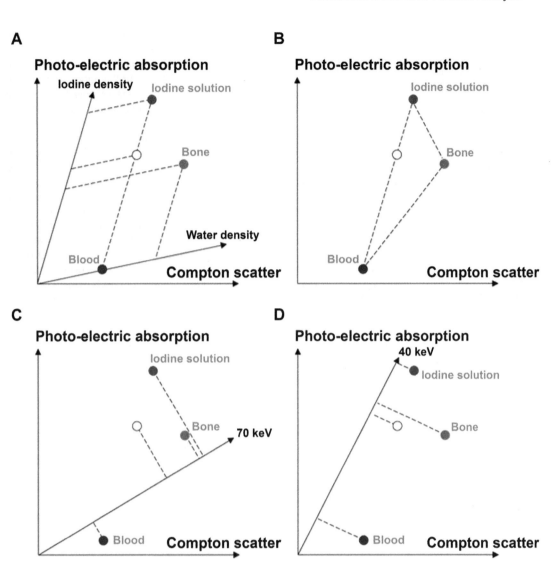

Fig. 6. BMD. In clinical CT scanning, tissue attenuation is fundamentally a combination of Compton scatter and photoelectric absorption (excluding the small contribution from Rayleigh scatter). Therefore, Compton scatter and the PE can form a *material basis pair* in which other materials can be expressed, although in DECT it is more common to express materials in material basis pairs that are more closely related to human tissues, such as water and iodine. In this figure, example graphs are shown that illustrate the principles and approach for (A) water-iodine BMD, (B) multimaterial decomposition, and (C, D) virtual monochromatic imaging at 70 keV and 40 keV. Please refer to the text for additional details and explanations. (*Courtesy of* Reza Forghani, MD, PhD, Montreal, Quebec, Canada; and Bruno De Man, PhD, Niskayuna, New York.)

their attenuation properties to that of known materials. For instance, in **Fig. 6**A, a voxel or region that is bright or has high "signal" on the iodine map but not on the water map is likely to be iodine containing blood (ie, iodine within the perfused blood volume or microvasculature within a tissue). Different tissues can have unique characteristics on these maps and if their characteristics are sufficiently different, and the relationships linear, then their presence, distribution, and tissue content may be estimated using this approach. This information

can then be used to create a visual map of the distribution and relative content of the material of interest, such as iodine on the iodine-water map shown in **Fig. 7**.

At the same time, when interpreting these maps, one must recall that they do not represent the actual physical distribution of a material, as was discussed earlier. For example, a region that is bright on both maps is probably bone or calcified tissue (see **Fig. 6**A). The very high "signal" of osseous or calcified structures on these maps,

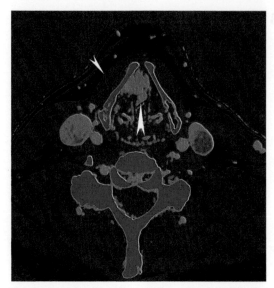

Fig. 7. Example of iodine (iodine-water) BMD map from a contrast-enhanced CT of the neck of a patient with laryngeal cancer (same patient as in **Fig. 4**). Iodine maps represent the distribution and relative content of iodine in different tissues. For example, note the much higher iodine "signal" in the tumor (large *arrowhead*) compared with normal prelaryngeal strap muscles (small *arrowhead*). ROI analysis of iodine-water maps can provide an estimate of iodine concentration within a tissue. This scan was acquired with a fast kVp switching scanner.

as seen in **Fig. 7**, should not be misinterpreted as iodine. Generally, this pitfall can be easily avoided by cross-correlating the map to the standard VMIs at 65 or 70 keV. In rare cases in which there is a diagnostic dilemma, other maps (virtual unenhanced or calcium maps) can be useful for additional characterization.

Even though in principle DECT provides only 2 independent measurements and is best suited for material decomposition of 2 constituent elements, DECT data also may be used to accurately characterize 3 or more materials (multimaterial decomposition) (see **Fig. 6**B). However, for this to be done, certain major assumptions have to be made. One method is based on the assumption of constant volume or mass and another is a semiempirical method used to estimate the effective density in the absence of volume conservation.[5,11] Each approach has its limitations, but practically, for multimaterial decomposition to be effective, the materials under investigation should have sufficiently different spectral or energy-dependent characteristics for reasonable discrimination. **Fig. 6**B illustrates an example of how a given voxel on a map can be expressed as a combination of a true physical material, and may even be used for

material labeling; that is, classification of a material into a predefined group.[12] **Fig. 6**C, D illustrate how materials may be projected on a respective VMI axis and interpreted in VMI images. These are meant to provide examples of how the spectral data acquired from a DECT scan may be used in different ways for tissue analysis.

When performing BMD, one must keep in mind certain fundamental limitations. For example, if the K-edge of a material of interest is in the range of "useful" X-ray energy spectrum, this will result in an attenuation discontinuity, making their energy dependence fundamentally different. In these cases, the material can no longer accurately be expressed as a combination of 2 basis materials *without* the K-edge. In such cases, a third basis material with the appropriate K-edge is needed to represent the position of that K-edge. For accurate material decomposition using DECT, the imaged materials should be *linearly* dependent on the chosen basis materials. Some of these limitations of DECT may be overcome with advanced spectral CT systems currently under development (such as photon counting scanners) that have the potential to accurately discriminate 3 or more basis materials simultaneously and allow K-edge imaging.

Another potential limitation that has to be kept in mind when performing BMD is that depending on the material pair of interest, there can be overlap in their spectral characteristics. Noise in X-ray measurements can also impact BMD maps, which introduces errors in the analysis. In addition, when performing tissue analysis in vivo, the pure solutions or ideal theoretical conditions in a laboratory or a phantom are not present. These additional and sometimes unpredictable factors can influence the maps and could affect the accuracy for detection or estimation of the concentration of a material of interest, such as overestimation or underestimation of a material of interest or oversubtraction or undersubtraction of a reference material basis pair. Therefore, although material decomposition maps can be powerful tools for tissue analysis, one must be aware of their potential limitations and rigorous validations should be performed when pertinent.

That these maps do not represent the actual physical distribution of a material was discussed earlier, and exemplified in the high "signal" of calcified tissue or bone on iodine maps. Another circumstance in which caution is required for interpretation of these maps is in the presence of significant artifact (such as significant beam-hardening artifact), which could result in misclassification on BMD maps. This again highlights the importance of interpreting these maps (or other specialized DECT reconstructions for that matter) in conjunction with the standard 65-keV or 70-keV VMIs.[3,4]

OTHER DUAL-ENERGY COMPUTED TOMOGRAPHY ANALYTICAL TOOLS OR RECONSTRUCTIONS

SHUACs, VMIs, and BMD are powerful and perhaps the most commonly used analytical tools or reconstructions with DECT. However, DECT data also can be evaluated and represented in other ways. One of these is calculation of the effective atomic number or effective Z of a voxel within the image. One study found that the effective Z of malignant lesions is significantly different from that of benign lesions or tissues in the neck.[8] Another study reported that there can be significant differences in the effective Z of parathyroid adenomas compared with thyroid tissue or lymph nodes on certain phases of 4-dimensional (4D)-CT performed in DECT mode.[13] The effective Z can be calculated within an ROI. It can also be displayed graphically (for example, as a scatterplot) based on ROI analysis (**Fig. 8**) or used to create images or maps (**Fig. 9**). The advanced processing capabilities of the Advantage workstation (GE Healthcare) also enables generation of other graphs,

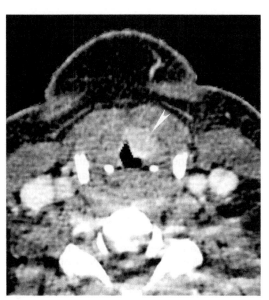

Fig. 9. Example of effective Z map from a contrast-enhanced CT of the neck of a patient with laryngeal cancer (*arrowhead*). Note the brighter or higher density of the tumor compared with adjacent muscle reflecting the higher effective Z of the tumor. ROI analysis of these maps can be used to determine the effective Z values within the tissue of interest. The scan was acquired with a fast kVp switching scanner.

such as histograms depicting the distribution of voxel attenuation within an ROI (**Fig. 10**) or calculation of "optimal" contrast-to-noise ratio for a selected ROI relative to another ROI used as a reference. These are interesting tools that could

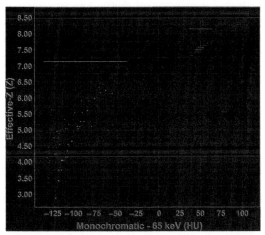

Fig. 8. Example of scatterplot of effective Z (Y-axis) and attenuation (X-axis) from ROI analysis of different tissues. The example shown is derived from the same ROIs as shown in **Fig. 2A**, with blue representing thyroid tissue, green representing muscle, and yellow representing subcutaneous fat. Note the separation of the values derived from within the ROI, represented by "dots" of different colors, into separate clusters based on the tissue analyzed. The lines with corresponding colors have been added to the top to help visualization of the range of spread for each cluster. The scan was acquired with a fast kVp switching scanner.

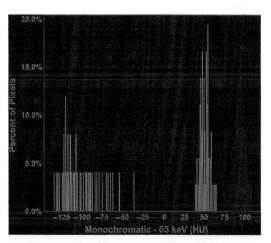

Fig. 10. Example of histogram analysis of percent distribution of attenuation of voxels from ROI analysis of different tissues. The example shown is derived from the same ROIs as shown in **Fig. 2A**, with blue representing thyroid tissue, green representing muscle, and yellow representing subcutaneous fat. The scan was acquired with a fast kVp switching scanner.

be explored in different clinical and research applications, although they need validation with clinical endpoints and should not be used "blindly."

ADVANCED QUANTITATIVE APPROACHES FOR THE EVALUATION OF SPECTRAL DATA

Like any curve, the SHUACs derived from different tissues lend themselves to a variety of quantitative analytical methods, including using nonlinear methods to fit the curves for derivation of different parameters. In one study comparing malignant neck pathology with benign posttreatment changes or lesions, the range of the curve, the asymptote, and the decay of the fitted curves were evaluated (**Fig. 11**).[8] The range represents the difference between the maximum Hounsfield unit (HU) value and the asymptote of the curve (the value the curve is approaching as the keV increases past 140). Decay was calculated using a formula for the fitted model. The investigators performed ROI analysis of malignant lesions, benign lesions, and the normal paraspinal muscle as an internal reference. Other than the previously mentioned parameters for the curves, the *differences* and *ratios* for these parameters were also calculated.

Logistic regression was used to determine whether a mass was malignant or benign. The investigators found that the best predictor for

identifying and distinguishing a malignant lesion was the *difference* in the range between the lesion and the normal paraspinal muscle.[8] A cutoff of a *difference between the ranges* of 75 or more between the lesion and the paraspinal muscle was found to be predictive of malignancy with 95% sensitivity, 89% specificity, and overall area under the curve of 91.8%. Although some other parameters, including effective Z, were also found to be significantly different between malignant and benign tissue, adding these other parameters had minimal effect on improving the model. The study demonstrated that certain parameters derived from the SHUACs, specifically the difference in range, were significantly different between malignant and benign tissues and, furthermore, the differences became more pronounced when internal standardization was performed using the normal paraspinal muscle within a given patient.[8]

Other groups have used different methods to analyze SHUACs and derive quantitative parameters of potential interest. One such parameter is the "slope" of the SHUAC, referred to as λHU, and calculated as the difference between the attenuation (HU) at 40 keV and another energy such as at 70 keV[14] or 90 keV,[15] divided by the energy difference (ie, 30 keV if 70 keV is used as the second point or 50 keV if 90 keV is used as the second point). Other studies have used iodine concentration derived from overlay maps (as an absolute value or normalized value, for example by dividing by the value in the carotid artery), to distinguish pathologic lymph nodes.[15,16] Yet another parameter that may be evaluated for distinction of different tissues is the area under the SHUAC curve.[13] These are just some examples of how the quantitative data obtained using DECT can be analyzed.

TEXTURE OR RADIOMIC ANALYSIS USING SPECTRAL DATA

In the earlier sections, the rich quantitative data available using DECT, and different methods of analysis, were discussed. Some of the observations made using quantitative analysis of DECT data can be translated to qualitative image sets to supplement the standard 65-keV or 70-keV reconstructions for lesion characterization.[3,4,9,10,17] Some examples are the use of iodine overlay maps for evaluation of thyroid cartilage invasion by HNSCC,[17] use of high-energy VMIs for distinction of nonossified thyroid cartilage from HNSCC,[9] and use of low-energy VMIs for improving HNSCC visibility and contour delineation,[10,18] among other applications discussed in detail in multiple accompanying articles in this issue.

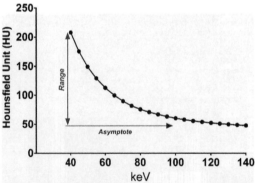

Spectral Hounsfield Unit Attenuation Curve

Fig. 11. Example of analysis of the SHUACs. Like any curve, SHUACs can be fitted using nonlinear modeling and analyzed in different ways. Some parameters that can be evaluated are the asymptote of the curve (the value the curve is approaching as the keV increases past 140) and the range (the difference between the maximum HU value and the asymptote of the curve). The decay of the curve can also be calculated using a formula for the fitted model, among other parameters. Please refer to the text for additional explanations.

Beyond predominantly qualitative approaches to image interpretation used during routine image interpretation, there is increasing interest in the use of sophisticated analytical tools and software for the evaluation of medical images to derive clinically relevant information that is not readily available or obtained during routine clinical interpretation. This is referred to as texture or radiomic analysis and is a growing area of investigation with the potential for a significant impact on the field of medical imaging. Texture or radiomic analysis has been used in different organ systems to predict different clinical features of interest, including but not limited to molecular features of tumors (sometimes referred to as radiogenomics), association with distant metastases, tumor response to treatment, and outcome.[19–26]

Despite numerous published investigations and applications of texture analysis in the literature in various organ systems, there is so far little to no published data using texture or radiomic analysis that take advantage of the rich quantitative datasets generated by DECT scans. Given the differences in energy-dependent attenuation characteristics of some pathologic entities and tissues, texture analysis could be used to take advantage of the information within these rich spectral datasets, and open new horizons for lesion or tissue characterization, biomarker development, and noninvasive assessment of different pathology for prediction of treatment response or prognostication. We therefore conclude this article with a brief discussion of potential approaches to texture or radiomic analysis of DECT data.

Preparation of Dual-Energy Computed Tomography Data for Texture Analysis

There is currently no established protocol for preparation of DECT data for texture analysis. However, conceptually, the main objective is to capture the energy-dependent attenuation characteristics of different tissues to help superior tissue classification or potentially improved prediction of tumor molecular features, response to treatment, or other associated clinical endpoints of interest. Building on principles of DECT material characterization and the DECT analytical tools or reconstructions discussed in the earlier sections, one attractive approach would be to use the image correlates of SHUACs for texture analysis, namely VMIs reconstructed at different energies. This approach is attractive, at least as a starting point, because it could capture the spectral or energy-dependent attenuation characteristics of tissues and can be applied to DECT acquisitions available from different vendors. This could potentially also

avoid the pitfall of relying on analysis of proprietary spectral datasets generated by each scanner type, making this approach more readily applicable across DECT platforms.

Looking at the examples of curves provided in this article, one would ideally want to cover the entire range of VMI energies; that is, 40 to 140 keV. Increments of 5 keV seem to capture the tissue attenuation characteristics well and therefore are a good starting point. One could consider smaller keV intervals, but this needs to be weighed against the significantly more labor involved, both in analyzing the large number of reconstructions as well as the additional demands on the mathematical analysis and prediction model creation. Using 5-keV intervals would result in a total of 21 image sets per scan acquisition ranging from 40 to 140 keV.

Whether performing standard ROI analysis or texture analysis, one of the challenges posed by multiple image sets is related to accurate registration between the different sets; however, this is not a problem with DECT. Because all the different energy VMI datasets are created from the same source spectral dataset, these are naturally coregistered. Therefore, ROI analysis can be performed on a single image set that demonstrates the lesion of interest best, and applied to all the different VMI energy datasets.

Mathematical Texture Data Analysis and Application of Machine Learning Methods for Generation of Prediction Models

A discussion of specific texture analysis software and approaches for feature extraction is beyond the scope of this article. Suffice it to say that currently there are a variety of programs and approaches for texture analysis, many of which have been built "in-house" at different institutions, while others are commercially available, such as TexRAD (TexRAD Ltd, Cambridge, UK). Once the first-order statistical parameters are generated using ROI analysis of image sets with image processing software such as TexRAD, the statistical parameters for each patient, along with the associated outcome for that patient, are fed into a classification algorithm, with the goal of building a prediction model. Using a supervised learning method, the texture features of images from patients with known outcomes are turned into prediction models that may determine different lesion characteristics or outcomes of clinical interest in other patients.

To build a prediction model, one of the many machine learning methods can be used. The goal is to build a model that is accurate and uses only the statistical parameters that are useful. To do this, a search is necessary for the tuning parameters of the machine learning method, as well as the set of predictors that matter. This is basically an optimization problem whose goal is to find the optimum prediction model; that is, one that would produce the most accurate prediction, given a set of input parameters. The optimization problem may be replaced by a simple grid search, but searching over the entire space of a high-dimensional dataset may be too time-consuming. An alternative approach would involve a careful examination of all the parameters before the search begins. If some of the input parameters are highly correlated, then there is redundancy, and if some of the parameters are not found to have any discriminating power for the classification problem at hand, then they are insignificant and can be removed from the set. As an example, in recent experiments involving building a model for predicting p16 status of head and neck cancer, the procedure started with an initial set of (21 energy levels × 6 filtered images × 6 statistical parameters), or a total of 756 predictors. However, in preliminary test runs, the number of useful predictors was found to be 7 and these were spread over different energy levels (R Forghani and colleagues, unpublished data, 2016). Perhaps not unexpected, this also implies the additional utility of rich quantitative or multienergy data generated by DECT. In this example, during the search for the optimum model, approximately 600 intermediate models were trained and tested for accuracy, taking several hours of computation. In practice, the time taken to find and train the optimum model is not very critical, as long as the prediction, using the resulting model, can be made in real time (as is most often the case with most machine learning methods).

There are a number of machine learning methods that can be used in building a diagnostic tool from the texture data obtained by image processing. The challenge in dealing with the "omics" data is that there are usually a large number of predictors compared with the number of samples, and often the number of samples is much smaller than the number of predictors (the so-called "curse of dimensionality"). Therefore, even though using DECT scans with VMIs created at multiple energy levels provides a much richer data set, at the same time, for building a prediction model, it makes finding an accurate model very difficult. In such cases, the prediction model obtained from a machine learning method often ends up overfitting the data, meaning that the model fits itself to the training data (including the noise in that data) so well that it is no longer capable of accurately predicting the outcome in new patients. Put in another way, the prediction model has a large generalization error. Therefore, when searching for an optimum model, measures should be taken to determine at what point during the search the resulting model may become prone to overfitting. Validating the models with an independent set of data is always the best way to determine when overfitting begins to take place. For example, before the search begins, 30% of the patients can be randomly selected and set aside for the validation. Note that this should not be confused with the cross-validation of every single model, which is required to determine its own accuracy.

The high-dimensional nature of the "omics" data also places a requirement on the machine learning method to be scalable; that is, a method that can deal with tens, hundreds, or even thousands of samples/predictors, with the same level of accuracy. Another challenge is that very often the classes that the samples belong to are not balanced and at times they are highly imbalanced. One example is when in a dichotomous outcome, the number of positive samples is very few compared with the number of negative samples. There are techniques, such as oversampling or undersampling, that could yield a reasonable prediction model; however, the bias in the resulting model may still be too large. In these cases, the accuracy parameter of the machine learning methods do not portray a true picture of the model's performance and often other criteria should be used for determining whether the model is good enough.

These are just some general concepts and challenges that should be kept in mind when using machine learning or artificial intelligence for evaluation of texture data, including the large datasets that can be generated using DECT scans. Although challenging, this is an exciting area of future research and development and represents another area in which the rich quantitative datasets generated by DECT approaches may represent a significant advantage over conventional SECT.

SUMMARY

DECT acquisitions provide rich spectral datasets that include information on the energy-dependent attenuation of tissues not available using conventional SECT scans. In this article, different DECT reconstructions and advanced analytical DECT tools were reviewed. In addition to enabling reconstructions and material maps not possible with SECT, ROI analysis of DECT spectral data can be used to generate rich quantitative data far beyond measurements of attenuation at a single energy with SECT. The different types of graphs generated, such as SHUACs, provide information on the energy-dependent attenuation of different tissues and lend themselves to even further mathematical analysis that can be used for more detailed and sophisticated tissue characterization. Last, advanced texture or radiomic analysis of the spectral data combined with machine learning methods could be used to generate prediction models for clinical endpoints of interest, and is an exciting new field of study. Although this article focused on the tools available for fast kVp switching scanners, many of the reconstructions and tools discussed are also available with other DECT scanner types. It is our hope that the article will help familiarize readers with the different advanced analytical tools available with DECT and stimulate interest in routine clinical use as well as research and development in this powerful technology.

REFERENCES

1. Johnson TRC, Kalender WA. Physical background. In: Johnson T, Fink C, Schönberg SO, et al, editors. Dual energy CT in clinical practice. Berlin: Springer-Verlag; 2011. p. 3–9.

2. Johnson TR. Dual-energy CT: general principles. AJR Am J Roentgenol 2012;199(5 Suppl):S3–8.

3. Forghani R. Advanced dual-energy CT for head and neck cancer imaging. Expert Rev Anticancer Ther 2015;15(12):1489–501.

4. Lam S, Gupta R, Kelly H, et al. Multiparametric evaluation of head and neck squamous cell carcinoma using a single-source dual-energy CT with fast kVp switching: state of the art. Cancers (Basel) 2015; 7(4):2201–16.

5. McCollough CH, Leng S, Yu L, et al. Dual- and multi-energy CT: principles, technical approaches, and clinical applications. Radiology 2015;276(3):637–53.

6. Alvarez RE, Macovski A. Energy-selective reconstructions in X-ray computerized tomography. Phys Med Biol 1976;21(5):733–44.

7. Michael GJ. Tissue analysis using dual energy CT. Australas Phys Eng Sci Med 1992;15(2):75–87.

8. Srinivasan A, Parker RA, Manjunathan A, et al. Differentiation of benign and malignant neck pathologies: preliminary experience using spectral computed tomography. J Comput Assist Tomogr 2013;37(5):666–72.

9. Forghani R, Levental M, Gupta R, et al. Different spectral Hounsfield unit curve and high-energy virtual monochromatic image characteristics of squamous cell carcinoma compared with nonossified thyroid cartilage. AJNR Am J Neuroradiol 2015; 36(6):1194–200.

10. Lam S, Gupta R, Levental M, et al. Optimal virtual monochromatic images for evaluation of normal tissues and head and neck cancer using dual-energy CT. AJNR Am J Neuroradiol 2015;36(8):1518–24.

11. McCollough CH, Schmidt B, Liu X, et al. Dual-energy algorithms and postprocessing techniques. In: Johnson T, Fink C, Schönberg SO, et al, editors. Dual energy CT in clinical practice. Berlin: Springer-Verlag; 2011. p. 43–51.

12. Krauss B, Schmidt B, Flohr TG. Dual source CT. In: Johnson T, Fink C, Schönberg SO, et al, editors. Dual energy CT in clinical practice. Berlin: Springer-Verlag; 2011. p. 10–20.

13. Forghani R, Roskies M, Liu X, et al. Dual-energy CT characteristics of parathyroid adenomas on 25-and 55-second 4D-CT acquisitions: preliminary experience. J Comput Assist Tomogr 2016;40(5):806–14.

14. Liu X, Ouyang D, Li H, et al. Papillary thyroid cancer: dual-energy spectral CT quantitative parameters for preoperative diagnosis of metastasis to the cervical lymph nodes. Radiology 2015;275(1):167–76.

15. Yang L, Luo D, Li L, et al. Differentiation of malignant cervical lymphadenopathy by dual-energy CT: a preliminary analysis. Sci Rep 2016;6:31020.

16. Tawfik AM, Razek AA, Kerl JM, et al. Comparison of dual-energy CT-derived iodine content and iodine overlay of normal, inflammatory and metastatic squamous cell carcinoma cervical lymph nodes. Eur Radiol 2014;24(3):574–80.

17. Kuno H, Onaya H, Iwata R, et al. Evaluation of cartilage invasion by laryngeal and hypopharyngeal squamous cell carcinoma with dual-energy CT. Radiology 2012;265(2):488–96.

18. Forghani R, Kelly H, Yu E, et al. Low-energy virtual monochromatic dual-energy computed tomography images for the evaluation of head and neck squamous cell carcinoma: a study of tumor visibility compared with single-energy computed tomography and user acceptance. J Comput Assist Tomogr 2017. http://dx.doi.org/10.1097/RCT.0000000000000571.

19. Zhang H, Graham CM, Elci O, et al. Locally advanced squamous cell carcinoma of the head and neck: CT texture and histogram analysis allow independent prediction of overall survival in patients treated with induction chemotherapy. Radiology 2013;269(3):801–9.

20. Cheng NM, Fang YH, Chang JT, et al. Textural features of pretreatment 18F-FDG PET/CT images: prognostic significance in patients with advanced T-stage oropharyngeal squamous cell carcinoma. J Nucl Med 2013;54(10):1703–9.

21. Buch K, Fujita A, Li B, et al. Using texture analysis to determine human papillomavirus status of oropharyngeal squamous cell carcinomas on CT. AJNR Am J Neuroradiol 2015;36(7):1343–8.

22. Fujita A, Buch K, Li B, et al. Difference between HPV-positive and HPV-negative non-oropharyngeal head and neck cancer: texture analysis features on CT. J Comput Assist Tomogr 2016;40(1):43–7.

23. Leijenaar RT, Carvalho S, Hoebers FJ, et al. External validation of a prognostic CT-based radiomic signature in oropharyngeal squamous cell carcinoma. Acta Oncol 2015;54(9):1423–9.

24. Liu J, Mao Y, Li Z, et al. Use of texture analysis based on contrast-enhanced MRI to predict treatment response to chemoradiotherapy in nasopharyngeal carcinoma. J Magn Reson Imaging 2016;44(2):445–55.

25. Parmar C, Leijenaar RT, Grossmann P, et al. Radiomic feature clusters and prognostic signatures specific for lung and head & neck cancer. Sci Rep 2015; 5:11044.

26. Vallieres M, Freeman CR, Skamene SR, et al. A radiomics model from joint FDG-PET and MRI texture features for the prediction of lung metastases in soft-tissue sarcomas of the extremities. Phys Med Biol 2015;60(14):5471–96.

Moving?

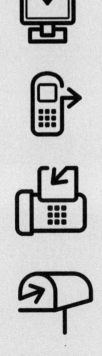

Moving?

Make sure your subscription moves with you!

To notify us of your new address, find your Clinics Account Number (located on your mailing label above your name), and contact customer service at:

Email: journalscustomerservice-usa@elsevier.com

800-654-2452 (subscribers in the U.S. & Canada)
314-447-8871 (subscribers outside of the U.S. & Canada)

Fax number: 314-447-8029

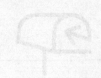

Elsevier Health Sciences Division
Subscription Customer Service
3251 Riverport Lane
Maryland Heights, MO 63043

*To ensure uninterrupted delivery of your subscription,
please notify us at least 4 weeks in advance of move.
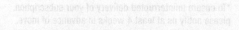

Printed and bound by CPI Group (UK) Ltd, Croydon, CR0 4YY

03/10/2024

01040302-0018